Urodynamics

Paul Abrams

Urodynamics

Third Edition

With 152 Figures

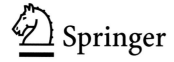 Springer

Paul Abrams, MD, FRCS
Bristol Urological Institute
Southmead Hospital
Bristol
UK

Artwork marked with ⬚ symbol throughout the book is original to the 2nd edition (Abrams
P. Urodynamics, second edition, Springer London Ltd. 1997) and is being republished in this
3rd edition.

A catalogue record for this book is available from the British Library

Library of Congress Control Number: 2005932032

ISBN-10: 1-85233-924-1
ISBN-13: 978-1-85233-924-1

Printed on acid-free paper.

Printed in Singapore.   (Expo/KYO)

9 8 7 6 5 4 3 2 1

Springer Science+Business Media
springeronline.com

Preface

Lower urinary tract dysfunction produces a huge burden on sufferers in particular and on society in general. Lower urinary tract symptoms have a high prevalence in the community: 5% of children aged 10 wet the bed, while 15% of women and 7% of men have troublesome incontinence; and in elderly men of 75, benign prostatic hyperplasia occurs in more than 80% of individuals, with benign prostatic enlargement coexisting in up to half this group and half of these having bladder outlet obstruction.

The confusion felt in many people's minds as to the role of urodynamics has receded for the most part. The need to support the clinical assessment with objective measurement has become accepted by most clinicians specialising in the care of patients with lower urinary tract symptoms (LUTS). Since the first edition of this book in 1983, urodynamics has become more widely accepted. In the last 20 years the number of urodynamic units in Britain and Europe has increased rapidly and almost every hospital of any significance embraces urodynamic investigations as an essential part of the diagnostic armamentarium of the urology and gynaecology departments. Further, specialists in geriatrics, paediatrics and neurology recognise the importance of urodynamics in the investigation of a significant minority of their patients.

Despite the technological innovations that have seen the introduction of computerised urodynamics, the development of neuro-physiological testing and the introduction of new techniques such as ambulatory monitoring, the objectives of this book remain unchanged. Urodynamics may appear complicated, and one of the objectives of this book is to put the subject over simply but in enough detail to allow urodynamic investigation to be accepted, on its own merit, as a fundamental contribution to the management of many patients. To do this means not only describing the tests but also showing in which clinical areas they help management and in which they are pointless. It means concentrating on the common clinical problems and on the presenting symptom complexes, not the diagnosis; and it means pointing out any limitations and possible artifacts of investigation.

We hope that a clinician with no previous experience in urodynamics will, after reading this book, appreciate both the value and limitations of the subject, and will have obtained the necessary practical advice on the use of the appropriate equipment in the correct situations. Because this book is based on personal experience, references in the text are relatively few.

The scientific basis of urodynamics does not change and the principle reason for producing the 3rd edition has been the publication in 2002 of the new ICS terminology report 2002 together with the ICS reports on "Good Urodynamic Practice" (2002).

Bristol Urological Institute   Paul Abrams
2005

References

Brocklehurst JC (1993). Urinary incontinence in the community – analysis of a MORI poll. Br Med J 306:832–834.

Burgio KL, Matthews KA, Engel BT (1991). Prevalence, incidence and correlates of urinary incontinence in healthy, middle-aged women. J Urol 146:1255–1259.

O'Brien J, Austin M, Sethi P, O'Boyle P (1991). Urinary incontinence: prevalence, need for treatment, and effectiveness of intervention by nurse. Br Med J 303:1308–1312.

Sandvik H, Hunskaar S, Seim A, Hermstad R, Vanvik A, Bratt H (1993). Validation of a severity index in female urinary incontinence and its implementation in an epidemiological survey. J Epidemiol Community Health 47:497–499.

Torrens MJ (1974). The control of the hyperactive bladder by selective sacral denervation. ChM Thesis, Bristol University.

Turner Warwick R, Milroy E (1979). A reappraisal of the value of routine urological procedures in the assessment of urodynamic function. Urol Clin N Am 6:63–70.

Whiteside CG (1979). Symptoms of micturition disorders in relation to dynamic function. Urol Clin N Am 6:55–62.

List of Abbreviations

AUDS	ambulatory urodynamic studies
BOO	bladder outlet obstruction
BPE	benign prostatic enlargement
BPH	benign prostatic hyperplasia
BPO	benign prostatic obstruction
DFV	dysfunctional voiding
DSD	detrusor sphincter dyssynergia
DUA	detrusor underactivity
GP	general practitioner (family physician)
ICS	International Continence Society
IDO	idiopathic detrusor overactivity
ISC	intermittent self-catheterisation
LUTD	lower urinary tract dysfunction
LUTS	lower urinary tract symptoms
MCUG	micturating cystourethrography
MUCP	maximum urethral closure pressure
NDO	neurogenic detrusor overactivity
p_{abd}	abdominal pressure
p_{det}	detrusor pressure
PFS	pressure-flow studies
p_{ves}	intravesical pressure
PVR	post-void residual
Q_{ave}	average flow rate
Q_{max}	maximum flow rate
TURP	transurethral resection of the prostate
UDS	urodynamic studies
UFS	urine flow studies
UPP	urethral pressure profile
USI	urodynamic stress incontinence
VUDS	videourodynamic studies
VUR	vesico-ureteric reflux

Measurement Units

Quantity	Unit	Symbol
volume	millilitre (ml)	V
time	second (s)	t
flow rate	millilitres/second (ml/s)	Q
pressure	centimetres of water (cmH$_2$O)	P

Urodynamic Qualifiers

Intra vesical (bladder)	ves
Intra urethral	ura
Detrusor	det
Abdominal (usually rectal)	abd

Contents

Chapter 1
Principles of Urodynamics

Urodynamics has two basic aims:

- To reproduce the patient's symptomatic complaints during urodynamics, and
- To provide a pathophysiological explanation by correlating the patient's symptoms with the urodynamic findings.

Implicit in these aims is the acceptance that whilst the patient's symptoms are important, because they bring the patient to the clinician, they are often misleading. Most patients with lower urinary tract dysfunction present to their doctor with symptoms, but in all branches of medicine symptoms have been shown to be misleading to a varying degree. Were symptoms reliable, further investigation would not need to precede active management. At one time, the elderly male patient with lower urinary tract symptoms (LUTS) would automatically have been offered a prostatectomy and, similarly, a woman with LUTS would have had an anterior repair with or without a hysterectomy. Most of the published literature indicates that the symptoms of lower urinary tract dysfunction (LUTD) are unreliable. Previously, clinicians appreciated the need for some investigations and chose to assess the lower urinary tract using "static" investigations, such as intravenous pyelography (IVP) and cystourethroscopy. However, the lower urinary tract, both during filling and emptying, is a dynamic system. Hence it is appropriate to use dynamic investigations for the investigation of lower urinary tract problems.

The statement "the bladder is an unreliable witness" was made by Bates in 1970 in one of the early papers on urodynamics (Bates et al., 1970). Two important papers appeared in 1980. One by a gynaecologist, Gerry Jarvis (1980) found that of 100 patients diagnosed by their symptoms as having stress incontinence, only 68 were shown to have urodynamic stress incontinence. This was supported by the findings of Powell (working in the Bristol unit; Powell et al., 1980) that only 50% could be shown to have urodynamic stress incontinence. Both authors also looked at patients with apparent overactive bladder symptoms presumed to be the result of detrusor overactivity. Jarvis confirmed this diagnosis in only 51% of cases, while Powell showed detrusor overactivity in only 33% of such patients. Further work in women has shown that in women presumed to have urodynamic stress incontinence, 12% had another cause for their stress incontinence. In most patients, factors such as change of posture, leading to the apparent stress incontinence, provoked detrusor overactivity, leading to the reported incontinence. Clearly in this group of patients, with apparent stress incontinence, surgery would have been unsuccessful in at least the 12% who were suffering from an altogether different type of problem. These papers illustrate the difficulty of assessing women with lower tract dysfunction by symptoms alone. As in women, LUTS in the males are of poor diagnostic value. Furthermore, the findings from IVP and cystoscopy have been shown to be poor indicators of bladder outlet obstruction. Both Abrams (1978) and Andersen (1979) have shown that the symptoms of apparent prostatic obstruction are misleading. Of the many symptoms that the textbooks attribute to prostatic outlet obstruction, they could show that only slow stream and hesitancy bore any correlation with the urodynamic findings of obstruction, that is, high voiding pressure and low urine flow rate. Because symptoms have been shown to lack diagnostic specificity in all clinical groups, it is not surprising to find that when surgery was based on symptoms alone the results were less than satisfactory. The decision to recommend prostatic surgery was previously indicated by an assessment of symptoms backed by the findings from IVP and cystourethroscopy. Early audit of prostatectomy assessed by these means showed a cure rate of only 72%, poor for an elective procedure. Urodynamic studies provided alternative explanations for many symptoms and, when dynamic investigations of function (urodynamics) rather than static investigations of structure (IVP and cystoscopy) were used in preoperative evaluation, the results of surgery improved to 88%.

The preceding discussion relates to men and women who are neurologically normal and therefore able to appreciate sensation from their lower urinary tract. In patients who have neurological conditions affecting the lower urinary tract, it is common for sensation to be absent or abnormal, making their symptomatic complaints even more difficult to interpret.

Faced with the unpalatable fact that patients submitted for surgery without objective confirmation of their condition did rather poorly, surgeons reacted in different ways. Some became ostrich-like, and dismissed those who published these results as poor surgeons bereft of clinical acumen and operative skills, while making no effort to assess their own results. Others, who had always been uneasy about patient assessment by symptoms and non-functional studies, such as intravenous pyelography, seized the opportunity to study these large groups of patients by urodynamic means. Hence in the 1970s there was a rapid expansion of clinical and research urodynamics. The wider acceptance of urodynamics has allowed us to look at LUTS from a different perspective.

The Urodynamic History

Despite the shortcomings of the patient's symptoms for diagnosis, they are important. They trouble the patient sufficiently for him or her to seek medical help, and LUTS should be assessed in a systematic way.

Some quarters have taken a nihilistic approach to urodynamic investigations because of the alleged inadequacy of this method of assessment and on the premise that if the patient's symptoms are improved by an intervention (e.g., an operation), then nothing else matters! However, because the patient's symptoms and the objective urodynamic findings bear little relationship to each other, this approach has several major drawbacks. Already mentioned are the less than adequate results from elective surgery, when only symptoms were considered in diagnosis. Second, there is a well- established, very large placebo effect in patients with LUTS. The symptoms of men with proven bladder outlet obstruction, secondary to benign prostatic hyperplasia, can be improved by placebo treatment to such an extent that 40% to 60% of men in the placebo arm of drug studies consider themselves considerably improved.

Nevertheless, doctors and nurses familiar with urodynamic techniques and with a functional appreciation of bladder and urethral physiology are able to take a history from a patient that gives a much more accurate picture of the patient's real problems. The significance of individual symptoms and groups of symptoms is discussed in detail in Chapter 4.

The Urodynamic Physical Examination

Patients referred for urodynamics will have been examined in a general way, either in the hospital clinic from which the referral emanated, or by the patient's general practitioner (primary care physician). Hence the urodynamic staff should concentrate its efforts on a physical examination that will shed light on the patient's symptomatic complaints and the underlying pathophysiological processes that could have caused these complains. One of the great advantages of the Bristol unit is that adequate time is given for close questioning, the relevant physical examination, an unhurried urodynamic investigation and practical advice. The importance of the urodynamic physical examination is discussed in detail in Chapter 4. Urine examination should be performed in all patients, and radiology and endoscopy have their indications, as will be discussed in Chapter 4. Urodynamic studies should follow only when careful investigations have been performed to exclude other pathologies that might mimic lower urinary tract dysfunction.

The Aims of Urodynamics

The objectives of any test can be achieved if the appropriate questions that the test is designed to address are posed. Therefore, at the outset, it is important to ask the following question:

"What do I want to know about this patient?"

Urodynamic studies have their limitations. It may be useful for the clinician to answer this question in terms of the filling and voiding phases of the micturition cycle and in terms of the bladder and the urethra. In this way, the urodynamicist can ask the next relevant question, which is:

"Which urodynamic investigations need to be performed to define this patient's problems?"

This question will concentrate the clinician's thought processes on eliminating those investigations which cannot help to make the diagnosis or indicate the line of management. For example, if a young male patient has had a urethral stricture and restricturing has to be excluded, then urine flow measurement will be the only required test.

Once the questions that need to be answered have been defined and the relevant urodynamic tests selected, the next question should be:

"Is the investigation likely to be of benefit to the patient?"

This question, again, can be answered by an analysis of the possible benefits to the patient, in terms of the increased knowledge generated by the test, and the influence this knowledge will have on his or her clinical management. Even when knowledge does not appear likely to improve the quality of life of that patient, there may still be an overall benefit to them if knowledge in a difficult area without effective treatment techniques can be increased. An increase in knowledge may, at a future date, result in the introduction of effective treatment. A good example would a young woman who cannot void adequately. When often normal voiding cannot be re-established, intermittent self-catheterisation is a good treatment, although it is resented by many patients. However, routine investigations usually contribute little to effective management, although neurophysiological testing may show abnormal sphincter activity. Hence investigations may show the cause, although the clinician does not have the means to reverse these abnormalities.

The benefits of the investigations must be set against the potential harm the tests could do. Fortunately, urodynamics are a relatively harmless investigation, although there is a small incidence of urinary tract infection (1% to 2%) and some discomfort. Then, there is the question of whether the information gained by the tests offsets their financial cost. Also important in deciding the benefit-risk analysis of the investigations will be the answers given to the following questions.

"Is urodynamics able to make a reliable diagnosis?"

This is a complex question within which the fundamental query is whether the tests themselves are reliable and reproducible. Three factors greatly influence the value of urodynamics:

- The urodynamic technique should be free of technical artefacts.
- The results of investigations should be reproducible.
- The clinician should be properly trained and able to interpret the results of urodynamics.

From a technical point of view, the tests must clearly be carried out in a careful way, eliminating all possible artefacts. This aspect of urodynamic studies is discussed extensively in Chapter 3. The patient's own bioconsistency is another problem. We know that symptoms vary considerably with time, but we do not have much information as to whether or not urodynamic findings vary. This problem is best dealt with at the end of the urodynamic tests by asking:

"Did the urodynamic studies reproduce the patient's complaints and did the complaints correlate with known urodynamic features?"

In the Bristol unit, we have always laid great emphasis on the clinician, who is aware of the therapeutic possibilities of subsequent treatment, being present during urodynamics. The clinician can then be sure whether the sensations felt by the patient and the findings demonstrated by urodynamics are typical of the patient's everyday symptoms and whether any urodynamic abnormalities can account for these. Occasionally during urodynamic studies either the patient complains of an unrepresentative symptom, for example, urgency, or there is a urodynamic abnormality noted which does not correlate with the patient's symptoms. These discrepancies can be detected and interpreted as artefacts, if the clinician is present. However, if the urodynamics is delegated to a technician they may be reported on their face value, leading to a possible bias in the report that may influence subsequent patient management.

In some instances more than one abnormality can be seen, therefore it is important to ask:

"Can urodynamics decide which is the most significant abnormality
if more than one is detected?"

Multiple abnormalities are commonly seen in patients with neurogenic vesicourethral dysfunction. They are also often seen in non-neurological patients, such as in women with mixed incontinence. Treatment should be directed to the most significant or troublesome abnormality. Hence, once again, the correlation between the patient's symptomatic complaint and the urodynamic findings are most important. This correlation allows the clinician to advise on which abnormality is the most significant and should therefore receive management priority.

As well as seeking answers to the above questions the urodynamicist needs to define the indications for urodynamic investigation, and these can be viewed in a slightly different way:

● To increase diagnostic accuracy above that which can be achieved by nonurodynamic means.

● To make a diagnosis on which a management plan can be based. Overactive bladder symptoms are usually treated empirically on the assumption that detrusor overactivity is the cause, if a patient fails conservative and medical therapy, urodynamic proof of detrusor overactivity is required prior to invasive surgery.

● If there are coexisting abnormalities, to provide evidence to determine which should be treated first. In female mixed incontinence, determining which form of incontinence is most bothersome can be difficult. By careful assessment of the patient during urodynamics, it is usually possible to decide which is the predominant problem and thereby establish the treatment priority.

● To define the current situation, knowing the likely abnormalities, as a baseline for future surveillance. In spinal cord trauma, it is usual to perform urodynamic after spinal shock has resolved. These baseline urodynamics establish whether there is a detrusor contraction in reaction to bladder filling and whether or not detrusor-sphincter-dyssynergia (DSD) has developed. DSD, as discussed later, is a dangerous condition that can lead to poor bladder compliance, upper tract dilatation and renal impairment.

● To predict problems that may follow treatment interventions. Elderly men with prostatic obstruction and co-existing detrusor overactivity (DO) should be warned that whilst their urine flows and other voiding symptoms will be improved by TURP, OAB symptoms due to DO may persist.

● To provide evidence that influences the timing of treatment. In patients with neurological disease (e.g., meningomyelocoele) being treated by antimuscarinics, ultrasound may show the development of upper tract dilatation. Urodynamics are vital to confirm whether or not poor bladder compliance is the cause. If so a procedure such as ileocystoplasty will be required.

● To exclude abnormalities which might interfere with the management of that patient. In neurological patients with stress incontinence, who are being considered for the implantation of an artificial sphincter, the urodynamic demonstration of poor bladder compliance would indicate the need for treatment of the bladder condition as well as implanting the sphincter. Failure to deal with the bladder would be likely to produce worsening bladder compliance with effects on upper tract drainage.

- To assess the natural history of lower urinary tract dysfunction. Our unit, by investigating men and women studied more than 10 years ago is providing important evidence as to the natural history of voiding dysfunction in men and OAB and DO in both men and women.

- To assess the results of treatments designed to affect lower urinary tract function. Simple urodynamics tests, such as urine flow studies, should be used to audit the result of surgeries to relieve bladder outlet obstruction, for example after optical urethrotomy for urethral stricture.

After a brief description of the anatomy and physiology of the lower urinary tract in Chapter 2, subsequent chapters discuss urodynamic techniques (Chapter 3) and their applications (Chapters 5 and 6).

References

Abrams PH, Feneley RCL (1978). The significance of the symptoms associated with bladder outflow obstruction. Urol Int 33:171–174.

Andersen JT, Nordling J, Walter S (1979). Prostatism 1. The correlation between symptoms, cystometric and urodynamic findings. Scand J Urol 13:229–236.

Bates CP, Whiteside CG, Turner Warwick R (1970). Synchronous urine pressure flow cystourethrography with special reference to stress and urge incontinence. Br J Urol 42:714–723.

Jarvis GJ, Hall S, Stamp S, Miller DR, Johansson A (1980). An assessment of urodynamic examination in incontinence women. Br J Obstet Gynaecol 87:873–896.

Powell PH, Shepherd AM, Lewis P, Feneley RCL (1980). The accuracy of clinical diagnosis assessed urodynamically. Proceedings 10th meeting ICS Los Angeles pp 3–4.

Chapter 2
Anatomy and Physiology

Introduction

Urodynamic investigations developed because of dissatisfaction with the assessment of patients and treatment results when management was based on symptom assessment and the definitions of anatomical abnormalities. Urodynamics attempts to relate physiology to anatomy, that is function to structure. A sound knowledge of anatomy and physiology form the basis for the effective assessment and treatment of patients. In addition, this knowledge can be used to critically evaluate the role of urodynamic studies in assessing patients with lower urinary tract symptoms (LUTS).

Although the bladder and urethra are described separately below, it should be remembered that they normally act as a reciprocal functional unit.

Urethral Structure and Function

Very often the urethra is considered only as a passive conduit for urine. The bladder is viewed as the more important and more active part of the lower urinary tract. One reason for this may have been the observation of Lapides that continence was maintained in the isolated bladder even when most of the urethra had been removed. Urethral function is here discussed first in an attempt to redress this balance. Indeed it would be possible to argue that the urethra is the controlling agent in the micturition cycle.

The urethral closure mechanism and hence urinary continence depends on active and passive factors. Its function may be classified as normal or incompetent on filling, and normal or obstructive on voiding.

Anatomy

It is always tempting to infer function from structure. In general, the following comments on anatomy give greater perspective to functional urodynamic observations. The terminology and general arrangement of the lower urinary tract are shown in Fig. 2.1.

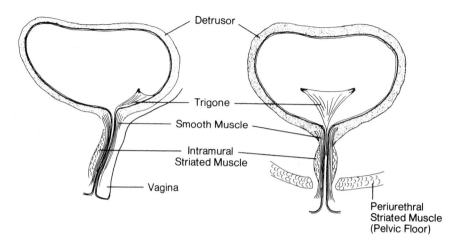

MALE

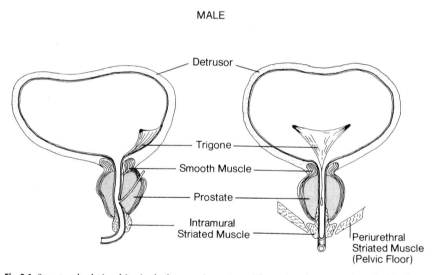

Fig. 2.1 Structural relationships in the lower urinary tract. The various layers are described in the text. (Modified from Gosling 1979) 📖

Mucosa

In both sexes, the mucosa is organised in longitudinal folds that give the urethral lumen a stellate appearance when closed. This arrangement allows considerable distensibility. The surface tension may be a factor in urethral closure.

Submucosa

The submucosal layer is a vascular plexus. Zinner (1976) discussed the role of this layer in relation to inner urethral wall softness. He suggested that the submucosa acts in a passive plastic way to "fill in" between the folds of mucosa as the urethra closes. This occurs as the tension increases in the muscular wall of the urethra, and its effect is to improve the efficiency of the seal of the urethral lumen.

There is an extensive submucosal vascular plexus which may have more than a passive role. Huisman (1979) has suggested that myoepithelial cells are found in association with arteriovenous shunts. This would provide a means of controlling submucosal pressure. Others suggest that the vascular element may be an important factor in the urethral closure in females where it is difficult to attribute all the occlusive forces to urethral muscle. This also explains the presence of urethral pressure changes synchronous with the arterial pulse and may be the reason for some postural and menstrual pressure changes. Gosling was unable to confirm the anatomical basis for this vascular control. In women after menopause, oestrogen deficiency is thought to lead to a reduction in the turgor of the vascular plexus and hence to be, in part, responsible for the increase in LUTS.

Urethral Muscle in Females

The smooth muscle of the female urethra is arranged longitudinally. Gosling (1979) showed from acetylcholinesterase analysis that the dominant innervation is cholinergic. Virtually no noradrenergic nerves are seen. This may appear confusing at first because the majority of the measurable resting urethral pressure depends on the alpha-adrenergic activity, if studies using alpha-blocking drugs are to be believed (Donker et al. 1972). This leads to a choice of conclusions:

- There are alpha-receptors on the smooth muscle, but no nerves to produce the trans-mitter (noradrenaline). This conclusion seems illogical.
- The urethral smooth muscle does not produce the urethral pressure. This is not as improb-able as it sounds, because the fibres are not circular, but longitudinal, and not very prolific.
- The alpha-adrenergic effects occur not on the muscle but at the level of the pelvic ganglia. This is the currently popular explanation.
- Alpha-blocking drugs have effects on the neuromuscular transmission that are not conventionally recognised.

There are two groups of striated muscle fibres in relation to the urethra, called intramural and peri-urethral by Gosling (1979). Intramural striated muscle bundles are found close to the urethral lumen, sometimes interdigitating with smooth muscle. In the female, these fibres are found in the greatest frequency anteriorly and laterally in the middle third of the urethra. In the adult female, they do not surround the urethra posteriorly to form a circular sphincter as in the male. The muscle is of a "slow twitch" type, rich in myosin ATPase, and adapted to maintain contraction over a relatively long period of time. No muscle spindles have been seen.

The pelvic floor is separated from the urethra by a layer of connective tissue and is histo-chemically and histologically different from the intraurethral striated sphincter.

Urethral Muscle in Males

The smooth muscle of the preprostatic urethra in males is histochemically distinct from that of the detrusor and from urethral muscle in females. This muscle also forms the

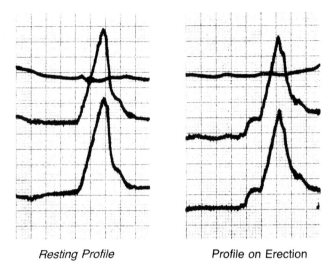

Resting Profile   Profile on Erection

Fig. 2.2 Urethral pressure profile demonstrating the elevation of the pressure in the region of the bladder neck/preprostatic sphincter during penile erection. 📖

prostatic capsule. It is richly provided with noradenergic terminals and little acetyl-cholinesterase has been found. It is agreed generally that this well-defined muscle represents the "prostatic or genital sphincter" designed to prevent reflux of ejaculate at the time of orgasm. Certainly we have observed changes in pressure in this part of the urethra during penile erection (Fig. 2.2), and these changes do not seem to occur during any part of the micturition cycle unless there is erection.

The striated muscles in the male can be divided into the same two groups described above for the female. The innervation is similar. The intramural striated muscle is orientated circularly around the postprostatic "membranous" urethra as a distinct sphincter.

Innervation of Striated Muscle

The innervation of the intramural striated muscle is usually predominately from S4, with a smaller S3 component. The muscle is probably innervated both from the pelvic nerve as well as from the pudendal nerve. The nerve cell bodies are located in Onuf's nucleus in the antero-lateral part of the sacral cord (S2-4). The pelvic floor itself, is innervated by the pudendal nerve and possibly branches of the pelvic nerves, on its inner (cephalad) surface.

Receptor Sites and Neurotransmitters

Much recent effort has been directed towards the analysis of receptors in the urinary tract. The distinction between experimentally demonstrable alpha- and beta-adrenergic receptor sites and innervation is not always clear. Alpha-adrenergic receptors, causing smooth muscle contraction when stimulated, produce their effects mainly in the bladder neck and the proximal 3 cm of urethra in both sexes. Beta-receptor activity is very weak in this area, although it is present over the bladder dome. Beta stimulation encourages bladder relaxation. Appreciation of these functions aids the understanding of the action of drugs on the urinary tract. However the appropriate sympathetic nerves may not even be present anatomically in the areas where receptors have been demonstrated.

The complex interrelation of nerves, transmitter substances and receptor sites has been the subject of controversy for years. Some of the reasons why progress is slow in this field are outlined below:

- Individual nerves may produce more than one neurotransmitter.
- Neurotransmitters may act on more than one type of receptor, producing different actions.
- Neurotransmitters may act in different ways at the same receptor site depending on their concentration.
- Neurotransmitters may interact with one another.
- There are considerable species differences in both neurotransmitters and receptors.

An example of fundamental controversy has been the question of the identity of the principal neurotransmitter to the detrusor muscle. The postganglionic parasympathetic fibres are presumed to be cholinergic in that they are associated with identifiable acetylcholinesterase. However if the transmitter is acetylcholine it should be blocked by atropine. Although some species are atropine-sensitive, the majority are not. This has led to the suggestion that another substance may be the principal neurotransmitter. Alternatively the receptor on the bladder muscle may have more nicotinic characteristics than muscarinic. Perhaps some receptors are not accessible to freely circulating atropine. Suggestions for alternative transmitters have included 5-hydroxytryptamine, purine nucleodes such as ATP, and prostaglandins. It is now believed that in normal function acetylcholine is the principal neurotransmitter, although the situation may be different in abnormal conditions, such as bladder outlet obstruction and detrusor overactivity, when ATP may be important. More work needs to be performed on human muscle preparations, so that a better understanding of bladder neuropharmacology emerges. Meanwhile the unpredictable response to the pharmacotherapy for detrusor overactivity merely emphasises our incomplete understanding of the pathophysiological processes involved in lower urinary tract dysfunction.

Central Nervous Activity

As seen in Fig. 2.3, the organisation of central control is a complex business. It can, however, be reduced to several relatively simple concepts. Sensation from the lower urinary tract must be appreciated centrally and consciously if normal cerebral control is to function. The sensation of bladder fullness and of bladder contraction ascends in the anterior half of the spinal cord. It may be affected by damage in that area of the cord, for example, in anterior spinal artery thrombosis and bilateral spinothalamic tractotomy, as well as other spinal cord lesions. Sensation of activity in the pelvic floor ascends in the posterior columns.

Sensation must not only reach the conscious level when the subject is awake; it must also, by its collateral effects on the reticular formation perhaps, be able to wake the subject from sleep or otherwise subconsciously to inhibit micturition. This may be the fundamental problem in nocturnal enuresis.

Assuming sensation is normal, the brain acts by balancing the various facilitatory and inhibitory effects suggested in Fig. 2.3, and the final common efferent pathway is through the "bladder centre" in the pontine reticular formation. This centre is essential for normally co-ordinated micturition. It acts on the sacral micturition centre in the conus medullaris, where the final integration of bladder and urethral activity takes place. Because the usual response of a bladder liberated from cerebral control is one of detrusor overactivity, it is assumed that the major cerebral output is one of tonic inhibition, hence the old term

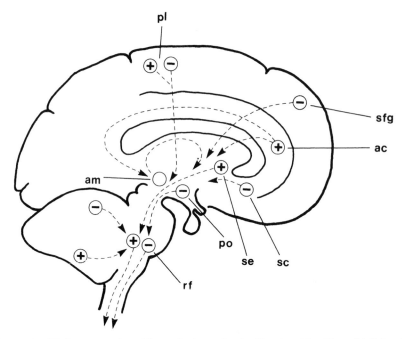

Fig. 2.3 Simplified representation of the cerebral areas involved in micturition. The multiplicity of inter-actions makes it easy to appreciate why the subject should be left to the research physiologist. +, facili-tation; –, inhibition; *ac*, anterior cingulate gyrus; *am*, amygdala; *pl*, paracentral lobule; *po*, preoptic nucleus; *rf*, pontine reticular formation; *sc*, subcallosal cingulate gyrus; *se*, septal area; *sfg*, superior frontal gyrus. (Torrens 1982)

"uninhibited bladder". However this is only an assumption, and prejudging the activity of the nervous system can only slow down the understanding of it. We suggest that terms which imply specific pathophysiology should be avoided as much as possible. The detailed neurological control of the bladder has been reviewed elsewhere (Nathan 1976; Fletcher and Bradley 1978; Torrens 1982; Blok 2002; Griffiths 2002).

Normal Urethral Function

The normal urethral closure mechanism maintains a positive urethral closure pressure during bladder filling, even in the presence of increased abdominal pressure. Continence can be seen to be maintained at the bladder neck in normal persons. This can be regarded as the proximal urethral closure mechanism. If the vesico-urethral junction (bladder neck) is incompetent, then continence may still be maintained at the high-pressure zone in the urethra, approximately 2 cm to 3 cm distally. This zone corresponds to the maximum condensation of muscle, both smooth and striated, and may be regarded as the distal urethral closure mechanism. Whether it is really valid to separate two parts of the urethra in this way from the physiological point of view is debatable; the normal urethra probably works as one unit. However from a practical standpoint it is useful because the urethral areas may not be abnormal simultaneously.

    Many factors have been thought to contribute to urethral closure; some are obvious, others less so. They are:

- Muscular occlusion by the intraurethral striated muscle.
- Transmission of abdominal pressure to the proximal urethra.
- Mucosal surface tension.
- Anatomical configuration at the bladder neck, including support from the endopelvic fascia and the pelvic floor muscles.
- Submucosal softness and vascularity.
- Inherent elasticity, particularly at the bladder neck.
- Urethral length.

While the relative importance of these various factors remains unknown, it is better to consider and describe only those that can be observed objectively: urethral closure pressure, electromyography (EMG) and videoscopic appearance of the urethra. Mechanical and hydrodynamic analogues, such as those quoted by Zinner et al. (1976), serve only to demonstrate how complicated the situation is. However the work of Delancey (1990) has helped us to understand the way in which the endopelvic fascia consisting of fascial sheets and condensations of fascia, around the urethra and bladder neck, are important in normal function. The attachments of the vagina to the pelvic floor provide a hammock under the proximal urethra and bladder base against which the bladder neck can be compressed when intra-abdominal pressure rises.

Typically urethral closure pressure decreases at or before the onset of micturition and is synchronous with bladder base descent seen by imaging and with the reduction of EMG activity from striated muscle of the intraurethral sphincter of the urethra, the pelvic floor or the external anal sphincter (Fig. 2.4, *overleaf*). It is a fallacy to consider that the urethra is forced open by a head of detrusor pressure. Micturition usually occurs at a voiding pressure less than the maximum resting intraurethral pressure; the decrease in urethral closure pressure represents an active relaxation process. Part of the pressure decrease can be attributed to the relaxation of the striated muscle of the pelvic floor, but part seems to be the result of active inhibition of the intraurethral striated sphincter. This can be reproduced by stimulation of the sacral nerves, especially S4 (Torrens 1978). Many women appear to void by relaxation and urethral opening only, no detrusor pressure rise being necessary. Undoubtedly urethral resistance in women is low, and the inner longitudinal smooth muscle may help reduce resistance by contracting and thereby making the urethra shorter and wider, thus facilitating micturition.

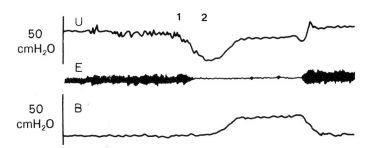

Fig. 2.4 Intravesical (*B*) and urethral (*U*) pressure and striated sphincter EMG (*E*) during volitional voiding. At the initiation of voiding (*1*), the urethral pressure falls to a minimum before the intravesical pressure starts to rise. Flow is initiated at (*2*), before an appreciable intravesical pressure has been generated. Flow is therefore a consequence of urethral relaxation in this female subject. At cessation of flow EMG activity returns after a period of silence, and the urethral pressure transiently rises while the proximal urethra is emptied back into the bladder. (McGuire 1978)

Detrusor Function

The urinary bladder is not a sphere even when contracting, and calculations of tension based on that premise must be to some extent erroneous. Its shape is more that of a three-sided pyramid, base posterior and apex at the urachus. The superior surface is covered by peritoneum and is pressed upon by the other viscera. The two inferior surfaces are supported by the pelvic floor and connected to the pelvic fascia by various condensations of fibroareolar tissue. Also important are the condensations of the endopelvic fascia, sometimes known as the "pubourethral ligaments". The functional adequacy of the bladder does depend on its correct anatomical position, so heavy viscera or inadequate pelvic support cause functional problems such as incontinence and prolapse. The detrusor is composed of an interlacing network of smooth muscle bundles. These are not layered, as has sometimes been described and as is the case in the intestine. It is not clear whether the detrusor around the bladder neck is involved in the mechanisms of closure and opening of the bladder neck, and the various mechanical theories of function that have been elaborated are presumptive and should be interpreted with great caution.

The golf enthusiast will readily understand the muscle fibre arrangement of the detrusor because it is similar to the structure of a golfball beneath its white coating. The muscle fibres run in all directions and change depth in the bladder wall. The detrusor muscle is relatively rich in acetylcholinesterase. As discussed, this is evidence for a dominant cholinergic innervation and very little noradrenergic activity can be demonstrated histochemically.

Innervation

Efferent motor nerves to the detrusor arise from the parasympathetic (cholinergic) ganglion cells in the pelvic plexus. The preganglionic fibres run in the sacral roots 2 to 4 within the pelvic nerves. The third root is the dominant nerve in most cases. The parasympathetic supply is excitatory. Preganglionic parasympathetic fibres and post-ganglionic sympathetic fibres both synapse with ganglion cells close to and within the bladder wall: it is believed that the sympathetic fibres act to inhibit the parasympathetic before being "switched off" at the onset of micturition.

Nerve-mediated detrusor inhibition has been described, occurring after stimulation of the pelvic floor or perianal area, and may be the mechanism by which some methods of nerve stimulation are effective in treating detrusor overactivity. Such inhibition may be mediated by the sympathetic nervous system (Sundin and Dahlstrom 1973). Bladder relaxation evoked by bladder wall stretch (accommodation) may be similarly mediated. Gosling (1979) has shown that little significant sympathetic innervation reaches the bladder dome in humans. As a result, it is suggested that inhibition occurs at the neurones in the pelvic ganglia where noradrenergic axosomatic terminals have been observed. The sympathetic supply to the pelvic ganglia arises at the T10 to T12 level and runs in the presacral nerves and hypogastric plexus. The muscle around the bladder neck in both sexes is similar to that of the rest of the bladder. Most nerve terminals are acetylcholinesterase-positive and almost no noradrenergic terminals are seen. (This is in contradistinction to certain species of animals.)

The sensory nerves from the bladder run with the motor supply. In general, the proprioceptive afferents related to tension enter the sacral segments, as do the greater proportion of enteroceptive afferents related to pain and temperature. Poorly localised sensations of pain and distension enter with the sympathetic fibres at a high level. The innervation of the bladder and urethra is summarised in Fig. 2.5.

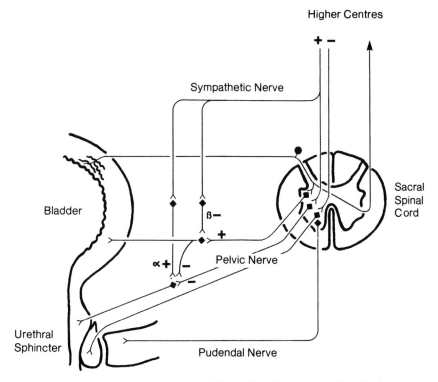

Fig. 2.5 Summary of the possible organisation of the peripheral nervous supply to the lower urinary tract. Preganglionic parasympathetic fibres and postganglionic sympathetic fibres both synapse with ganglion cells close to, and within, the bladder wall. The arrangement in relation to the urethra may be morphologically similar but functionally different. The periurethral striated muscle (pelvic floor) is supplied by the pudendal nerve. The somatic nerve supply to the intramural urethral striated muscle runs with the pelvic nerve and is vulnerable during pelvic surgery. (Torrens 1982)

References

Andersson KE (1996). Prostatic and extraprostatic adrenoceptors – contributions to the lower urinary tract symptoms in benign prostatic hyperplasia. Scand J Urol Nephrol 30 suppl. 179.

Andersson KE, Persson K (1993). The L-arginine nitric oxide pathway and non-adrenergic, non-cholinergic relaxation of the lower urinary tract. Gen Pharmacol 24:833–839.

Blok BFM (2002). Brain control of the lower urinary tract. Scand J Urol Nephrol 210(Suppl 210):21-26.

Chapple C R (1995). Selective ?l-adrenoceptor antagonists in benign prostatic hyperplasia. Br J Urol 75:265–270.

Delancy JOL (1990). Anatomy and physiology of urinary continence. Clin Obstet Gynaecol 33:298–307.

Donker PJ, Ivanovici F, Noach EL (1972). Analysis of the urethral pressure profile by means of electromyography and the administration of drugs. Br J Urol 44:180–193.

Fletcher TF, Bradley WB (1978). Neuroanatomy of the bladder/urethra. J Urol 119:153–160.

Gosling JA (1979). The structure of the bladder and urethra in relation to function. Urol Clin N Am 6:31–38.

Gosling JA, Dixon JS, Critchley HOD, Thomson SA (1981). A comparative study of the human external sphincter and periurethral levator ani muscles. Br J Urol 53:35.

Griffiths DJ (2002). The Pontine Micturition Centres. Scan J Urol Nephrol 210(Suppl 210):21-26.

Huisman AB (1979). Morfologie van de vrouwelijke urethra. Thesis, Groningen, The Netherlands.

Lapides J, Freind CR, Ajemian EP, Reus WS (1962). Denervation supersensitivity as a test for neurogenic bladder. Surg Gynecol Obstet 114:241.

McGuire FJ (1978) Reflex urethral instability. Br J Urol 50:200–204.

Moriyama N, Kurimoto S, Horie S, Kameyama S, Nasu K, Tanaka T, Yano J, Sagehashi Y, Yamaguchi T, Tsujmoto G, Kawabe K (1996). Quantification of a 1-adrenoceptor subtype mRNAs in hypertrophic and non-hypertrophic prostates. J Urol 155–331A (abstract 82).

Muramatsu I, Oshita M, Ohmura T, Kigoshi S, Akino H, Okada K (1994). Pharmacological characterisation of ?l adreno-ceptor subtypes in the human prostate: functional and binding studies. Br J Urol 74:572–578.

Nathan PW (1976). The central nervous connections of the bladder. In: Williams DI, Chisholm GD (eds). Scientific foundations of urology. London, Heineman pp 51–58.

Nilvebrant L, Sundquist S, Gilberg PG (1996). Neurourology and Urodynamics. Athens abstract 34 p 310.

Sundin T, Dahlstrom A (1973). The sympathetic innervation of the urinary bladder and urethra in the normal state and after parasympathetic denervation at the spinal root level. Scand J Urol Nephrol 7:131–149.

Torrens MJ (1978). Urethral sphincteric responses to stimulation of the sacral nerves in the human female. Urol Int 33:22–26.

Torrens MJ (1982). Neurophysiology. In: Stanton SL (ed.) Gynaecological urology. St Louis, Mosby.

Torrens M, Morrison JFB (1987). The physiology of the lower urinary tract. London, Springer-Verlag.

Zinner NR, Ritter RC, Sterling AM (1976). The mechanism of micturition. In: Williams DI, Chisholm GD (eds). Scientific foundations of urology. London: Heinemann pp 39–50.

Chapter 3
Urodynamic Techniques

Introduction

The evolution of urodynamic units may be traced to the interest in the hydrodynamics of micturition which had been simmering since the early cystometric studies of the nineteenth century, but it was the advent of electronics that acted as the catalyst for modern urodynamic studies. In 1956 von Garrelts described a simple practical apparatus, using a pressure transducer, to record the volume of urine voided as a function of time. By derivation, urine flow rates could be calculated. His work stimulated a revival of interest in cystometry because it was then possible to record the bladder pressure and the urine flow rate simultaneously during voiding. As a result, normal and obstructed micturition could be defined in terms of these measurements (Claridge 1966), and a formula was applied to express urethral resistance (Smith 1968). Enhorning (1961) measured bladder and urethral pressures simultaneously with a specially designed catheter, and he termed the pressure difference between them the "urethral closure pressure". He demonstrated that a reduction of intraurethral pressure occurred several seconds prior to detrusor contraction at the initiation of voiding. This appeared to be related to the relaxation of the pelvic floor, thus confirming the EMG studies of Franksson and Peterson (1955).

These original research studies led rapidly to the application of urodynamic investigations in the clinical field. Radiological studies of the lower urinary tract, using the image intensifier and cine or videotape recordings, were already established, and their value in the assessment of micturition disorders had been described (Turner Warwick and Whiteside 1970). Thus it was a relatively simple step to combine cystourethrography with pressure flow measurements (Bates et al. 1970) Later, more sophisticated techniques, using EMG recordings of the pelvic floor, were employed, particularly for neurogenic bladder problems (Thomas et al. 1975). These clinical studies during the 1970s emphasised the need to investigate the function as well as the anatomical structure of the lower urinary tract, when evaluating micturition disorders. Urodynamics was established as a necessary service commitment, rather than a research tool.

Simulaneous with these technical developments was an increasing awareness of the clinical problem of urinary incontinence. Caldwell (1967), working in Exeter, initiated considerable interest in the subject because he approached the treatment of incontinent patients with electronic implants. In his sphincter research unit, a small receiver was developed that could be placed subcutaneously in the abdominal wall and activated by a small external radio-frequency transmitter. Platinum iridium electrodes led down to the pelvic floor muscles, which could be stimulated. Other new techniques advocated at this time included pelvic floor faradism applied under general anaesthetic (Moore and Schofield 1967) and a variety of external electronic devices which could be placed in the anal canal or vagina to stimulate pelvic floor contraction (Hopkinson and Lightwood 1967; Alexander and Rowan 1968)

Through the 1980s and 1990s the principles of urodynamics remained unchanged. As microchip technology has advanced, so urodynamic equipment has become computerised, although this has not always been for the best, as discussed later. New techniques became available, such as the measurement of bladder neck electrical conductance, a technique devised by Plevnik. Computerisation has allowed the development of more complex and sophisticated neurological investigations, such as cortical evoked responses, although these techniques are used only in specialist centres. James introduced long-term (ambulatory) techniques to study bladder and urethral function. His work became the focus of increased attention in the early 1990s, and, with computerisation, the patient has been set free from the fixed urodynamic recording apparatus. Ambulatory studies, which represent a more physiological approach, have become established as a secondary method of investigation in more specialist units.

This chapter discusses the technical aspects of urodynamics. The indications of urodynamics are mentioned here only briefly, as their clinical role is discussed fully in Chapter 5.

Principles of Urodynamic Technique

Investigations must be carried out in a safe and scientific manner. The investigator is responsible for ensuring the privacy and comfort of the patient. Micturition is a private matter, and unless this is respected, urodynamics will be less than satisfactory. Proper care must be applied to the infection control aspects of investigation and the principles of sterility followed.

The investigations themselves must be free of technical errors, and, just as the grand prix driver must be familiar with the mechanics of his car, the urodynamacist must be familiar with the technical aspects of the tests they are using. This applies particularly to the measurement of pressure. The investigator must also be satisfied as to the reproducibility of urodynamic results, so that at the end of the investigation the patient can be offered explanations for his or her symptoms and the clinician can be given advice as to how the patient should be managed.

Standardisation of Techniques

Both technique and terminology should be standardised. Of course, techniques must evolve, but not on an unplanned basis. Each department's individual technique should be standard to allow for interpretation of findings. So that others may understand and interpret the results from any urodynamic unit, standardised terminology to describe the technique and the results obtained is essential. To facilitate this, the International Continence Society in 1973 set up a standardisation committee, which has produced reports on the terminology of lower urinary tract function (Appendix 1, Part I). The first six reports were collated in 1988 and comprehensively rewritten in 2002. The subjects covered include:

- Procedures related to the evaluation of urine storage.
- Procedures related to the evaluation of micturition.
- Procedures related to the neurological investigations of the urinary tract during filling and voiding.
- A classification of lower urinary tract dysfunction.
- Pelvic floor and pelvic organ prolapse assessment
- Ambulatory urodynamics
- Pressure-flow studies of voiding, urethral resistance and urethral obstruction.
- Good urodynamic practices.

These standards are proposed to facilitate comparison of results by investigators who use urodynamic methods. It has been recommended that written publications acknowledge the use of these standards with a footnote stating: "Methods, definitions and units conform to the standards proposed by the International Continence Society except where specifically noted." The author has accepted these standards and used them in this book. They are repeated and explained in the relevant chapters; the reports are listed and published in full in Appendix 1.

This chapter forms the core of the book. Urodynamic studies are described at three levels: uroflowmetry, basic urodynamics (inflow cystometry, pressure-flow studies and pad testing) and complex urodynamics (urethral pressure profilometry, videourodynamics, ambulatory studies and various aspects of neurophysiological testing).

References

Alexander S, Rowan D (1968). An electric pessary for stress incontinence. Lancet 1:728.

Bates CP, Whiteside CG, Turner Warwick R (1970). Synchronous urine pressure flow cystourethrography with special reference to stress and urge incontinence. Br J Urol 42:714–723.

Caldwell KPS (1967). The treatment of incontinence by electronic implants. Ann R Coll Surg 41:447–459.

Claridge M (1966). Analyses of obstructed micturition. Ann R Coll Surg 39:30–53.

Enhorning G (1961). Simultaneous recording of intravesical and intra-urethral pressure. Acta Chir Scand [Suppl] 276:1–68.

Franksson C, Petersen I (1955). Electromyographic investigation of disturbances in the striated muscle of the urethral sphincter. Br J Urol 27:154–161.

Hopkinson BR, Lightwood R (1967). Electrical treatment of incontinence. Br J Surg 54:802–805.

Moore T, Schofield PF (1997). Treatment of stress incontinence by maximum perineal electrical stimulation. Br Med J iii:150–151.

Smith JC (1968). Urethral resistance to micturition. Br J Urol 40:125–156.

Thomas DG, Smallwood R, Graham D (1975). Urodynamic observations following spinal trauma. Br J Urol 47:161–175.

Turner Warwick R, Whiteside CG (1970). Investigation and management of bladder neck dysfunction. In: Riches Sir Eric (ed) Modern trends in urology 3. London: Butterworth pp 295–311.

Yalla SV, Sharma GVRK, Barsamian EM (1980). Micturitional static urethral pressure profile. A method of recording urethral pressure profile during voiding and the implications. J Urol 124:649.

Uroflowmetry

Urine flow studies are the simplest of urodynamic techniques, because they are noninvasive and the the necessary equipment is simple and relatively inexpensive. Before reliable recording apparatus was commercially available, some clinicians made a habit of watching the patient void. Any such semi-objective observation is valuable. However, for any flow rate assessment to be meaningful, the bladder should be reasonably full, an uncommon event in the outpatient clinic. In addition, the patient may find it embarrassing to have the voiding observed. Further, in most circumstances, it is not practical in women. The advantage of modern urine flowmeters is that a permanent graphic recording is obtained. Flowmeters had been available for many years, but not until von Garrelts developed his flowmeter in 1956 was equipment sufficiently accurate for the recordings to be clinically useful. If, despite the availability of commercially produced apparatus, the clinician has no flowmeter, the patient can be asked to time his urinary stream with a stopwatch and to record the voided volume by calculating the average flow. In the normal patient, average flow is approximately half the maximum flow, although in patients with bladder outlet obstruction the average flow may almost equal the maximum flow. We found it impractical to obtain adequate urine flow measurements in the routine urological clinic and therefore established the urine flow clinic (see later).

Definitions

Urine flow may be described in terms of flow rate and flow pattern, and may be continuous or intermittent.

- *Flow rate* is the volume of fluid expelled via the urethra per unit time and is expressed in millilitres per second (ml/s). The basic information necessary in interpreting the flow trace includes the volume voided, the environment in which the patient passed urine and the position, that is lying, sitting or standing. It should also be stated whether the bladder filled naturally or if diuresis was stimulated by fluid or diuretics, or whether the bladder was filled by a catheter (either urethral or suprapubic). If filling was by a catheter, then the type of fluid used should be stated, as should whether the flow study was part of another investigation (e.g. a pressure-flow study).
- *Maximum flow rate* (Q_{max}) is the maximum measured value of the flow rate.
- *Voided volume* (*VV*) is the total volume expelled via the urethra.
- *Flow time* is the time over which measurable flow occurs (Fig. 3.1).
- *Average flow rate* (Q_{ave}) is voided volume divided by flow time.
- *Time to maximum flow* is the elapsed time from onset of flow to maximum flow.
- *Intermittent flow* The same measurements are used as for describing a continuous flow curve. However, flow time must be measured carefully, as the time intervals between flow episodes are disregarded. Voiding time is the total duration of micturition, including the interruptions (Fig. 3.2). Where flow is continuous, voiding time is equal to flow time. The area beneath the curve or curves represents the volume voided.

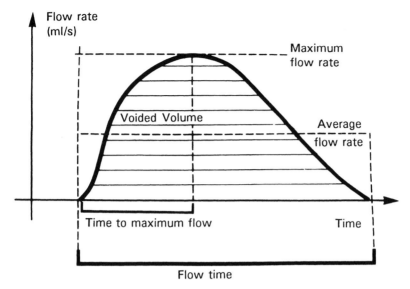

Fig. 3.1 Terminology relating to the description of urinary flow (International Continence Society report (1988) Standardisation of terminology of lower urinary tract function; see Appendix 1, Part 2). 📖

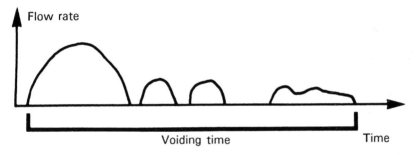

Fig. 3.2 Terminology relating to an intermittent flow rate tracing (see Appendix 1, Part 2). 📖

Urine Flow Clinic

Urine flow studies should be performed in privacy when the patient has a normal desire to void and is relaxed. In our experience, it is difficult to get an adequate flow study in the routine outpatient clinic, as it is essential that the bladder is adequately full. Furthermore, a sterile urine sample is often required for bacteriology, necessitating a second void.

To facilitate good-quality flow studies, we established a flow clinic in 1981. Following this, Carter showed that the proportion of patients who failed to void 150 ml fell from 59% to 21%. The principal objective of the urine flow clinic is to screen for bladder outlet obstruction. With a flow clinic appointment, each patient is sent a seven-day frequency – volume chart to complete before the appointment. Patients are also asked to drink normally before they leave home on the day of their appointments. On arrival, the clinic nurse checks that each patient has had adequate intake. If for any reason the patient is not adequately hydrated, additional fluid is administered. Every patient is asked to drink one litre of fluid on arrival. The clinic letter informs patients that the clinic stay is likely to last two to three hours during which time they will be asked to pass urine on at least three occasions. The patients are asked to hold their water until comfortably full. At that point, they find the nurse and are led into the flow room, having already been made familiar with the equipment. The door is then closed, and they are left to pass their urine in privacy. The flow room contains a couch and, after voiding, the patient's bladder is scanned ultrasonically to assess residual urine (see Fig. 3.3). When the patient has performed three flow rates and three ultrasound estimates of residual urine have been made, the results are presented on a flow rate nomogram. A variety of nomograms are available and these relate maximum flow rate to voided volume taking sex and age into account. Various authorities have produced such nomograms, including Von Garrelts (1958); Backman (1965); Gierup (1970); Siroky et al. (1979); Kadow et al. (1985) and Haylen (1990). In children and older subjects, the voided volume may not reach 150 ml. In these patients. the shape of the flow trace may be helpful in deciding whether or not outlet obstruction is present. Marshal et al. (1983) suggested that by measuring the initial slope of the flow trace when the voided volume was less than 150 ml, it was possible to make a reliable diagnosis of obstruction or no obstruction. In contrast, Gleason suggested that studying the stream velocity in the last 30 ml of the void would allow similar deductions to be made. The work of the above authors, together with that of Rollema (1981), shows that there is more information in flow traces than is appreciated. However, it would be true to say that most investigators use only the maximum flow rate values, together with a subjective evaluation of the shape of the trace in association with a flow rate nomogram, to make a clinical diagnosis. Based on the results from the flow clinic the patient may be referred on for pressure-flow studies of micturition or videourodynamics.

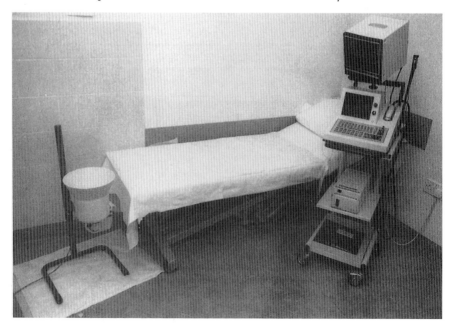

Fig. 3.3 Urine flow clinic: room layout. The flowmeter and commode are at the foot of the couch with the ultrasound machine at the head of the bed. 📖

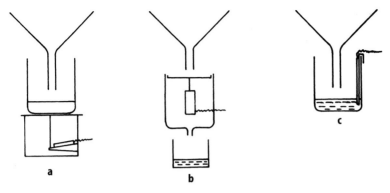

Fig. 3.4 Urine flowmeters: using the weight transducer (**a**), spinning disc (**b**) and capacitance methods (**c**). 📖

Equipment

The available flowmeters (Fig. 3.4) use several different principles, as follows:

- The weight transducer flowmeter involves weighing the urine voided, thereby measuring the volume of urine voided. It also calculates the urine flow rate by differentiation with respect to time.
- The rotating-disc flow meter has a spinning disc on which the urine falls. The disc is kept rotating at the same speed by a servomotor, in spite of changes in the urine flow rate; the weight of the urine tends to slow the rotation of the disc. The differing power needed to keep disc rotation constant is proportional to the urine flow rate. The flow signal is electronically integrated to record the volume voided.
- It is also possible to "weigh" urine by measuring the hydrostatic pressure exerted by a column of urine, using an ordinary pressure transducer.

Most commercially available flowmeters have acceptable accuracy. However, the buyer should always seek independent information on the machine's performance and, in particular, the accuracy (errors should be less than 5%), the linearity of response over the range 0 ml/s to 50 ml/s, the reliability of the apparatus, the compatibility with any existing equipment, the safety of the flowmeter, and its ease of cleaning. It is wise to check the performance of the flowmeter at regular intervals and a simple flowmeter tester has been described (Fig. 3.5, *overleaf*). Most manufacturers also produce a chart recorder, which is marketed as a package with the flowmeter. Because changes in flow rate are relatively slow in electronic terms, an inexpensive pen recorder is adequate for uroflowmetry. In the last five years, the flowmeter package has included an automatic printout of the major measurements listed above. This development is the cause of many problems, however. The software within these flowmeters is not adequately intelligent to distinguish physiological flow changes from flow changes produced by artefact (Fig. 3.6, *overleaf*). Hence the flowmeter will often record an artefactually high maximum flow rate, and if the nurse or doctor interpreting the trace is not sufficiently trained then a falsely high maximum flow rate will be recorded, and this may influence the patient's management. In a large study, 23 857 flow curves were reviewed and the machine readout compared with a manual assessment: there was a difference of more than 1 ml/s in 62% and a difference of more than 3 ml/s in 9% (Grino 1993). As flowmeter

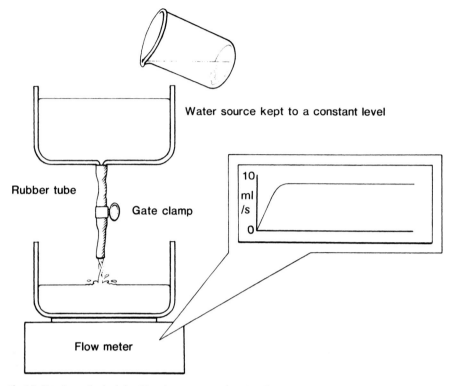

Water source kept to a constant level

Rubber tube

Gate clamp

10
ml
/s
0

Flow meter

Fig. 3.5 Simple method of checking the accuracy of a urine flowmeter: gateclamp is adjusted to give a constant flow of a given volume of 100 ml in 10 s. 📖

accuracy is limited flow rate should be expressed to the nearest whole millilitre (15 ml/s rather than 14.8 ml/s). The rapid changes in flow can be eliminated by using a sliding average over 2 seconds (see Appendix 1 Part 6). This process smooths the trace to remove positive and negative spikes. Volumes should be rounded to the nearest 10 ml. Results from the flow clinic should be expressed as Maximum Flow Rate voided Volume/Residual Volume (e.g., 12 ml/s/210 ml/30 ml).

Normal Flow Patterns

When considering the normality of flow rates, the patient's age and sex and the voided volume should be taken into account. In addition to the numerical data derived from any flow trace, the shape of the trace is also important.

In *normal flow*, the flow curve has a "bell" shape. Maximum flow is reached in the first 30% of any trace and within 5 seconds from the start of flow. The flow rate varies according to the volume voided (Fig. 3.8, *overleaf*). Figure 3.9 (*overleaf*) shows how different traces can look quite different in the same unobstructed individual voiding different volumes. Although the traces look superficially different, they all have similar first and final phases. The final phase of a normal flow trace shows a rapid fall from high flow, together with a sharp cutoff at the termination of flow (two similar Q_{max} readings in different patients can

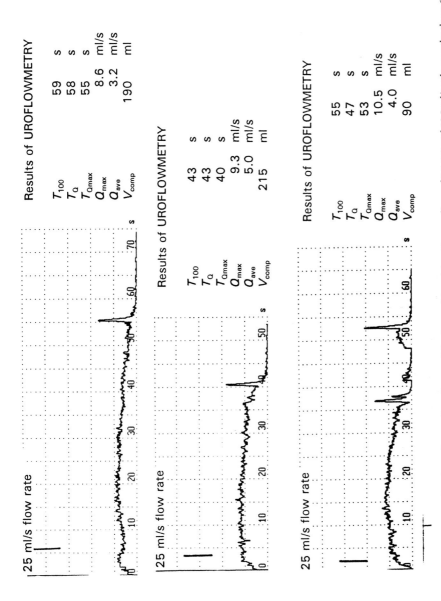

Fig. 3.6 Traces from the flow rate clinic showing spike artefacts that result in the machine giving Q_{max} readings of 8.6, 9.3 and 10.5 ml/s, whereas the three Q_{max} values are 4, 6 and 6 ml/s respectively.

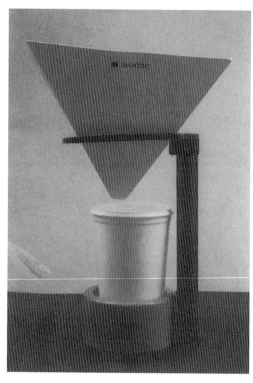

Fig. 3.7 Home flowmeters: battery-powered flowmeter with a disposable paper funnel. 📖

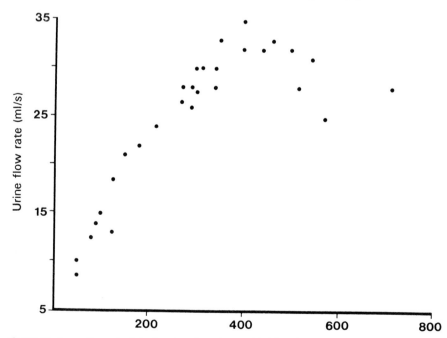

Fig. 3.8 Maximum flow rate plotted against the volume voided for a large number of voids in one individual normal case. 📖

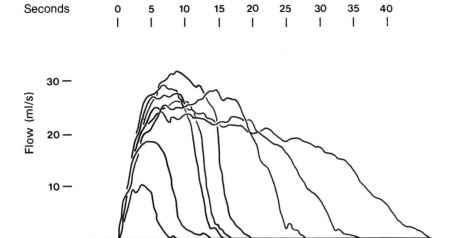

Fig. 3.9 Superimposition of various flow rate tracings; the examples are taken from the same case as in Fig 3.8. This is a very useful way to display multiple flow rate tracings. 📖

give quite different flow curve shapes owing to the different voided volumes) (Fig. 3.10). The appearance of the trace also depends on the paper speed of the recorder. If this is very slow then flow will appear as a vertical line; if it is faster then the flow curve will be elongated. A paper speed of 0.25 cm/s is practical and allows easy interpretation of the shape of the curve.

Urine flow rate is highly dependent on the volume voided. Detrusor muscle when stretched achieves an optimal performance, but if stretched further it becomes inefficient.

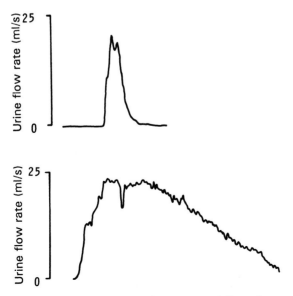

Fig. 3.10 Similar Q_{max} readings of 21 ml/s and 23 ml/s giving very different flow curve shapes due to different voided volumes of 80 ml and 550 ml respectively. 📖

Table 3.1. Lowest acceptable maximum urine flow rates according to age and sex for minimum voided volumes[a]

Age years	Minimum Volume ml	Male ml/s	Female ml/s
4–7	100	10	10
8–13	100	12	15
14–45	200	21	18
46–65	200	12	15
66–80	200	9	10

[a]Values given are taken from personal experience and relevant literature. In general the values are one standard deviation below the mean for the maximum flow. Values below those given may not be abnormal, but need further consideration.

At more than 400 ml, the efficiency of the detrusor begins to decrease and Q_{max} is lower (Fig. 3.8). Flow rates are highest and most predictable in the volume range between 200 ml and 400 ml. Through this range the maximum flow tends to be constant. In practice, the definition of normality can be considered in two ways. The simplest is to have a minimum acceptable flow rate for any sex and age group. Because of the dependence on volume voided this is relatively inaccurate, but may be acceptable provided that the volume voided is in the range 200 ml to 500 ml. Such values are given in Table 3.1.

Much work has been devoted to the construction of flow rate nomograms. Nomograms have been described for boys, girls, men under 55, men over 55 and women. In our unit we use the Siroky nomogram for men under 55 (Fig. 3.11) and the Bristol nomogram for men over 55 (Fig. 3.12, *overleaf*).

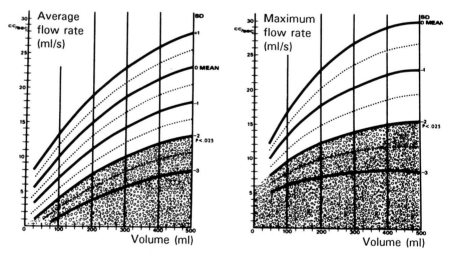

Fig. 3.11 Nomogram for flow rate in male subjects, allowing an estimate for the probability of normality. Three standard deviations below the mean are plotted. The *stippled zone* indicates flow rates that occur in less than 2.5% of the normal male population. (Siroky et al. 1979).

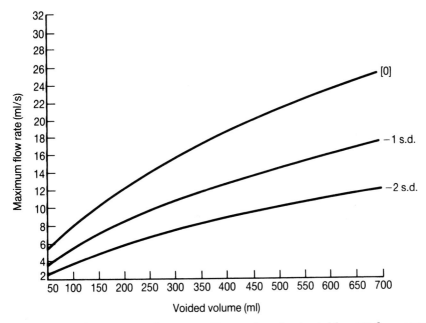

Fig. 3.12 Bristol uroflow nomogram for men over 55 years of age. Constructed from 286 flow measurements from 123 asymptomatic men. 📖

Abnormal Flow Patterns – Classification and Interpretation

Urine flow results from the interaction between the expressive forces (detrusor contraction plus any abdominal straining) and urethral resistance. Hence urine flow rates have limitations which must be appreciated.

Although male patients fit into two main patterns–normal flow and normal pressure, and low flow and high pressure (obstructed, as in Fig. 3.6)–the information from urine flow traces, without simultaneous pressure recording, must be interpreted with care. Two examples of misleading situations are shown in Table 3.2, which indicates that patients with normal flow can have bladder outlet obstruction when a normal maximum flow rate is maintained by abnormally high voiding pressures (Fig. 3.13, *overleaf*). The other misleading group comprises patients whose low flow rates are due to detrusor underactivity rather than to bladder outlet obstruction. This situation is relatively common in older women.

Table 3.2. Flow and pressure combinations giving different diagnoses

Flow	Pressure	Diagnosis
NORMAL	Normal/low	UNOBSTRUCTED
Normal	High	Obstructed
LOW	High	OBSTRUCTED
Low	Normal	Equivocal
Low	Low	Unobstructed

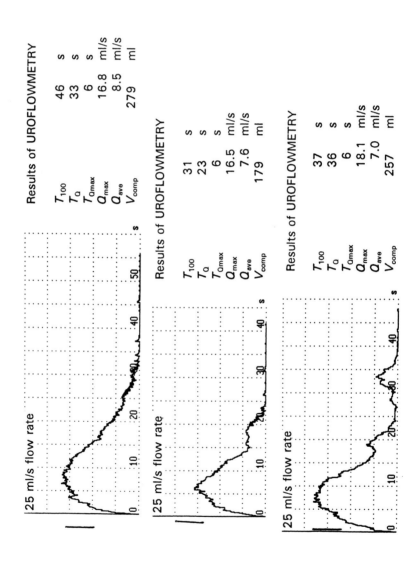

Fig. 3.13 Flow clinic data from a man of 80 with normal Q_{max} readings but who on pressure flow studies was shown to be obstructed.

Continuous Flow Curves

Normal. As already described, the normal flow curve is bell-shaped but its appearance will differ quite markedly according to the volume of urine voided (Fig. 3.9). Maximum flow is normally reached within 3 s to 10 s from the onset of micturition.

Detrusor Overactivity. Strictly speaking, the pattern sometimes seen in idiopathic detrusor overactivity is not abnormal, but is supranormal (Fig. 3.14). Very high maximum flow rates may be achieved by patients who have s detrusor muscle with high contraction velocities, giving a flow trace that shows a very rapid increase in flow to a high maximum reached in an abnormally short time (1 s-3 s). The reduction in time to maximum flow is achieved because the detrusor contraction has already opened the bladder neck widely, hence reducing the urethral resistance. Thus when the patient starts to void he or she has only to relax the distal sphincter which has previously prevented the involuntary contraction from producing incontinence.

Bladder Outlet Obstruction (BOO). Flow curves in obstructed patients are characterised by a low maximum and reduced average flow, with the average flow greater than half the maximum flow rate. Maximum flow is usually obtained relatively quickly (3–10 secs), but the flow rate then decreases slowly (Fig. 3.15). In outlet obstruction the flow rate is expected to be continuous, although it may end in a terminal dribble.

Obstruction may be "compressive", for example in benign prostatic obstruction, or "constrictive" as in a urethral stricture. The two types of obstruction give different types of trace. The "constrictive" obstruction gives a "plateau"-shaped trace with little change in flow rate and little difference between Q_{max} and Q_{ave} (Fig. 3.16). In compressive obstruction, the

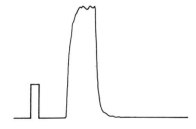

Fig. 3.14 Flow trace in a case of detrusor overactivity. In this and subsequent figures the height of the calibration mark indicates 10 ml/s flow rate and the width of the mark is 2 s. In this case supranormal flow is established almost immediately and cessation of flow is equally rapid as the bladder neck closes suddenly.

Fig. 3.15 Flow trace in a case of bladder outlet obstruction. Maximum flow is established soon after the onset of voiding. 📖

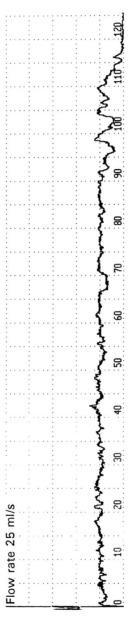

Fig. 3.16 Flow trace from a man of 50 with a 10-year history of bulbar urethral stricture: the characteristic "plateau"-shaped trace is shown ($Q_{max} = 5$ ml/s).

first third of the flow trace may appear relatively normal, although the Q_{max} will be reduced, but the latter part of the trace usually is elongated into a pronounced "tail" of reducing flow rate (Figs. 3.13, part 1, and 3.15).

Detrusor Underactivity (DUA). This diagnosis is discussed later in this chapter under "Cystometry". However, it can be suspected if a symmetrical trace with a low maximum flow rate is seen (Fig. 3.17). The characteristic in detrusor underactivity is that the time to reach maximum flow is very variable, and the maximum flow may occur in the second half of the trace. However, there is considerable overlap between the flow traces of the obstructed and the underactive detrusor group, and therefore the diagnosis can only be suspected: proof comes from a pressure-flow study.

Interrupted Flow Patterns

Irregular Trace Secondary to Straining. Some patients are in the habit of using, or need to use, their diaphragmatic and abdominal muscles to increase urine flow. Straining makes the flow trace irregular (Fig. 3.18). With straining the changes in flow tend to be relatively slow and the stream is usually continuous. Straining flow traces are very variable in appearance, because they may occur in the presence or absence of obstruction and in the presence or absence of a detrusor contraction. In general the flow increases as the patient strains, although this is not the case in men with bladder outlet obstruction (Reynard 1995). The situation often needs further elucidation by a pressure-flow study that includes detrusor pressure recording.

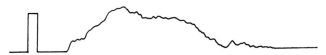

Fig. 3.17 Flow trace in a case of detrusor underactivity. Maximum flow is established near the middle of the voiding time. 📖

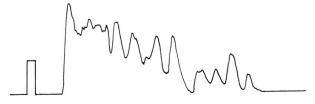

Fig. 3.18 Straining producing an irregular tracing. 📖

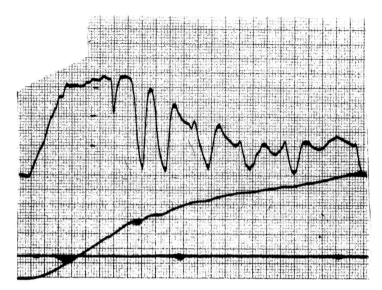

Fig. 3.19 Dysfunctional voiding in a man of 63 with LUTS. The irregularity of flow was due to anxiety resulting in pelvic floor overactivity: subsequent flows had a smooth pattern (Q_{max} is 17 ml/s and VV 360 ml). 📖

Irregular Trace Secondary to Urethral Overactivity. In neurologically abnormal patients, involuntary contraction of the distal urethral sphincter mechanism is termed detrusor sphincter dyssynergia. It is also seen in patients without neurological abnormality, where it may merely be the result of anxiety in unfamiliar surroundings. However, an abnormal trace found on repeat investigation in neurologically normal patients is due to a pattern termed dysfunctional voiding. As with straining, the appearances are variable, but in general flow rate changes are faster than those due to straining (Fig. 3.19).

Irregular Trace Due to Poor Sustained or Fluctuating Detrusor Contractions. This abnormality is generally seen in patients with a neurological problem, most commonly multiple sclerosis. The detrusor contraction, instead of producing an approximately constant pressure throughout voiding, fluctuates. This produces either a continuous but varying flow or, more commonly, an interrupted flow (Fig. 3.20).

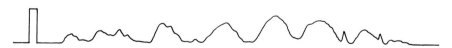

Fig. 3.20 Intermittent flow due to fluctuating detrusor contraction. The changes in flow rate are relatively slow. 📖

Irregular Trace Secondary to Artefacts

There are a number of artefacts that may trick the urodynamicist.

"Cruising". The most potent is caused by the patient, usually a man, moving their stream in relation to the central exit from the collecting funnel; Fig. 3.21 is a good example. The "peaks" occur when the point of impact of the stream is moving down the side of the funnel towards the central exit; that is, the urine being passed is catching up with the urine passed immediately before. The "valleys" occur when the impact point is moving away from the exit. Usually the "peaks" will fit into the "valleys" in this type of tracing. Manufacturers have attempted to minimise this phenomenon by complex baffles in the funnel, although a better solution might be to paint a target onto the funnel for the patient to aim at! Whereas this artefact is almost exclusive to men, the next one described is entirely so.

"Squeezing". Perhaps in an effort to deny the onset of age (and reducing urine flow), some men have the habit of squeezing the tip of their penis or foreskin during voiding (Fig. 3.22). This leads to a series of peaks, as shown in the upper diagram (Fig. 3.23). When the patient is asked to stop this practice, the flow trace usually becomes classically obstructed, and the flow rate is no longer within the normal range (lower trace). These artefacts are not detected by the computerised analysis of flow, which potentially misleads the clinician. (Q_{max} in Fig 3.22 is measured at 25 ml/s but is probably closer to 11 ml/s)

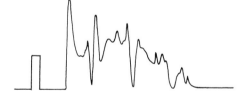

Fig. 3.21 "Cruising": the irregular trace resulting from a male patient moving his stream backwards and forwards across the neck of the collecting funnel. The changes in flow are rapid and biphasic in type. 📖

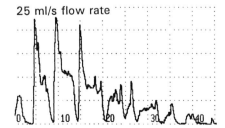

25 ml/s flow rate

Results of UROFLOWMETRY

T_{100}	65	s
T_Q	49	s
T_{Qmax}	10	s
Q_{max}	25.0	ml/s
Q_{ave}	4.9	ml/s
V_{comp}	240	ml

Fig. 3.22 "Squeezing" artefact due to the patient intermittently compressing the end of the penis during voids. The peaks of flow are due to urine building up in the penile urethra to give spurts as the man releases his grip. 📖

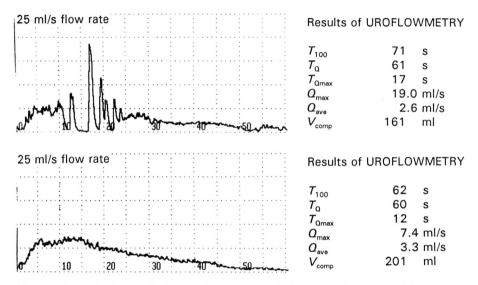

Fig. 3.23 A "squeezing" artefact is shown in the upper trace. The lower trace shows a smooth "obstructed" curve after the patient has been asked not to hold the penis during voiding. 📖

Uroflowmetry and the Recording of Residual Urine

In our flow clinic, we routinely measure the residual urine after voiding by ultrasound. The formula, $D_1 \times D_2 \times D_3 \times 0.7$ gives an approximation of the residual volume in millilitres. D_1, D_2 and D_3 are three different diameters (of the bladder). The diameters D_1 and D_2 are measured in the saggital plane (D_1 is bladder neck to fundus and D_2 is anterior to posterior wall) and D_3 is measured in the coronal plane (D_3 is right side to left side). Such measurements are subject to considerable observer error in particular because the bladder assumes an irregular shape at the end of voiding; sometimes it looks rather more like a squashed football, being much wider in the transverse plane than it is from the bladder neck to the fundus. Nevertheless, from the clinical point of view an adequate degree of accuracy can be obtained from relatively inexpensive ultrasound machines, one of which is handheld (Fig. 3.24). However, it should be noted that there is some conflict as to the significance of increased residual urine. It had been assumed to indicate obstruction, but Abrams and Griffiths (1979) and others have suggested that it may represent detrusor underactivity rather than bladder outlet obstruction. Despite this, many or perhaps most clinicians allow the quantity of residual urine to influence their management of patients. In our urodynamic unit, the residual urine is stated both on the results from the flow clinic and after pressure-flow studies.

Indications for Uroflowmetry

Urine flow studies are an excellent screening study in a wide variety of patients, but frequently they must be followed by pressure-flow studies which allow more precise definition of bladder and urethral function. Uroflow is used to investigate possible bladder outlet obstruction and can also give a guide to detrusor contractility. It should be used for patients of all ages and for both sexes.

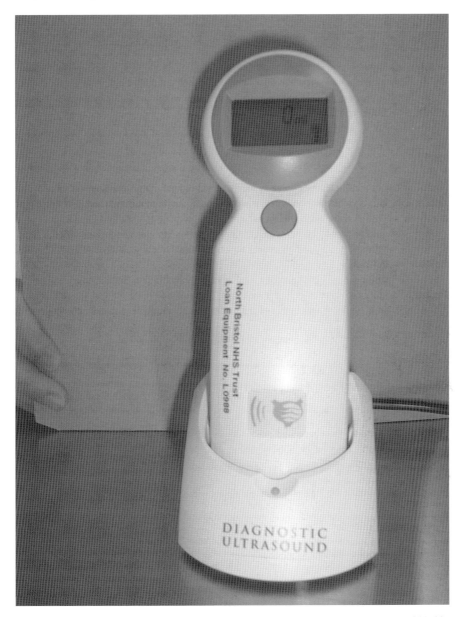

Fig. 3.24 Hand-held or patient-worn ultrasound machine which allows easy recording of bladder volume/post void residual, in clinic, on the ward or in the patient's home. The photo shows the ultrasound head, with display.

Children

Uroflow is the screening test for all neurologically normal children with possible functional outlet obstruction (see "Voiding Cystometry").

Women

When surgery for stress incontinence is planned, uroflow provides evidence of normal detrusor voiding function if flow rates are excellent. Reduced flows may lead to post-operative voiding problems as they are indicative of abnormal voiding function. In elderly women, uroflow is useful in excluding residual urine, which may be the cause of recurrent urinary tract infections.

Men

Uroflow is the screening test of choice in men of all ages with symptoms suggestive of outlet obstruction. This applies to those men who have less classic symptoms, such as recurrent infections, as well as those with the classic symptoms of poor stream and hesitancy.

Uroflow should be measured before and after any procedure designed to modify the function of the outflow tract, e.g. for urethral stricture, bladder neck obstruction and benign prostatic obstruction.

Note: All urine flow curves should be evaluated by the clinician, so that artefacts can be eliminated and a true value of Q_{max} derived.

The indications for uroflowmetry are further dealt with in Chapter 5 under patient groups.

References

Abrams P (1991). The urine flow clinic. In Fitzpatrick JN (ed) Conservative treatment of BPH Edinburgh: Churchill Livingstone pp 33–43.

Abrams P (1977). Prostatism and prostatectomy: The value of urine flow rate measurement in the preoperative assessment for operation. J Urol 117:70–71.

Backman KA (1965). Urinary flow during micturition in normal women. Acta Chir Scand 130:357–370.

Backman KA, von Garrelts B, Sundblad R (1966). Micturition in normal women. Studies of pressure and flow. Acta Chir Scand 132:403–412.

Chancellor MB, Blaivas JG, Kaplan SA, Axelrod S (1991). Bladder outlet obstruction versus impaired detrusor contractility: the role of uroflow. J Urol 145:810–812.

Drach GW, Steinbronn DV (1986). Clinical evaluation of patients with prostatic obstruction; correlation of flow rates with voided, residual or total bladder volume. J Urol 135:737–740.

Garrelts B von (1956). Analysis of micturition. A new method of recording the voiding of the bladder. Acta Chir Scand 112:326–340.

Garrelts B von (1958). Micturition in the normal male. Acta Chir Scand 114:197–210.

Gierup T (1970) Micturition studies in infants and children. Scand J Urol Nephrol 4:217–230.

Gleason DM, Bottaccini MR, Perling D, Lattimer JK (1967). A challenge to current urodynamic thought. J Urol 97:935.

Golomb J, Linder A, Siegel Y, Korezah D (1992). Variability and circadian changes in home uroflowmetry in patients with benign prostatic hyperplasia compared to normal controls. J Urol 147:1044–1047.

Griffiths CJ, Murray A, Ramsden PD (1983). A simple uroflowmeter tester. Br J Urol 55:21–24.

Griffiths DJ, Scholtmeijer RJ (1984). Place of the free flow curve in the urodynamic investigation of children. Br J Urol 56:474–477.

Grino PB, Bruskewitz R, Blaivas JG, Siroky MB, Andersen JT, Cook T, Stower E (1993). Maximum urinary flow rate by uroflowmetry: Automatic or visual interpretation. J Urol 149:339–341.

Haylen BT, Parys BT, Anyaegbunam WI, Ashby D, West CR (1990). Urine flow rates in male and female urodynamic patients compared with Liverpool nomograms. Br J Urol 65:483–487.

Jensen KM-E, Jørgensen JB, Mogensen P (1985). Reproducibility of uroflowmetry variable in elderly males. Urol Res. 13:237–239.

Jørgensen JB, Jensen KM-E, Bille-Brahe NE, Morgensen P (1986). Uroflowmetry in asymptomatic elderly males. Br J Urol 58:390–395.

Jørgensen JB, Jensen KM-E, Morgensen P (1993). Longitudinal observations on normal and abnormal voiding in men over the age of 50 years. Uroflowmetry and symptoms of prostatism. Br J Urol 72:413–420.

Kadow C, Howells S, Lewis P, Abrams P (1985). A flow rate nomogram for normal males over the age of 50. Proc. ICS 15th Annual meeting, London 138–139.

Renard JM, Lim C, Swami S, Abrams P. (1996). The obstructive effect of a urethral catheter. J Urol 155:901-3.

Reynard JM, Peters TJ, Lamond E, Abrams P. (1995). The significance of abdominal straining in men with lower urinary tract symptoms. Br J Utol 75:148-53.

Rollema HJ (1981). Uroflowmetry in males. Reference values and clinical application in benign prostatic hypertrophy. Rijksuniveriteit te Groningen, Druk-kerij van Denderen BV, Groningen.

Ryall RR, Marshall VR (1982). Normal peak urinary flow rates obtained from small voided volumes can provide a reliable assessment of bladder function. J Urol 127:484–488.

Siroky MB, Olsson CA, Krane RJ (1979). The flow rate nomogram. I. Development. J Urol 122:665–668.

Sullivan J, Swithinbank L, Abrams P (2003). An audit of urodynamic standardisation in the West Midlands, UK. Br J Urol Int 91:430.

Szabo L, Fegyverneki S (1995). Maximum and average urine flow rates in normal children – the miskolc nomograms. Br J Urol 76:16–20.

Cystometry

Introduction

The previous section on uroflowmetry examined the role of urine flow studies in defining bladder and urethral function. We concluded that its role is limited because flow is a product of the forces of expulsion against the resistance given by the urethra. Whilst urine flow rate gives an idea as to whether voiding is normal, it tells us little about the storage phase of micturition. It also cannot offer a precise diagnosis because it cannot distinguish between obstruction and detrusor underactivity, as the cause of reduced flow rate.

Cystometry is used to study both the storage and the voiding phase of micturition to make a diagnosis which enables effective treatment to be given. Cystometry is the method by which the pressure-volume relationship of the bladder is measured. Cystometrograms have been performed for many years using incremental filling and intermittent pressure measurement by water manometer (Fig. 3.25). However, since the introduction of reliable

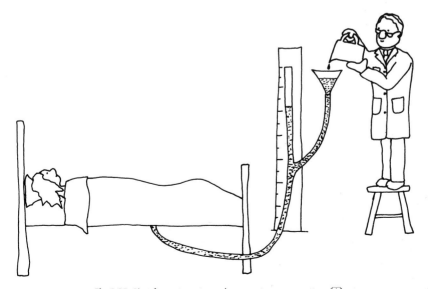

Fig. 3.25 Simple cystometry using a water manometer. 📖

Table 3.3. Normal and abnormal lower urinary tract function described in terms of bladder and urethral behaviour during the storage and voiding phases

Normal function			Abnormal function	
	STORAGE	VODING	STORAGE	VOIDING
BLADDER	Relaxed	Contracts	Overactive	Underactive
				Acontractile
URETHRA	Contracted	Relaxes	Incompetent under stress	Functional obstruction
			Inappropriate relaxation	Anatomic obstruction

pressure transducers, which have allowed the continuous measurement of pressure during bladder filling, new cystometric patterns have been recognised.

When thinking about the diagnosis and treatment of micturition disorders, it is useful to separate bladder and urethral function by defining the behaviour of each during the storage phase and during the voiding phase. In normal micturition, the bladder is relaxed and the urethra is contracted during the storage phase, whereas the bladder contracts and the urethra relaxes during voiding (Table 3.3). It therefore follows that abnormal function must be a failure of either the bladder or the urethra to behave normally during storage or voiding (Table 3.3). During storage, the bladder cannot be described as underactive, because in normal function it should be relaxed; during voiding, it cannot be described as overactive, because its function is to contract with maximal efficiency to empty the bladder.

Similarly, the urethra cannot be described as overactive during storage or as underactive during voiding, because its function is to give total continence during storage and total "incontinence" during voiding. Newcomers to urodynamics find the subject easier to understand if bladder and urethral function is viewed in this way and by asking themselves four simple questions:

- Is the bladder relaxed during storage?
- Is the urethra contracted during storage?
- Does the bladder contract adequately during voiding?
- Does the urethra open properly during voiding?

Although cystometry seems a simple technique, a number of areas present difficulties and limitations that must be appreciated. First, the measurement of pressure is subject to numerous artefacts, so precise scientific method is vital in ensuring that valid data is obtained. Second, there is increasing evidence that the technique used for cystometry will have a bearing on the results obtained. Both these points are discussed in full below.

Principles of Cystometry

Cystometry is used to study bladder and urethral function during the micturition cycle, that is during bladder filling and during voiding. During standard cystometry, the pressure within the bladder (intravesical pressure) is measured together with the pressure within the abdominal cavity (abdominal pressure is almost always by measuring the pressure in the rectum). Intravesical pressure measurement reflects both detrusor activity and any changes in abdominal pressure. The abdominal pressure may be affected by contraction of the diaphragmatic and abdominal wall muscles.

The measurement of both bladder and abdominal pressure allows the investigator to assess whether changes seen in intravesical pressure are due to contraction of the bladder alone or whether they are due to abdominal straining.

Bladder pressure (p_{ves}) and rectal pressure (p_{abd}) are measured by catheters, and by electronically subtracting abdominal pressure from intravesical pressure, the detrusor pressure (p_{det}) can be calculated: $p_{det} = p_{ves} - p_{abd}$. Fig. 3.26 (*overleaf*) illustrates a series of changes during the measurement of bladder pressure. Without the measurement of abdominal pressure, it is difficult to know what has produced these changes. However, when p_{abd} is also measured, the changes can readily be defined as the result of detrusor activity, raised abdominal pressure or a combination of both.

The pressure changes seen on the p_{ves} trace of Fig. 3.26 allow simple rules to be devised:

- If a pressure change is seen in both p_{ves} and p_{abd} but not in p_{det} then it is due to raised abdominal pressure (event S).
- If a pressure change is seen on p_{ves} and p_{det} but not on p_{abd} then it is due to a detrusor contraction (event U).
- If a pressure change is seen on p_{ves} p_{abd} and p_{det} then there is both a detrusor contraction and increased abdominal pressure (event C + U).
- If a pressure change is seen on p_{abd} with no change in p_{ves} and a consequent fall in p_{det} then this due to a rectal contraction (Fig. 3.44).

Whilst detrusor function can be assessed directly by observation of the pressure changes, urethral function is usually inferred from the pressure changes within the bladder and by measuring any urine leakage during filling, and by measuring urine flow during voiding.

Aims of Cystometry

The principal aim of UDS is to reproduce the patient's symptoms and to relate them to any synchronous urodynamic events. Other aims are to define detrusor function and urethral function during both filling and voiding. This will give four possible diagnoses during cystometry, for example, on filling, detrusor function normal, urethra incompetent (patient leaked, urodynamic stress incontinence.); on voiding, detrusor underactive (low flow rate, patient strained to void), and urethra normal. It is essential that the clinician relates these diagnoses to the symptomatic complaints of the patient and any abnormal physical findings. In this way, the relevance of the results can be assessed and, should the clinical problems not have been answered, further investigations can be planned.

Measurement of Pressure

The principles and practice discussed below apply to the measurement of pressure at any site, be it the bladder, the urethra, or the rectum. There are certain key elements to the process of pressure measurement and the investigator needs to understand the principles of pressure measurement. Pressure can be measured simply by a water column (Fig. 3.27) with a catheter placed in the bladder. The height of the water column in centimetres above the

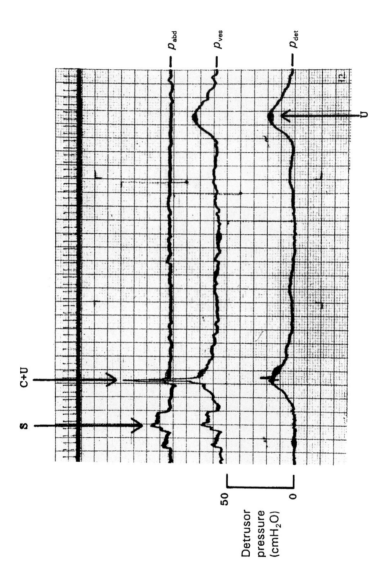

Fig. 3.26 Cystometry trace showing the patient straining (*S*), a cough superimposed on an involuntary detrusor contraction (*C* + *U*) and an involuntary detrusor contraction (*U*). 🖳

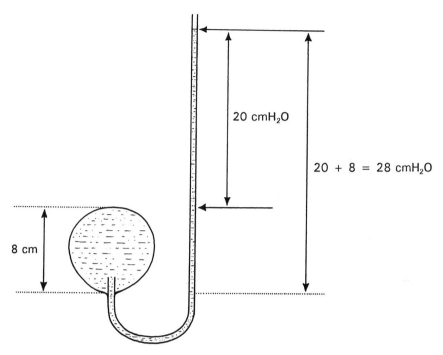

20 cmH₂O

20 + 8 = 28 cmH₂O

8 cm

Fig. 3.27 Bladder pressure can be measured by a simple, vertically held water manometer: the bladder pressure equals the height of the bladder plus the height of the water column above the bladder (8 cm + 20 cm) or the height from the bladder outlet to the top of the column. The pressure measured depends as the reference height used: The ICS standard is at the upper border of the symphysis pubis. 📖

bottom of the bladder gives the pressure within the bladder, measured in centimetres of water. However, modern urodynamic systems utilise transducers for the accurate measurement of pressure.

Pressure Transducers

A pressure transducer is a device which converts (transduces) a change in pressure, occurring, for example in the bladder, into a change in electrical signal. The change in electrical signal can then be magnified (amplified) until it is large enough for a recorder to register the change on a paper trace. Pressure transducers used in urodynamics are of two main types, the first is the conventional external strain gauge transducer mounted on a stand and connected to the patient by a water-filled tube (Fig. 3.28) down which passes a pressure wave that bends a thin metal diaphragm (Fig. 3.29). Attached to the back of the diaphragm is a strain gauge manufactured from a metal alloy which when bent changes its electrical resistance. A "large" pressure change will produce a "large" movement of the transducer diaphragm, and will produce a "large" degree of bend in the strain gauge, producing a "large" change in electrical signal (Fig. 3.29c). This type of transducer is relatively cheap, robust and easy to handle. However, the tube by which it is linked to the patient can itself introduce artefacts (see later).

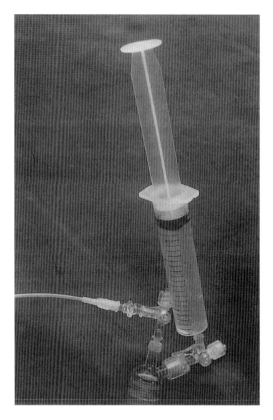

Fig. 3.28 External stand-mounted pressure transducer showing the syringe used to flush the transducer and tubing. 📖

The second type of transducer is the catheter tip (catheter-mounted) transducer. The principle of measurement is identical to that employed in the previous device, but the diaphragm and strain gauge are sited on the catheter (Fig. 3.30, *overleaf*) and therefore within the bladder or rectum. By using slightly larger catheters, additional transducers can be used, and even a filling channel built into the catheter. The advantages of catheter-mounted transducers are the elimination of the artefacts arising from the fluid-filled connecting line which links the patient to a transducer of the external type. Their disadvantages include the relatively high cost, their greater fragility and the fact that they are more difficult to handle. However, they are especially useful if rapid changes in pressure need to be measured, for example during stress urethral profilometry (see p. 107) and are essential in ambulatory urodynamics. (see p. 94)

It has to be remembered that transducers of these two types measure pressure differently. The actual measurement of p_{ves} by an external transducer depends on the vertical level of the transducer in relation to the bladder (Fig. 3.31, *overleaf*). On the other hand the pressure measured by a catheter tip transducer depends on the position of the transducer *within* the bladder (Fig. 3.32, *overleaf*).

Transducer should be able to measure in the range -20 to + 250 cmH$_2$O with an accuracy of ± 1 cmH$_2$O.

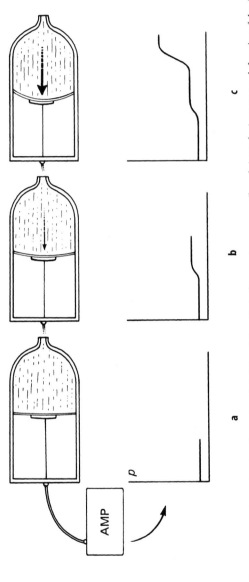

Fig. 3.29 External pressure transducer showing the resting state (a) and the effect of increasing pressure (b and c) producing greater deformity of the diaphragm and the strain gauge mounted behind the diaphragm. The resultant increased electrical charge is amplified (AMP) and recorded as increased pressure (p) on graphs b and c. ▯

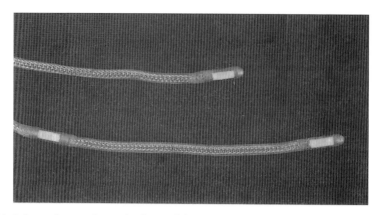

Fig. 3.30 Catheter tip transducers: in these solid-state devices the transducer(s) is mounted on a catheter; dual and single transducers are shown. 📖

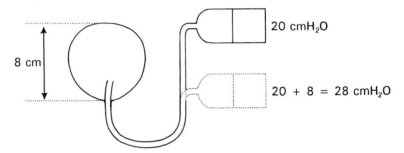

Fig. 3.31 External pressure transducers measure pressure according to their position (outside the body) in relation to the bladder: the lower position (dotted lines) [??046] records a pressure of 28 cmH$_2$O (20 cmH$_2$O represents the pressure generated by the detrusor, and 8 cmH$_2$O by the additional pressure lead due to its lower position). The position of the end of the catheter in the bladder does not change the pressure measurement. 📖

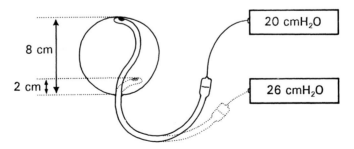

Fig. 3.32 Catheter tip transducers measure pressure according to the position of the transducer within the bladder. When the transducer is high in the bladder (solid lines) the pressure is lower (20 cmH$_2$O); when the transducer is lower in the bladder the pressure is higher (26 cmH$_2$O = 20 cmH$_2$O *plus* the 6-cm column of urine on top of the transducer). 📖

Measuring Pressure Correctly

There are three fundamental and vital steps:

- Set zero.
- Calibrate the transducers.
- Establish the pressure reference level.

Step 1: Setting Zero

The International Continence Society (ICS) has published a technical report which established the convention that *zero pressure is the surrounding atmospheric pressure*. The zero is *never* set with the transducer exposed to intravesical pressure after the catheter is passed into the bladder. Figure 3.33 shows a typical arrangement of a transducer (T) linked by two three-way taps to the manometer tubing that connects the transducers to the bladder and rectal catheters, and to a syringe (S) used to flush fluid through the system to eliminate bubbles and check for leaks. The transducer can either be held vertically, or horizontally as shown in Fig. 3.34, *overleaf*. In both systems the zero level is taken as the open end of the

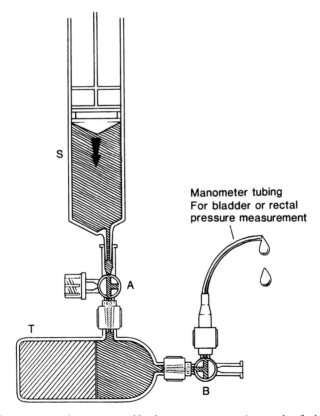

Fig. 3.33 External pressure transducer connected by three-way tap to a syringe used to flush the transducer and manometer connected to the transducer via tap B.

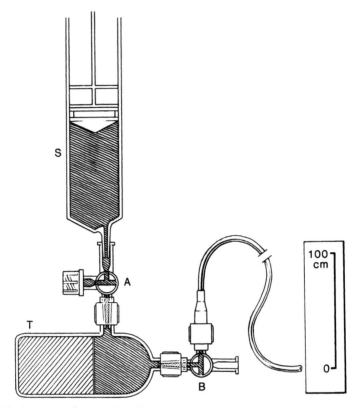

Fig. 3.34 Setting zero: with tap A selected to isolate the syringe, the end of the manometer tube is positioned at the same horizontal level as the transducer. 📖

manometer tubing (connected to the three-way tap B) when the open end is held at the same horizontal level as the transducer (Fig. 3.34). Before zero is set the manometer tubing connected to the two transducers should be flushed.

Step 2: Calibrating the Transducer

Most urodynamic systems have the facility for the electronic calibration of the pressure transducers, but it is wise to check this manually from time to time. This is easiest with a machine which supplies a stand with transducers attached and two identified points 100 cm apart. If no such system is available, then a 100-cm ruler should be employed as follows:

- With the open end of the manometer tubing at the 0-cm mark, the machine should read zero and the trace on the paper should be at the zero point (see above).
- The open end of the catheter is now raised to the 100-cm mark, whereupon the machine should read 100 and the trace should have moved up the paper from the 0-cm to 100-cmH$_2$O level (Fig. 3.35).

Catheter tip transducers can be calibrated by submerging them in a water column of measured depth.

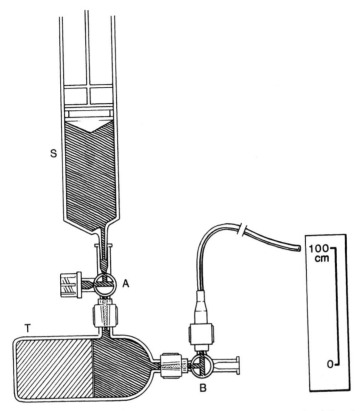

Fig. 3.35 Calibrating the transducer: the open end of the manometer tubing is levated to the 100-cm mark on the vertical scale. 📖

Step 3: Establishing a Reference Level for Pressure

The ICS has defined the reference level (or height) for external transducers and fluid-filled catheters as the superior edge of the symphysis pubis. Hence it is essential to level the transducers to this horizontal plane. Catheter tip transducers do not need a reference level in this way.

Sterility of Transducers and Tubing

AIDS and the frequency of hospital-acquired infections has changed sterility practices. It has become necessary to change the tubing linking the infusion pump to the patient, as well as the tubing linking the patient to the external transducers, after each patient. The external transducers need not be sterilised, but should be flushed through with chlorhexidine solution (0.2%). If the transducers are not being used regularly, the domes should be removed and sterilised with Cidex (gluteraldehyde). Catheter tip transducers must be kept sterile using Cidex. Controversy surrounds the use of gluteraldehyde because the staff have to be protected as far as possible from exposure, it must not get into the transducer connection, and the transducer must be washed well before use, for which sterile water or saline is suitable. Local regulations may determine urodynamic practice.

Recording Equipment

The first edition of this book dealt at length with various types of recorders, but such an exposition is unnecessary because all manufacturers of urodynamic equipment supply a recorder as part of their system. However, certain principles remain important and, unfortunately, some of these have come under threat from so-called "developments":

- The printout must be clear. Some modern recorders have a much narrower paper width, which necessitates the traces crossing each other on occasions during investigation. This can make a trace very difficult to read (Fig. 3.36). Manufacturers need to learn from this mistake and produce better printers in the future. The minimum vertical scaling should be 50 cmH$_2$O/cm.

- The printout must be based on an adequate sampling rate. In each of the new computerised systems, the data is sampled at rates unique to that urodynamic system. A minimum sampling rate of 10 data points per second is necessary for a good-quality trace (10 Hz). Failure to sample at this rate may mean the loss of important data when fast changes are seen, particularly in pressure recording (e.g., when the patient coughs) (Fig. 3.36).

- The recorder must have an adequate frequency response for the intended use. Hence in more sophisticated electrophysiological testing, such as single-fibre electromyography, a very rapid response is needed. This can only be met by systems such as UV recorders or oscilloscopes that use light to record the signals.

The paper speed should be such that the clinician can identify important events during filling and voiding. In computerised systems, to minimise the use of paper, different paper speeds may be used according to the phase of urodynamic measurement. Hence the paper speed for the filling phase tends to be slower than that used during voiding; the minimum time axis should be 50 s/cm to 60 s/cm for filling and a 25 s/cm for voiding. For urethral pressure measurements the paper speed of some recorders is matched to the rate of withdrawal of the urethral profile catheter during profilometry (see later). Where the intent is to

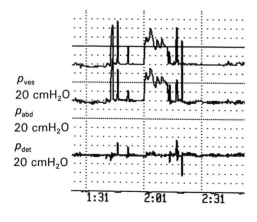

p_{ves}
20 cmH$_2$O

p_{abd}
20 cmH$_2$O

p_{det}
20 cmH$_2$O

1:31   2:01   2:31

Fig. 3.36 Recording artefacts: the figure shows a series of three coughs before the patient was asked to perform a Valsalva manoeuvre (strain) and two coughs afterwards. There are positive deflections on p_{det} for coughs two and three indicating defective electronic subtraction due to inadequate measurement sampling. The strain shows perfect subtraction because the changes are slower and the machine can record them; coughs one and five are difficult to interpret as the p_{ves} and p_{det} traces overlap. 📖

"custom build" a system, expert medical physics advice should be sought. Expense, reliability and the appropriateness of design will be important factors in the choice of equipment. Whilst most companies are extremely helpful in ensuring that pieces of equipment will connect to each other, local medical physics advice can be invaluable.

Technique of Filling Cystometry

Performing Filling Cystometry

To evaluate the storage phase of filling cystometry, four essential measurements must be made throughout filling:

- Intravesical pressure (p_{ves}).
- Abdominal pressure (p_{abd}).
- Detrusor pressure ($p_{det} = p_{ves} - p_{abd}$) – calculated electronically.
- Urine flow rate to detect leaks.

Other optional measurements may be made during cystometry:

- Bladder volume.
- Simultaneous video cystography.
- Electromyography.
- Urethral pressure measurement.

Intravesical Pressure (p_{ves}) Measurement

p_{ves} is the pressure measured within the bladder. Usually it is measured continuously, although sometimes in children the technique needs to be changed so that only intermittent pressure measurement is performed (see "Urodynamics in Children" in Chapter 5).

Unfortunately it is essential to pass a catheter into the bladder in order to measure p_{ves} and access may be via the perurethral or percutaneous (suprapubic) route. In the adult patient, the bladder rises to the upper border of the pubis when the bladder volume is approximately 300 ml; it only becomes easily palpable in a thin patient when the bladder volume is approximately 500 ml, so the routine use of the suprapubic route can present practical difficulties. Further, the suprapubic route is relatively contra-indicated in the presence of lower abdominal scars, which may tether intraperitoneal contents to the lower part of the abdominal wall. It is also more difficult in obese patients. However, the suprapubic route for intravesical pressure measurement remains the ideal, because it avoids the unphysiological effects of a catheter in the urethra and the possible effects of urethral anaesthesia. The recent availability of portable ultrasound machines allows a suprapubic catheter to be introduced with more confidence than before. Some workers put in a urethral catheter in order to fill the bladder prior to insertion of a suprapubic catheter, but this in some part compromises the advantages of a suprapubic catheter as outlined above. However, most units still use urethral catheters routinely.

If p_{ves} is measured using external strain gauge transducers, the transducer must be linked to the patient by a fluid-filled tube. The fluid in the tube is usually water, because the use of solutions (such as saline) may lead to the deposition of crystals in the transducer, thereby affecting its performance. James has pioneered the use of air-filled tubes, although these are still not commercially available. When a water-filled tube (known as manometer tubing) is used to conduct pressure changes from the bladder to the transducer then certain physical characteristics of the tubing are important:

- The tubing must be flexible, yet the walls must not be elastic. If the tubing was elastic, the pressure measured would be lower than the true pressure, because part of the energy of the pressure wave would be used to stretch the elastic walls of the connecting tube.
- The manometer tubing should not be excessively long, narrow or wide.
- There should be no marked changes in the calibre of the tubing where the tubing joins the catheter or the transducer.

Anaesthesia for Urethral Catheterisation

In a female patient with a short, straight urethra, local anaesthetic is probably unnecessary; adequate lubrication may be all that is needed to ensure patient comfort. Occasionally the urethra may be extremely sensitive. If so, use local anaesthetic rather than upset the patient and risk unusual stimulation of the bladder. Some would state that male patients also require only adequate lubrication, but it is the current practice of the author to use local anaesthetic gel. Investigations in our unit have shown that urethral anaesthesia has no effect on the measurements recorded during filling cystometry or pressure-flow studies. In most men, the anaesthetic jelly does not pass through the pelvic floor region into the prostatic urethra.

Introducing the Catheter(s)

The system we have used for twenty years to measure p_{ves} works well. An epidural catheter is used to measure pressure and is passed *per urethram* into the bladder together with an 8 Fr filling catheter. In women this is quite straightforward, but in men the epidural catheter needs to be "railroaded" into the bladder on the filling catheter.

- First the epidural catheter is introduced into the eyehole of the filling catheter.
- Both catheters are then passed into the bladder, until the urine drips from the filling catheter (Fig. 3.37, *top left*).
- Both catheters are then withdrawn until the urine flow just stops. The catheters will then be just below the bladder neck (Fig. 3.37, *top right*).
- The catheters are then advanced by 1 cm until urine drips again. The catheters will now be lying in the bladder just above the bladder neck. Whilst the filling catheter is gripped so it cannot move, the epidural catheter is pulled gently until it is felt to disengage from the eyehole of the filling catheter, which is possible with a little experience (Fig. 3.37, *bottom left*).
- Both catheters are now advanced together so that the epidural passes into the bladder with the filling catheter (Fig. 3.37, *bottom right*).
- The epidural catheter is next held and the filling catheter partly withdrawn (approximately 10 cm), so that the epidural is left within the lumen of the bladder (Fig. 3.37, *top left*).

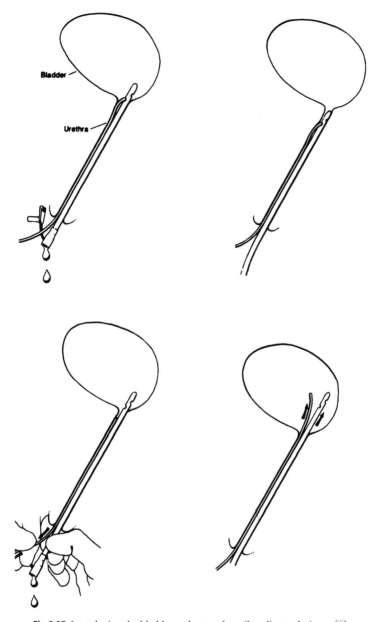

Fig. 3.37 Introducing the bladder catheters: the railroading technique.

- Both catheters are now advanced together so that the epidural is railroaded into the bladder and begins to curl up. The epidural catheter has convenient markings on the side to show the length that has been introduced into the bladder (Fig. 3.38, *top right*).
- The process is repeated until the epidural catheter has been fully advanced into the bladder, leaving only 15 cm outside the urethra (Fig. 3.38). This precise technique

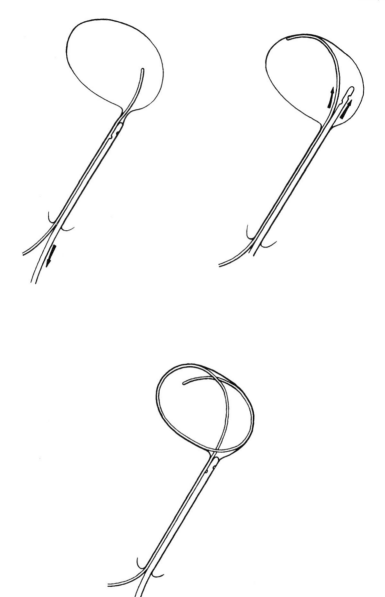

Fig. 3.38 Advancing the bladder catheter. 📖

prevents the annoyance (for both the patient and the doctor) of the pressure-measuring catheter being inadvertently withdrawn when the filling catheter is removed prior to voiding, which may occur if the epidural catheter has not been dislodged from the eyehole of the filling catheter (Fig. 3.39, *overleaf*).

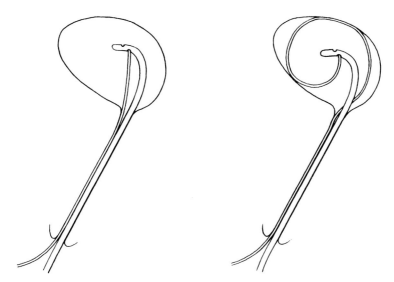

Fig. 3.39 If the technique described in Figs 3.37 and 3.38 is not followed then the epidural catheter may fail to disengage. It will then be pulled out when the filling catheter is removed at the end of the filling phase. 📖

Fixing the Catheters

We have used a two-catheter technique for many years. It is cheap, and after the filling catheter is removed, the epidural catheter will not cause obstruction during voiding.

In the male patient, the epidural catheter should be taped back over the shaft of the penis, ensuring that the tape does not compress the urethra on the underside of the penis (Fig. 3.40). The filling catheter should be passed well into the bladder, so that at least 10 cm protrudes into the lumen. The filling catheter should also be taped to the penis, leaving no gap between the external urinary meatus and the point at which the catheter is attached to the tape. The tape should be folded back over the dorsum of the glans penis and the shaft of the penis, as shown (Fig. 3.41, *overleaf*).

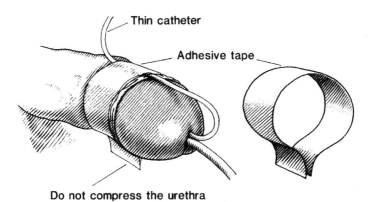

Thin catheter

Adhesive tape

Do not compress the urethra

Fig. 3.40 Fixing the epidural catheter. 📖

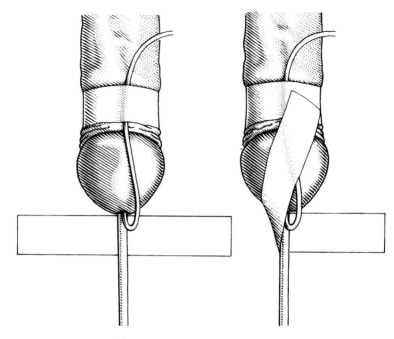

Fig. 3.41 Fixing the filling catheter. 📖

In the female patient, the epidural catheter should be taped as close as possible to the external urethral meatus on the inside of the thigh.

An alternative technique is to use a single catheter which has two channels, one for the measurement of p_{ves} and the other for bladder filling. Catheters are now available in size 6 Fr and allow a filling speed of 50 ml/min using a peristatic pump. A 6 Fr catheter does not cause obstruction in adults except in exceptional circumstances (e.g., a very tight urethral stricture). The catheter should be secured by tying a silk thread around the catheter junction box and sandwiching the silk ties between two layers of tape attached to the shaft of the penis (Fig. 3.42). As in the two-catheter technique, the tape must not obstruct the urethra on the underside of the penis. In women, the single-catheter technique can be used: the catheter must be taped as close to the urethral meatus as possible on the inside of the thigh.

The key to success in fixing the urethral catheters is to be sure that there is not a loop of catheter between the external meatus and the point of tape fixation. If the above technique is used then there should be only minimal problems with catheters being voided during micturition or being displaced or falling out during bladder-filling.

Measurement of Abdominal Pressure (p_{abd})

Abdominal pressure (p_{abd}) is the pressure surrounding the bladder. Currently, it is estimated from rectal pressure or less commonly by intraperitoneal pressure. It is also possible to measure abdominal pressure vaginally, from the stomach or from the pre-peritoneal space. Only vaginal measurement of p_{abd} is a widely used alternative to rectal pressure measurement.

The purpose of measuring p_{abd} simultaneously during bladder or urethral pressure recordings is to aid interpretation of the observed pressure changes. If pressure rises in the

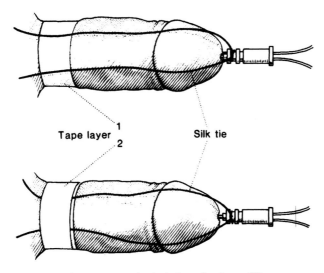

Fig. 3.42 Fixing the dual-channel catheter. 📖

bladder, then the increase may be due to contraction of the detrusor or to changes in extravesical pressure (p_{abd}) transmitted to the bladder. In the normal person, changes in p_{abd} are transmitted to the whole of the bladder and that part of the proximal urethra that lies above the pelvic floor. Figure 3.43 illustrates the importance of measuring p_{ves} and p_{abd}. If only p_{ves} were to be measured, then the changes seen on the trace would be very difficult to interpret. However the addition of the p_{abd} pressure trace, together with the electronic subtraction to produce detrusor pressure, will clarify the traces enormously. Certain artefacts may arise as a direct result of using the rectal pressure as an approximation of p_{abd}, and these must be appreciated. Rectal contractions may be recorded in the rectum particularly if there is faecal loading (Fig. 3.44, *overleaf*), and a patient noted to have a full rectum should be asked to empty his or her bowels.

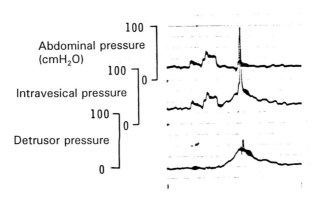

Fig. 3.43 Multi-channel trace showing, from the left, a short period of straining (pressure increases on the p_{abd} and p_{ves} traces but *not* on the p_{det} trace) followed by an involuntary detrusor contraction during which the patient has coughed (the involuntary detrusor wave is recorded on p_{ves} and p_{det} but *not* on p_{abd}; the coughs record only on p_{abd} and p_{ves}). 📖

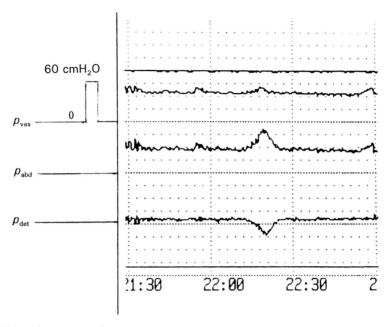

Fig. 3.44 Rectal contraction: characterised by a positive wave on the p_{abd} trace and a negative artefact on the p_{det} trace. 📖

The rectal recording line can be made cheaply from manometer tubing protected at its rectal end by a finger cot cut from a thin disposable plastic glove (Fig. 3.45). The finger cot is used to avoid blockage of the line with faeces. Prior to recording, the tubing needs to be flushed from the transducer end. To avoid distending the finger cot, make a small cut to allow excess air or fluid to escape. If a commercially supplied rectal catheter is used, then make a small hole in the balloon for the same reason.

The rectal catheter is introduced, using lubricant, through the anus so that the tip is positioned 10 cm to 15 cm above the anal verge. The perianal area should be dried and the catheter taped as close as possible to the anal verge (Fig. 3.46).

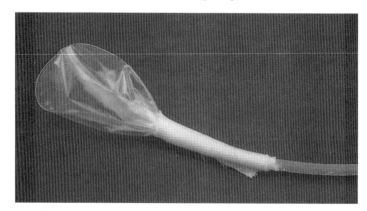

Fig. 3.45 "Home-made" rectal catheter constructed from manometer tubing protected at its end by a plastic glove finger. 📖

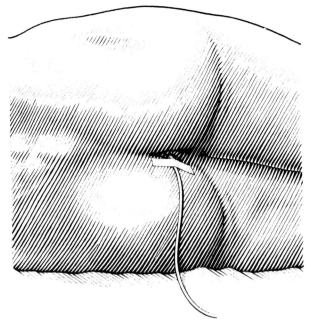

Fig. 3.46 The rectal catheter should be taped as close as possible to the anal verge. 📖

Detrusor Pressure (p_{det}) Measurement

Detrusor pressure (p_{det}) is that component of intravesical pressure that is created by forces in the bladder wall (passive and active). It is estimated by the electronic subtraction of p_{abd} from p_{ves} ($p_{det} = p_{ves} - p_{abd}$). The simultaneous measurement of p_{abd} is essential in allowing the continuous calculation of p_{det}, and all modern urodynamic systems have the electronic equipment which allows this calculation.

The accurate measurement of p_{det} is entirely dependent on the accuracy with which p_{abd} and p_{ves} are measured. These can be readily assessed during urodynamics. In Fig. 3.47 the patient has been asked to cough. The cough should be identical on the p_{ves} and p_{abd} traces (*upper traces*). However, if the p_{abd} line has not been flushed properly, the cough is not properly transmitted (*lower traces*). After flushing, the p_{abd} trace should show equal cough transmission and the resultant p_{det} trace no significant deflection. To get equal transmission, the tubing used for the p_{abd} and p_{ves} lines should be similar. However, transmission can never be identical if fluid-filled lines are used, and therefore the small biphasic deflection seen on the p_{det} trace (Fig. 3.47, *upper traces*) is acceptable. If transmission of pressure reading is not similar then adjustments should be made during cystometry to ensure accurate pressure recording, for example, to tighten a joint if a leak of fluid has developed.

Media Used for Bladder Filling

Water or physiological saline are the most commonly used media in urodynamics, together with radiographic contrast material if videourodynamics is being performed. Following the

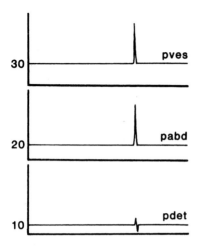

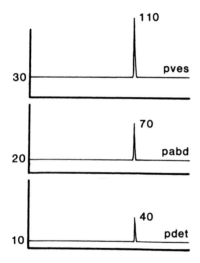

Fig. 3.47 Quality control: upper traces show good subtraction of a single cough with a small (acceptable) artefact on the p_{det} trace; lower traces show inadequate subtraction with a large cough artefact on p_{det}, which necessitates a check of the transducers and recording lines. 📖

introduction of gas cystometry (Merrill 1971) there was a vogue for the use of carbon dioxide as a filling medium. While water or saline can have the obvious advantage that they mimic urine, carbon dioxide can have no such pretension and is no longer used.

Temperature of Filling Fluid

Formerly, we heated our infusion fluid to body temperature (37°C), but we now use fluid at room temperature (70°F or 22°C). There has been no perceptable change in the results we obtain, although this has not been analysed scientifically. It is important not to use cold fluid (lower than 20°C) because, as has been shown, the use of cold infusion fluid stimulates detrusor contractility at low bladder volumes. The ice water test remains a research investigation and is used only as a routine at one or two centres.

Patient Position During Cystometry

The patient is catheterised when supine, but our practice is to fill the patient either sitting (in the case of women) or standing (in the case of male patients) because the supine position does not reflect the everyday stresses to which the bladder is subjected and most patients complain of bladder symptoms only when they are active (erect). Some patients complain of symptoms when they change posture, for example when rising from a sitting position. If the patient has symptoms related to change of posture, this should be tested during the urodynamic studies. Investigators who use videourodynamics as their investigation of choice tend to fill the patient in the supine position and then tilt the X-ray table so they stand to void. To us, this practice fails to adequately mimic the stresses on the bladder imposed by the vertical position. The sitting and standing positions result in an increase in intravesical pressure compared with when the patient is lying. Therefore changing the patient's position during investigation may cause an artefact if pressure transmission to the bladder or rectum is affected. If the patient's position is changed then the transducer's position must be readjusted to the pressure reference level of the upper border of the symphysis pubis.

- With some patient, it is may be impossible to fill the bladder in any position but supine. Patients who are severely disabled by neurological disease may have to be investigated in the lying position. In this situation, it is desirable to attempt to measure their flow rate. In men this can be done by the use of a plastic drain pipe (D. Thomas, personal communication), though in women this is clearly not practical.
- If there is gross detrusor overactivity preventing proper filling, then slow filling in the supine position may help.

Rate of Bladder Filling

Currently the ICS recommends that the exact filling rate is stated for each test, although the ICS formerly defined three categories of filling rate:

- *Slow-fill cystometry:* up to 10 ml/min.
- *Medium-fill cystometry:* between 10 ml/min and 100 ml/min.
- *Fast-fill cystometry:* when the rate is greater than 100 ml/min.

The rate of bladder filling has considerable influence on the resulting measurements. The faster the bladder is filled, the lower the bladder compliance, as defined below (see p. 00). A series of cystometrograms repeated one after the other with a medium or rapid filling rate will show a gradually increasing capacity – the phenomenon of hysteresis. This has been shown not to occur at more physiological rates of filling (Klevmark 1974). The rate of filling chosen depends on whether the investigator is attempting to reproduce normal physiological events, although some investigators use fast filling to provoke the bladder into involuntary contraction whenever possible. Often the filling rate chosen will be a compromise between these two extremes, and a convenient rate, which does not prolong the test unduly, is 50 ml/min to 60 ml/min. In children and patients with neurological abnormalities, and in particular patients with detrusor overactivity secondary to spinal trauma, the bladder should be filled very slowly (less than 10 ml/min) because faster flow rates may produce artefactual low compliance (Thomas 1979). This is discussed further in Chapter 5. The fastest physiological urine production for any individual can be calculated by dividing the body weight (in KG) by four (e.g., 20 ml/min for an 80-KG man).

What to Do About Residual Urine?

Prior to catheterisation the patient is asked to empty the bladder as fully as possible. If the patient self-catheterises, then the patient is asked to do this before urodynamics commences and to empty the bladder. However if the patient has neurological disease and does not self-catheterise, the bladder should *not* be emptied. In these patients, the post-void residual (PVR) can be measured by passing a catheter after the voiding phase of urodynamic studies. If a patient without neurological abnormalities has evidence of hydronephrosis, which could be secondary to elevated bladder pressure, the bladder should not be drained at the beginning of the filling phase of urodynamic studies. Removing the PVR and/or filling too quickly can fundamentally change the results, particularly in respect of bladder compliance, detrusor overactivity and cystometric capacity. In patients with neurological disease and/or upper tract dilatation, the artefacts of low compliance and reduced capacity are likely to be produced if the standard technique is used.

Ensuring a High-Quality Recording from the Patient

Before starting recording and after the patient is catheterised, both the bladder and rectal lines should be flushed again to ensure that all bubbles and leaks have been removed. Once the catheters are in place and connected to the transducers, the tubing must be flushed to ensure that all bubbles are removed. In addition to bubbles in the tubing, bubbles close to the transducer diaphragm must be removed. Failure to remove bubbles will lead to errors in measurement. Similarly the connections between the catheters and the manometer tubing and the tubing and the transducer should be tight; any leak will cause errors in the pressure measurement. Leaks, bubbles or elastic-sided tubing will tend to lead to the recording of lower values of pressure.

Quality control is ensured by two principle means: by feasible initial pressure recordings and by asking the patient to cough at regular intervals during the investigation.

There are a range of feasible pressures for pves and p_{abd} in the supine, sitting and standing positions. The 2002 ICS report (Appendix 1, Part 6) gives these as, for p_{ves}, supine 10 cmH_2O to 20 cmH_2O, sitting 15 cmH_2O to 40 cmH_2O, and standing 30 cmH_2O to 50 cmH_2O. The report says that after derivation, pdet is 0 cmH_2O to 6 cmH_2O in 80% of cases, and in rare cases up to 10 cmH_2O. However this data is not exactly the same as others, (Sullivan 2004). Our p_{det} data is evenly distributed around zero (-5 cmH_2O to +5 cmH_2O for 90% of prospectively evaluated patients). This is perhaps to be expected unless, for some reasons the bladder has a higher baseline pressure than the rectum. The ICS report gives useful examples of artefacts (p_{abd} too low or too high, p_{ves} too low or too high), and how to solve these artefactual problems.

Before recording starts, the patient should be asked to cough and the p_{ves} and p_{abd} traces observed. There should be an equal rise in pressure when the patient coughs (Fig. 3.47, *upper traces*). The patient should be asked to give a cough that produces a deflection of approximately 100 cmH_2O. The deflection should show a rapid increase to the peak, and then a rapid fall, as shown in the figure. On the p_{det} line there may well be a small biphasic

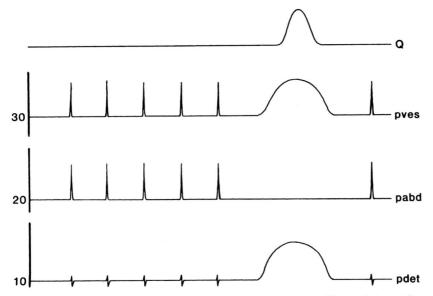

Fig. 3.48 Quality control: the patient is asked to cough every minute during filling *and* after voiding to ensure that the catheters have not become displaced during micturition. 📖

blip, but this does not matter: what is crucial is that the height of the spikes on the p_{ves} and the p_{abd} lines are identical.

If the spikes are not identical, as shown in Fig. 3.47, *lower traces*, then the explanation may be that there are bubbles or leaks, that the catheters are malpositioned or that there is interference with the measurement of p_{abd} due to faecal loading. All these points must be checked and the cough repeated until the proper pattern is observed.

Once the initial cough gives a good-quality signal, bladder filling can commence. Throughout bladder filling, the patient should be asked to cough every minute (Fig. 3.48). If at any stage the quality deteriorates, then the investigation must be stopped and the cause of the poor pressure transmission investigated. Once the fault is corrected then the filling can recommence.

After filling, the patient must cough again to ensure that the catheters have not moved during micturition. Failure to show an equal transmission of pressure after voiding means that the results of voiding cannot be confidently interpreted, and the investigation needs to be repeated if the voiding phase is vital for patient diagnosis.

Performing Filling Cystometry

The investigator should approach cystometry with two of the principles of urodynamics at the front of his or her mind, namely that "The role of urodynamics is to reproduce the patients symptoms", and "The role of urodynamics is to provide a pathophysiological explanation for the patient's complaints".

This means there should be a continuous dialogue between the investigator and the patient *throughout* the investigation. It is particularly important when assessing the sensations the patient experiences during cystometry.

During bladder filling the following should be assessed:

- Bladder sensation
- Detrusor activity
- Bladder compliance
- Urethral function
- Bladder capacity

Bladder Sensation

Certain terms have been accepted, but it should be emphasised that relating a precise bladder volume to one of them is subjective and is likely to vary considerably. These terms are:

- *First sensation of filling (FSF)*. This sensation is often difficult to interpret during cystometry because the mere presence of the urethral catheter is often interpreted as a desire to void. It occurs at approximately 50% of cystometric capacity.
- *Normal desire to void (NDV)*. This is defined as the feeling that leads the patient to pass urine at the next convenient moment, but voiding can be delayed if necessary. It is felt at about 75% of cystometric capacity.
- *Strong desire to void (SDV)*. This is defined as a persistent desire to void without the fear of leakage. It is felt at approximately 90% capacity.
- *Urgency*. This is defined as a sudden compelling persistent desire to void which is difficult to defer (ICS 2002).
- *Pain*. The site and character should be specified. Pain during bladder filling or micturition is abnormal.

A person with normal bladder function may occasionally feel urgency: bladder pain would only be felt in exceptional circumstances, for example if prevented from passing urine when trapped in a lift (elevator).

Abnormal sensation

Sensation can be said to be abnormal if it is one of the following:

- *Increased (hypersensitive)*. *Bladder hypersensitivity* is a term we have used and found useful. We define it as the condition of a bladder in which there is an early first sensation of filling (FSF) at less than 100 ml which, instead of passing away until the normal desire to void (NDV) occurs, persists and increases, limiting the cystometric capacity to less than 250 ml.
- *Reduced*. Reduced sensation is characterised by a later FSF and NDV, with the patient never experiencing a strong desire to void (SDV) or urgency.
- *Absent*. Absent sensation necessitates the patient passing urine "by the clock" and is usually indicative of a neurological condition such as spinal cord trauma or meningomyelocele.

Detrusor Activity

During bladder filling this can be either normal or increased (overactivity).

The normal detrusor remains quiescent during filling and detrusor overactivity does not occur under any circumstances (e.g., during the provocation tests used in an effort to uncover detrusor overactivity (DO)). In normal function the detrusor relaxes and stretches to allow the bladder to increase in size without any change in pressure (accommodation) (Fig. 3.49). This ability is essential for two reasons. The first is to allow normal urine transport from the kidneys; ureteric muscle is relatively weak, being capable of generating a maximum pressure of approximately 30 cmH$_2$O. The second is that increased bladder pressures during filling would be likely to compromise continence.

Detrusor overactivity exists when, during the filling phase, there are involuntary detrusor contractions. These contractions may be spontaneous or else may occur only on provocation as described above. The term, "detrusor overactivity incontinence" may be used when there is incontinence in voiding due to contraction, or when a voluntary contraction cannot be suppressed. At present this last category, impaired suppression, is not commonly recognised. Various special terms have been used to describe these features and they are defined as follows.

- *The overactive detrusor* is one that is shown objectively to contract spontaneously or on provocation, during the filling phase. The overactive detrusor may be asymptomatic, and its presence does not necessarily imply a neurological disorder. Idiopathic DO is the commonest form of detrusor overactivity.

- Neurogenic detrusor overactivity (NDO) is overactivity as a result of disturbance of the nervous control mechanisms. It must be confirmed by objective evidence of a neurological disorder. NDO occurs frequently in neurological conditions such as multiple sclerosis and cerebrovascular disease, as well as in conditions such as meningomyelocele and after spinal cord trauma. The cystometric trace in NDO is very variable and highly dependent on urodynamic technique. In the neuropathic patient, the difference between

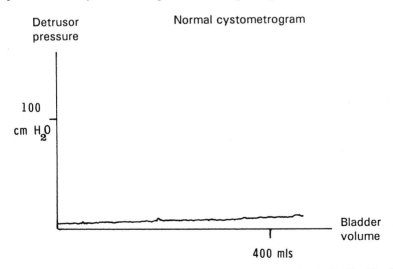

Fig. 3.49 Normal filling cystometrogram with almost no increase in p_{det} as the bladder fills. 📖

detrusor overactivity and low bladder compliance can become blurred (see later). Other conceptual and undefined terms should be avoided, such as hypertonic, systolic, spastic, automatic and uninhibited.

There has been considerable confusion over the applied definition of DO, with some investigators labelling patients as having DO if there is an increase of p_{det} greater than 15 cmH$_2$O during filling. However the ICS standardisation document of 1988 makes it clear that DO is characterised by phasic contractions in which the pressure rises and then falls. The ICS definition does not specify a minimum change in p_{det}, although waves of an amplitude of less than 5 cmH$_2$O are difficult to detect using most modern urodynamic equipment. However it is undoubtedly true that low-pressure DO waves (5 cmH$_2$O-15 cmH$_2$O) can and do produce troublesome symptoms of urgency and urgency incontinence, particularly in women with poor urethral function.

Is DO Normal or Abnormal?

The answer is that probably it is not abnormal and that most of us will have an occasional involuntary detrusor contraction. DO is abnormal when it produces troublesome symptoms; this illustrates the fundamental principle of urodynamics, that is, the need to relate urodynamic findings to the patient's symptoms.

If an involuntary contraction is seen then the investigator should ask the patient a series of questions as follows:

"Do you feel anything now?"

If an involuntary contraction has occurred but the patient either is unaware of the contraction or feels the contraction as a normal desire to void, then the DO is probably not clinically significant. If the patient answers "yes" and feels the contraction as an urgency or discomfort then a follow-up question should be asked:

"Is this the feeling that gives you trouble in your everyday life?"

If the patient answers "no" then the DO may be an artefact of the investigation. Artefactual contractions usually occur at the beginning of filling, after which the bladder settles down. If the patient answers "yes" then the association between symptoms and the urodynamic finding of DO has been made and the diagnosis confirmed.

DO occurs in different patterns. In general, involuntary contractions become more frequent and of greater amplitude as bladder filling proceeds (Fig. 3.50). DO during cystometry may or may not be accompanied by leakage (urgency incontinence), as in Fig. 3.51, *overleaf*. DO is often described as spontaneous or provoked.

Spontaneous DO means that the overactivity had no particular trigger (Fig. 3.51, *overleaf*), whereas provocation detrusor overactivity is usually qualified by the provoking factor, the commonest of which are:

- Changing position, for example, rising from sitting or lying, to standing.
- Coughing; Fig. 3.52 (page 69) shows cough-induced DO.
- Hand-washing or putting the hands in cold water, for example, whilst gardening on a cold day.
- "Latchkey incontinence" where a patient wishing to pass urine reaches their front door but before they can turn the key has extreme urgency and leaks.

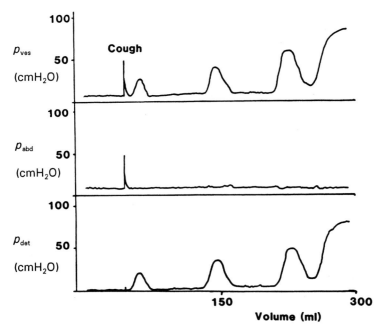

Fig. 3.50 Diagram to show involuntary detrusor contractions occurring at increasing frequency and with increasing pressure as the bladder fills. 📖

- "Telephone urgency" is a terrifying disease of the post-industrial world where telephone conversations lead to urgency and even, in the case of one of the author's children, the need to attempt to interrupt the conversation to pass urine.

The recognition that DO may develop in response to certain triggers has led some urodynamicists to advocate "provocative cystometry" in an effort to uncover "latent DO". In the author's view, provocation should be used if the patient gives a history suggestive of provoked DO. If not, then the patient should only be asked to cough during bladder filling. Coughing is of course also useful for quality control purposes, and in women as a means of demonstrating urodynamic stress incontinence (USI). There has been considerable work attempting to quantify DO, and Fig. 3.53 (*overleaf*) shows a DO index based on the number and height of the DO waves; other indices have measured the area under the p_{det} curve (Abrams 2004).

Bladder Compliance

In normal bladder function, intravesical pressure should change little from empty to full. Bladder compliance describes the relationship between bladder volume and bladder pressure ($\Delta v/\Delta p$) and is expressed as: increase in bladder volume per centimetre of water increase in pressure (ml/cmH$_2$O).

In the normal bladder with a capacity of 400 ml the change in pressure from empty to full should be less than 10 cmH$_2$O, giving a figure for normal compliance of greater than 40 ml/cmH$_2$O. Bladder compliance is dependent on the rate of bladder filling, on bladder function, and on the neurological state of the patient. Klevmark showed that if bladders are filled

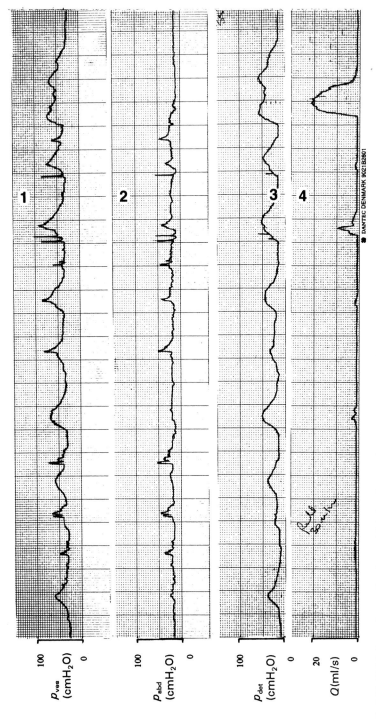

Fig. 3.51 Multi-channel trace showing multiple involuntary detrusor contractions, four of which cause leakage detected on the flow rate trace (bottom trace, Q (ml/s)). A normal void occurs at the extreme right-hand end of the recording.

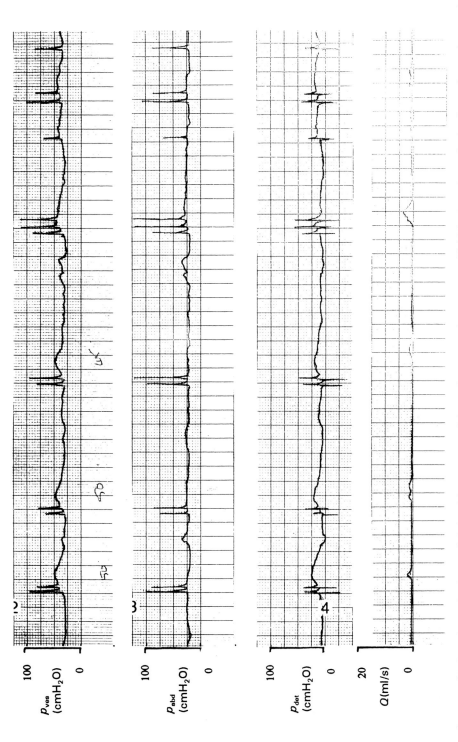

Fig. 3.52 Multi-channel trace showing cough-induced detrusor overactivity. On the p_{det} trace there are acceptable biphasic artefacts reflecting the coughs seen in p_{ves} and p_{det}. The flow trace detects leaks with most of the DO waves.

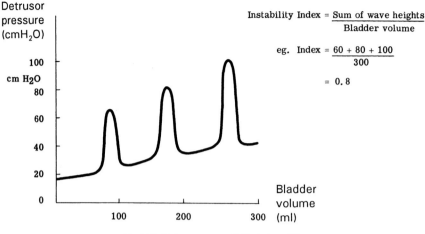

Fig. 3.53 Detrusor overactivity index. 📖

at physiological rates, there is little or no change in bladder pressure on filling. Figure 3.54 demonstrates how to determine whether or not low compliance is due to fast filling. When there is evidence of low compliance with a gradual increase in p_{ves}, then bladder filling should stop for at least two minutes. If the intravesical pressure falls (see Fig. 3.54c), then the reduced compliance was, at least in part, due to filling too fast. Once the pressure has stabilised then filling should be restarted, but at a significantly slower rate: if initial filling was at 50 ml/min then it should be reduced to 10 ml/min.

In theory, bladder compliance has a passive and an active component. The passive component depends on bladder wall composition. If the bladder wall has significant quan-

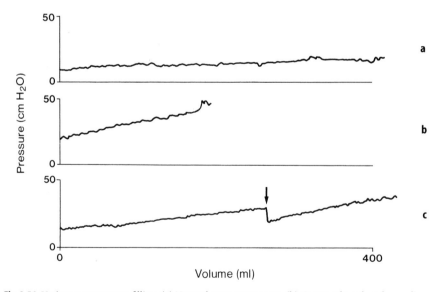

Fig. 3.54 Various responses to filling. (a) Normal cystometrogram. (b) Constantly reduced compliance. (c) Reduced compliance due to fast filling. When infusion is stopped (at the arrow) the pressure falls immediately, to increase again when infusion is restarted. 📖

tities of fibrous tissue, compliance may be reduced. In fact, even in interstitial cystitis or after radiotherapy it is unusual to see compliance changes. This may be because pain limits the degree to which the bladder can be filled. As we have said, the normal bladder distends without significant change in pressure; hence if the pressure rises gradually throughout bladder filling, this can be assumed to be an active process, at least in so far as the detrusor muscle is not relaxing normally. This view is supported by the fact that reduced compliance can be partly abolished by the use of intravenous anticholinergic agents.

In a small number of male patients with benign prostatic obstruction, chronic retention may lead to upper tract dilatation. This has been termed "high-pressure chronic retention", and it has been shown that these men have reduced bladder compliance. However it was later demonstrated that low compliance in this group of patients was largely artefactual and that, if filled at physiological rates, low compliance was replaced with phasic detrusor over-activity, albeit with a related underlying increased pressure (Fig. 3.55). In this author's view, detrusor overactivity and low compliance, in most cases, should both be viewed as part of the spectrum of detrusor overactivity on filling.

The first edition of this book (1983) discussed detrusor underactivity in the section on filling cystometry. Since then, the ICS report of 2002, reprinted as Appendix 1 Part 5, has been published and reasonably states that the detrusor can only be normal or overactive

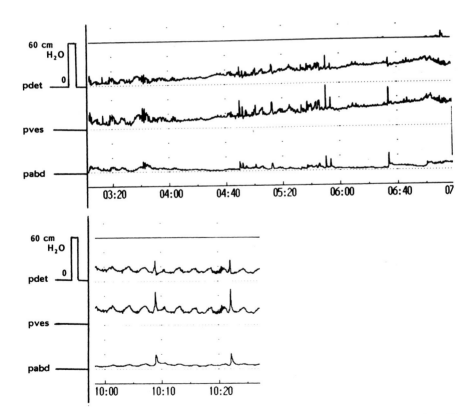

Fig. 3.55 Effect of filling rate on bladder compliance; the upper trace shows a conventional medium fill CMG in a man with prostatic obstruction and demonstrating reduced compliance; the lower trace is recorded during natural-fill cystometry and now demonstrates DO, masked during faster filling. 📖

during filling. *Detrusor underactivity can only be diagnosed during the voiding phase.* Patients with detrusor underactivity during voiding will often have a large cystometric capacity, although this is by no means the rule (see p. 77).

Urethral Function During Filling

During the storage phase the urethral closure mechanism function is either normal or incompetent:

- The *normal urethral closure mechanism* maintains a positive urethral closure pressure during filling, even in the presence of increased abdominal pressure. Immediately prior to micturition, the normal closure pressure decreases to allow flow.
- *Incompetent urethral closure mechanism.* An incompetent urethral closure mechanism is one which allows leakage of urine in the absence of a detrusor contraction. Leakage may occur whenever intravesical pressure exceeds intraurethral pressure (urodynamic stress incontinence) or when there is an involuntary fall in urethral pressure.

Incontinence has several causes and incompetence of the urethral sphincter mechanism leading to urodynamic stress incontinence is an important one. However if incontinence occurs due to an involuntary detrusor contraction, the urethral closure mechanism is not thought of as incompetent. In this case, urethral relaxation is a reflex action occurring as part of normal micturition. This begs the question, "Can an involuntary contraction be viewed as the premature activation of the micturition reflex?" During an involuntary detrusor contraction, with urethral relaxation, continence can be maintained by voluntary pelvic floor contractions until the individual can inhibit the involuntary detrusor contraction. But urgency incontinence due to DO is seen more frequently in women because urethral function and pelvic floor function, particularly after childbirth, is less powerful.

Urodynamic stress incontinence (USI)   is the involuntary leakage of urine during increased abdominal pressure in the absence of a detrusor contraction. The demonstration of (USI) is straightforward in most patients. The standard procedure is to ask the patient to cough and/or to perform the Valsalva test. USI is easier to show with the patient in the vertical position, either sitting or standing, and with a full bladder. If the patient has the symptom of stress urinary incontinence (SUI) and no leakage has been demonstrated by the time the bladder is full, then two of the following manoeuvres can be tried. First, remove the filling catheter and repeat the provocative tests. Second, USI is more easily provoked in women if they are asked to separate their legs widely, presumably because leg abduction weakens pelvic floor support to the sphincter mechanism (Fig. 3.56). If standard urodynamics are used without simultaneous lower urinary tract imaging, then the external meatus must be viewed when the patient coughs. Women in particular may become embarrassed and must be reassured and put at their ease.

Inappropriate Urethral Relaxation Incontinence   is leakage due to urethral relaxation in the absence of raised abdominal pressure or a detrusor contraction. The "unstable urethra" was the urodynamic diagnosis of the 1980s and was defined as a change

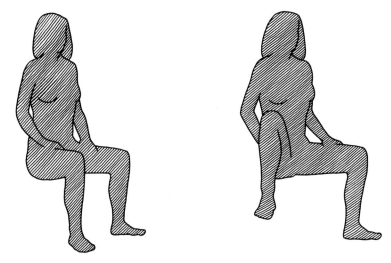

Fig. 3.56 Testing for GSI: ask the woman to flex and abduct one hip if GSI is not demonstrated in the usual more dignified position! 📖

in maximum urethral closure pressure of greater than 15 cmH$_2$O measured on urethral pressure profilometry; the term is no longer recommended. Urethral relaxation alone is an unusual cause of incontinence and it is not clear whether or not it is a variant of a prematurely activated micturition reflex, in which the rise in detrusor pressure due to an involuntary contraction is too small to see. This may be the case, because the phenomenon is seen only in women, and as many continent women void normally, apparently by relaxing their urethra without a measurable detrusor contraction, unless a "stop test" is done (see "Voiding Cystometry" later).

Bladder Capacity

In describing bladder capacity the ICS has recommended the following terms:

- Cystometric capacity is the bladder volume at the end of the filling cystometrogram, when the patient has a normal desire to void and "permission to void" has been given. Cystometric capacity is volume voided plus any residual urine.

- *Maximum cystometric capacity (MCC)* is the volume at which the patient feels that he or she can no longer delay micturition. MCC is difficult to define if the patient's sensation is absent or reduced. In deciding how far to fill the bladder in these circumstances, the urodynamicist should be guided by evidence of the functional bladder capacity from the frequency-volume chart.

- The *voided volume* is assessed from the frequency-volume chart completed by all patients before urodynamic studies (see "Analysis of Symptoms" in Chapter 4). When the urodynamicist uses voided volume to determine how full to fill the bladder, any residual urine should be added to the average voided volume taken from the frequency volume chart.

- *Maximum anaesthetic bladder capacity* is the volume to which the bladder can be filled under either deep general or spinal anaesthetic and may often be very different from the maximum cystometric capacity, particularly in conditions such as DO or bladder hypersensitivity.

Artefacts During Cystometry

The urodynamicist is aware that urodynamics even with natural filling rates is not physiological. This is due not only to the need for bladder filling and pressure measuring catherters, but also because, even with ambulatory UDS, the patient is being observed. These limitations must be accepted and appreciated but not ignored. We have already discussed how technique must be adapted in the light of particular findings such as low compliance; further adaptations aimed at minimising artefacts are discussed in later chapters.

The artefacts seen during cystometry can be divided into measurement and "physiological" artefacts.

Measurement Artefacts. This book tries to give sufficient practical detail to enable the urodynamicist to generate high-quality traces and avoid measurement artefacts. Measurement artefacts are produced by problems in the equipment, somewhere between the tip of the catheters and the writing mechanism of the recorder. Setting up the equipment will uncover and deal with most of these problems. Modern electronic equipment is reliable, but if there are problems with the transducers or the urodynamic equipment after proper calibration and setting zero procedures have been followed, then the agent or manufacturer will have to help. As filling cystometry is largely concerned with pressure measurement, this area produces most artefacts. Bubbles and leaks will alter the transmission of pressure from the patient to the transducer. The cough test is designed to eliminate this problem; hence the importance of asking the patient to cough *every minute*. If there is unequal transmission of pressure on the p_{ves} and p_{abd} traces, then the catheters and lines should be flushed from the syringes attached to the transducer as described above and the connections between catheter, tubing and transducer checked for leaks (see pages 56–58).

If unequal transmission of coughs continues, then catheter positions must be checked. Either the bladder or the rectal catheter may have slipped down into the sphincter region causing a pressure transmission problem. This is rather more common with the rectal catheter, which in patients with poor anal function can be difficult to keep in position. A gradual slippage of the rectal catheter can produce a confusing picture, with p_{abd} falling gradually, leading to an apparent increase in $p_{det.}$ However, examination of the p_{ves} line shows that intravesical pressure is constant and uncovers the cause of the artefact.

"Physiological" Artefacts. Rectal contractions are a cause of problems in interpretation and may lead to the misdiagnosis of DO. Rectal contractions are seen relatively frequently during urodynamic studies, and may be single or multiple. If single they should not create confusion, because there is then a single fall in p_{det} at the time of the rectal contraction (Fig. 3.44). However when they are repetitive then the effect on the p_{det} trace can give the illusion of phasic DO. Rectal contractions cannot be prevented other than in patients

who come for urodynamics with a loaded rectum. Such patients should be asked to visit the toilet before the start of urodynamic studies, because this can avoid a lot of trouble (and mess)!

Voiding Cystometry

Introduction

The improvements in electronic equipment that led to the increased acceptance and practice of cystometry were essential in the development of techniques for the accurate measurement of intravesical pressure and urine flow rate during voiding. These studies represent a natural progression from urine flow studies. As discussed, urine flow studies can only provide limited information. Flow rate is dependent both on the outlet resistance and on the contractile properties of the detrusor. A low flow rate may be associated with a high voiding pressure, or with a voiding pressure that is below normal. Similarly, the finding of a normal flow rate does not exclude bladder outlet obstruction (BOO), because normal flow may be maintained by a high voiding pressure in the presence of BOO. In the female, normal flow may occur despite no increase in intravesical pressure. Pressure-flow studies (PFS) are essential for a complete functional classification of lower urinary tract disorders, although personal experience of PFS allows greatly improved interpretation of isolated urine flow rate tracings.

Definitions

During a pressure-flow study of voiding, intravesical pressure and flow rate are measured continuously.

- *Premicturition pressure* is the pressure recorded immediately before the initial iso-volumetric contraction. It will be the same as the full resting pressure if the patient position has not been changed following the filling cystometrogram (Appendix 1, Part 3, Fig. A.1.6.1).
- *Opening time* is the time elapsed from the initial rise in detrusor pressure to the onset of flow. This is the initial isovolumetric contraction period of micturition.
- *Opening pressure* is the pressure recorded at the onset of measured flow. It should be remembered that there is a delay in the recording of flow because of the time taken for urine to reach the flowmeter. The delay is of the order of 0.5 s to 1.0 s and must be allowed for when interpreting the pressure-flow relationship.
- *Maximum voiding pressure* is the maximum value of the measured pressure during voiding.
- *Pressure at maximum flow* is the pressure recorded at the time of maximum flow rate. Again, allow for any delay in the recording of flow rate.
- *Contraction pressure at maximum flow* is the difference between the pressure at maximum flow and the premicturition pressure.
- *After-contraction* describes the common findings of a pressure increase after flow ceases at the end of micturition. The significance of this event is not understood (Fig. 3.57).

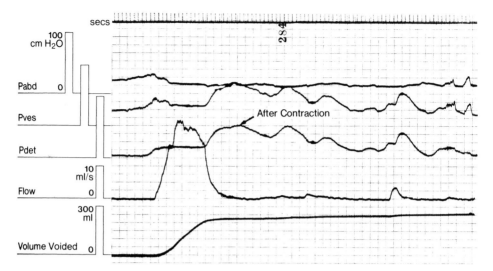

Fig. 3.57 Pressure-flow study of micturition demonstrating the phenomenon known as an after-contraction. This is sometimes associated with detrusor overactivity but has not been shown to be abnormal. ▢

These pressure may be expressed as p_{ves} or p_{det}.

The Concept of Urethral Resistance

The bladder and urethra have independent functional properties and in combination these characteristics determine the pressure-flow relationships of micturition. By knowing both factors and relating them to the normal values of each it is possible to ascertain whether voiding function itself is normal. This can be done more accurately than from either measurement alone. To formalise the relationship of pressure and flow, various urethral resistance factors have been elaborated. At one stage urethral resistance (UR) was defined according to the equation $UR = p_{ves}/Q_{max}^2$. However this calculation of resistance fell into disrepute largely because it was based on the hydrodynamics of laminar flow through rigid straight tubes; the urethra is neither rigid nor straight and flow is often turbulent and not laminar. In 1987 the ICS recommended that pressure-flow data should be presented graphically plotting one quantity against the other (Appendix 1, Part 3, Fig. A.1.6.3). From this basic idea have developed the nomograms used in the diagnosis of bladder outlet obstruction (see Chapter 5).

Performing Voiding Cystometry

In most patients it is quite clear when bladder filling should be stopped. But if the patient has little sensation it is important to use the functional bladder capacity from the frequency-volume chart as a guide to cystometric capacity, remembering to add on the patient's residual volume if present. Once filling has stopped, the filling catheter is removed with care being taken not to dislodge the strapping holding the epidural catheter in place. Prior to allowing the patient to void they should be asked to cough to ensure that proper pressure transmission is occurring. The patient is then instructed to void to completion if possible.

It is even more important during the voiding phase to respect the patient's privacy. Few women have ever voided in the presence of others and, therefore, it may be necessary to leave the room in order that patients can initiate voiding. It is also important to allow the patient to void in a position that is natural for them: for women sitting and for most men standing.

Interpretation of Voiding Cystometry

Detrusor activity and urethral function should be defined separately whilst remembering that urethral characteristics will define the precise voiding pressure.

Detrusor Activity

This can be classified as follows:

- Normal when the detrusor contracts to empty the bladder with a normal flow rate (Fig. 3.57).
- Underactive when either the detrusor contraction is unable to empty the bladder or the bladder empties at a lower than normal speed (Fig. 3.58).
- Acontractile when no measured detrusor pressure change occurs during voiding (Fig. 3.59).

These categories are easy to understand and use if there is no increase in outlet resistance, but they become more difficult to use if there is a coexisting bladder outlet obstruction. For example, in benign prostatic obstruction (BPO), failure of the detrusor contraction to fully

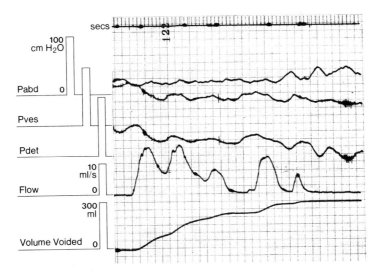

Fig. 3.58 Detrusor underactivity: a poor detrusor contraction results in a fluctuating and interrupted flow wave. 📖

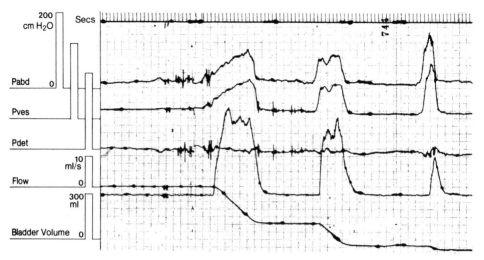

Fig. 3.59 Acontractile detrusor: PFS in a male patient who voids by straining without any sign of detrusor contraction. ▣

empty the bladder does not mean that contractility is abnormal. In BPO voiding pressures are higher than would be expected than if no bladder outlet obstruction existed, and most patients will show normal detrusor activity, with complete bladder emptying, after the BPO has been surgically resected.

It is not the intention of the author to enter into the complexities and controversies of measuring detrusor contractility. However the urodynamicist can make a simple assessment of detrusor contractility by using the "stop test" (Fig. 3.60). Once the patient is voiding and when the observer judges that Q_{max} has been reached, the patient is asked to stop

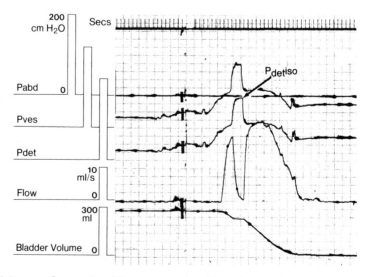

Fig. 3.60 Pressure-flow study of interrupted micturition showing the isovolumetric pressure increase generated by a normal bladder on interruption of flow. In this case the pressure increase is 66 cmH$_2$O. ▣

voiding. The patient achieves this by contracting the pelvic floor muscles and possibly the intrinsic striated muscle of the urethra. However the detrusor is not immediately inhibited and continues to contract. As the contraction is now against a closed outlet it becomes an isometric (isovolumetric) contraction and the intravesical pressure increases sharply to a new maximum. After 2 s to 5 s, the patient is asked to continue voiding and the p_{ves} falls to its previous level. The height of the increase in p_{det} is known as the $p_{det,iso}$ and gives some idea of detrusor contractility. This test can be performed only if the patient is able to interrupt flow instantaneously. However in many patients in whom an assessment of detrusor contractility would be useful, for example in women prior to stress incontinence surgery where post-operative voiding difficulty is common, it is not possible. This is because many older women have lost the ability to interrupt their urine flow. This inability can be circumvented if a Foley balloon catheter is left *in situ* during voiding and when Q_{max} is achieved the catheter is pulled down so that the bladder outlet is blocked; this variant of the stop test has not found favour in the urodynamic community! Figure 3.61 shows the stop test in a woman where a much lower $p_{det,iso}$ results than the one seen in the male patient (Fig 3.60). This does not mean that the woman has detrusor underactivity, but it may be indicative of the fact that women have less powerful bladders than men.

Detrusor Underactivity

This cannot be diagnosed from a filling cystometrogram; a voiding study is necessary. Problems arise when the patient cannot initiate micturition and it is unclear whether this inhibition is psychogenic or neurogenic. If synchronous urethral pressure or sphincter EMG is being recorded then it may be evident that the urethra cannot, or will not, relax. In such a case the inability to void is either psychogenic or, if neurogenic, due to a lesion above the sacral spinal cord. Psychogenic suppression of detrusor contraction is less common if the patient is put at ease by the investigator and the investigation environment.

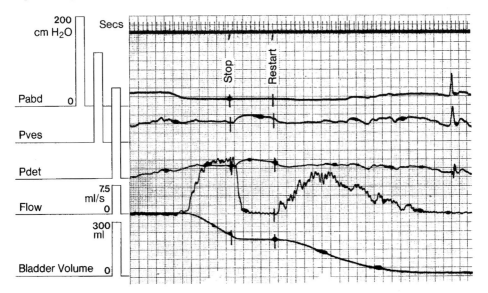

Fig. 3.61 Stop test: small increase in P_{det},iso (20 cmH$_2$O) in a female patient.

In other cases it may be difficult to distinguish between neurogenic and myogenic causes for detrusor underactivity. If the urethral function is quite normal then neuropathy is unlikely; if urethral function is abnormal then the sacral reflex arc can be tested using an evoked response and a denervation supersensitivity test may be performed.

Urethral Function During Voiding

During voiding the urethra may be either normal or obstructive. A *normal* urethra is relaxed throughout voiding. An *obstructive* urethra is most commonly due to *mechanical obstruction*. If there is a mechanical obstruction, such as an enlarged prostate, then sphincter relaxation is likely to be normal but prostatic enlargement will interfere, resulting in limited opening of the proximal urethra. Mechanical obstruction may occur at any site from the bladder neck to the external urinary meatus. Urethral obstruction for whatever reason leads to increased voiding pressures. In mechanical obstruction, the voiding pressures are constantly elevated (Fig. 3.61) whereas if the obstruction is due to urethral overactivity then the voiding pressures may fluctuate as in detrusor-sphincter dyssynergia (Fig. 3.62).

Urethral obstruction due to *urethral overactivity* is characterised by the urethra contracting during voiding or the urethra failing to relax. Urethral overactivity can be divided into:

● *Detrusor-sphincter dyssynergia (DSD)* is seen only in patients with neurological disease and most classically in high-level (cervical) spinal cord injury. It is characterised by phasic contractions of the intrinsic urethral striated muscle during detrusor contraction (Fig. 3.63). This produces a very high voiding pressure and an interrupted flow. The urodynamic characteristic of this type of urethral overactivity is a falling flow rate accompanied by a rising detrusor pressure which then falls when the urethra relaxes, leading to resumption of urine flow.

● *Dysfunctional voiding (DFV)* produces the same urodynamic pattern as DSD but occurs in a different group of patients and has a different cause. DFV occurs, most characteris-

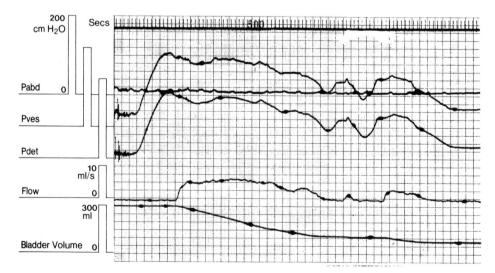

Fig. 3.62 Pressure-flow study in a man of 62 with bladder outlet obstruction. 📖

tically, in children who are neurologically normal but present with urinary incontinence and/or infections. The interrupted flow in these children is due to pelvic floor overactivity rather than to intrinsic striated muscle as in DSD. Figure 3.64 is from a man who showed some inhibition in the urodynamic room.

Nonrelaxing urethral sphincter obstruction is seen in classical form in meningomyelocele patients. In this condition, there is a failure of urethral relaxation rather than urethral contractions during attempted micturition. The urethra opens except for the area of the striated muscle sphincter, at pelvic floor level. This condition produces a continuous obstruction with reduced flow rates. Patients often suffer from stress incontinence owing to

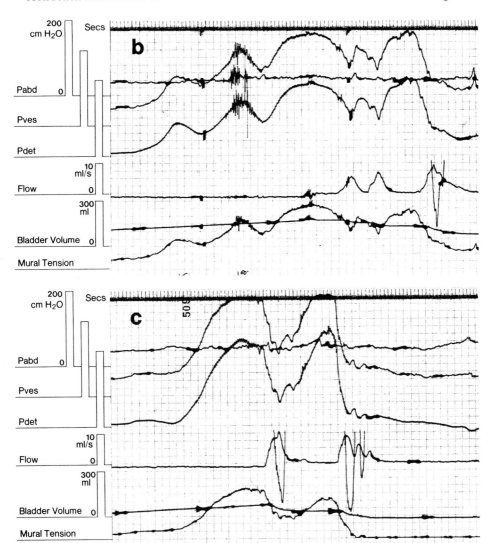

Fig. 3.63 Detrusor-sphincter dyssynergia: two examples both showing a high pre-voiding pressure (greater than 200 cmH$_2$O) which falls as voiding starts but increases rapidly as the urethra closes between urine spurts. 📖

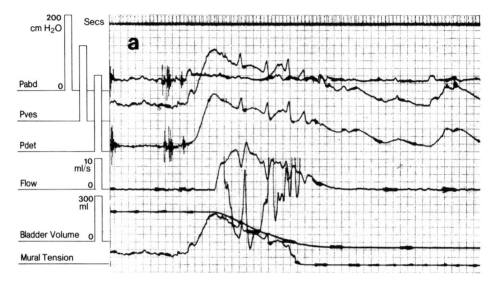

Fig. 3.64 Dysfunctional voiding: the flow curve shows dips which correspond to spikes on the p_{det} trace. This indicates that the patient is not properly relaxed and that the pelvic floor is partially contracted at intervals. 📖

sphincter incompetence during bladder filling, as well as from obstructed voiding due to the failure of urethral relaxation.

Artefacts During Voiding Cystometry

It is important that the limitations of voiding cystometry are understood and that any differences between the patient's performance during urodynamics and his or her normal voiding are appreciated. This is best judged by asking the patient and also by comparing the free urine flow rate with the flow rate during PFS.

Mechanical Artefacts

If p_{ves} is measured by an epidermal catheter, by a 6 Fr dual channel catheter or by a suprapubic catheter, there should be no obstructive effect due to the catheter itself. However catheter problems can make the interpretation of the voiding phase difficult or impossible. Even when the catheter is attached, as described earlier, either the urethral or the rectal catheter may move during voiding. The urethral catheter may slip down into the sphincter area or it may be voided with the urine stream. If it is voided then a characteristic trace results (Fig. 3.65). If it has slipped down into the sphincter area, when the patient coughs after voiding in order for a check to be made of pressure-measuring quality, then unequal transmission will be seen, with p_{abd} being greater than p_{ves}. If, on the other hand, the rectal catheter falls out or slips into the anal sphincter area, then the p_{abd} cough spike will be absent or reduced. If the urethral catheter is voided at the beginning of voiding, the test will have to be repeated. However, if the catheter moves after the maximum flow rate is achieved, a

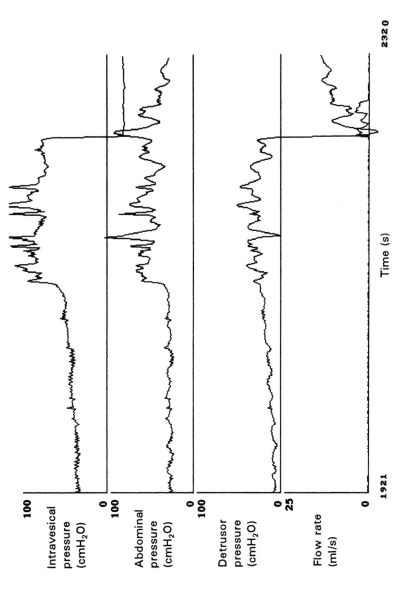

Fig. 3.65 Multi-channel recording showing a sharp decrease in p_{ves} and p_{det} at the start of voiding due to displacement of the p_{ves} catheter.

repeat test is probably not necessary. If problems occur with the rectal catheter, careful inspection of the p_{ves} trace is needed to assess whether a repeat test is required. If the cough spike on the p_{ves} trace, after voiding is similar to that preceding voiding, then it is likely that p_{ves} has been accurately measured. However if the p_{abd} recording is unreliable, it will not be possible to exclude straining as a significant part of the expressive force used by that individual patient to void. Indeed if the rectal catheter has slipped down or come out this is quite likely to be due in part, at least, to the patient straining: it may be necessary to repeat the PFS.

"Physiological" Artefacts

Voiding in the urodynamic laboratory is likely to be affected by a variety of factors:

- The *environment* may result in a patient who voids without problems at home finding it very difficult to void in the test situation. It has been estimated that 30% of women asked to void during videourodynamics carried out in the X-ray department cannot do so. This is hardly surprising if they are surrounded by complex equipment, and if asked to void in an unnatural position, watched by strangers!

- *Technique* used may also be important. Overfilling of the bladder generally makes normal voiding difficult. The effect of relatively fast filling may also be significant, because most studies which compare ambulatory urodynamics (with natural bladder filling) and conventional urodynamics show that voiding pressures are higher with natural filling, suggesting that the detrusor may be incompletely stimulated, partially inhibited or mechanically less efficient after being filled at a supraphysiological rate.

- *Abdominal straining* during voiding may be either a habit or a necessity for the patient. The effect of straining on the voiding trace needs to be understood. The patient should always be asked to void normally and in as relaxed a way as possible. If the patient has an acontractile detrusor then voiding can only be achieved by straining as in Fig. 3.59. If the detrusor contracts during voiding but the patient also strains then the trace can be difficult to interpret. It is also difficult to know precisely what effect straining has on urine flow: in patients without obstruction straining increases flow, but it does not produce the same increase in flow as that achieved by a detrusor pressure rise of the same magnitude (Fig. 3.66). In obstructed patients straining does not increase flow. This may be because the narrow, obstructed urethra is squeezed from outside by the same force that is raising the intravesical pressure and trying to open the bladder neck: hence there is no effect of straining on flow in this situation (Fig. 3.67, *overleaf*).

- *Detrusor overactivity* may produce a misleading trace. Because premicturition pressure may be very high, the patient may appear to be obstructed. Careful inspection reveals a normal voiding pressure and Q_{max} (Fig. 3.68).

The indications for cystometry are dealt with in Chapter 5 under patient groups.

References

Abrams P, Bruskewitz R, de la Rossette J, Griffiths D, Koyanagi T, Nordling J, Park YC, Schafer W, Zimmern P (1995). The diagnosis of bladder outlet obstruction: Urodynamics. The 3rd International Consultation on BPH p 297.

Abrams P, Griffiths DJ (1979). The assessment of prostatic obstruction from urodynamic measurements and from residual urine. Br J Urol 51:129–134.

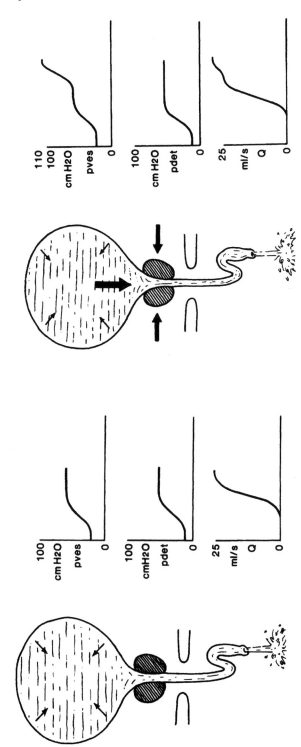

Fig. 3.66 Effect of straining in unobstructed voiding: flow is increased when intra-abdominal pressure increases (heavy arrows indicate straining forces).

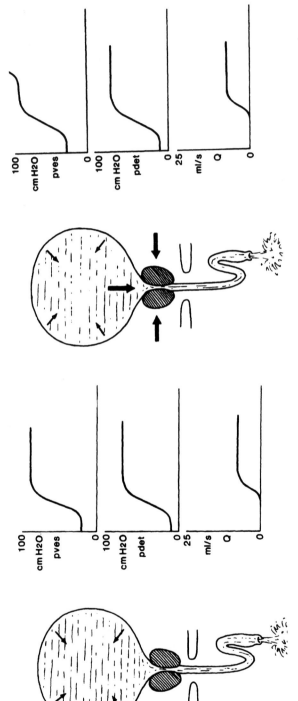

Fig. 3.67 Effect of straining in obstructed voiding: straining produces no effect on the flow rate.

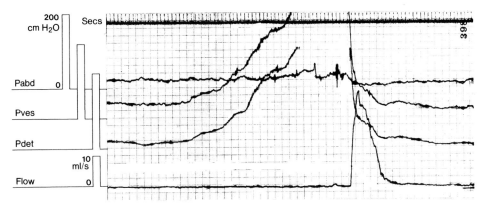

Fig. 3.68 Pressure-flow study in a case of detrusor overactivity in a man of 28. Involuntary contraction of the detrusor is producing a pressure of more than 260 cmH$_2$O; this pressure falls suddenly as soon as flow starts. The voided volume on this occasion was only 150 ml; the flow rate being achieved was 33 ml/s. The pressure at Qmax is 60cmH$_2$O.

Cannon A, Tamnela T, Barrett D, Abrams P, Schafer W, Malice MP and the UDS study group (1996). Repeat pressure flow studies (pQS) in patients with benign prostatic obstruction (BPO). Neurourol Urodyn 15:387–390.

Coolsaet BL (1985). Bladder compliance and detrusor activity during collection phase. Neurourol Urodyn 4:263.

Coolsaet BL, Van Duyl WA, Van Mastright R, van der Zwart (1973). Stepwise cystometry of the urinary bladder. Urology II:255.

Griffiths DJ (1973). The mechanics of the urethra and micturition. Br J Urol 45:497–507.

Griffiths DJ, Van Mastrigt R, Bosch R (1989). Quantification of urethral resistance and bladder function during voiding, with special reference to the effects of prostate size reduction on urethral obstruction due to benign prostatic hyperplasia. Neurourol Urodyn 8:17–27.

Hellstrom PA, Tammela TLJ (1993). The bladder cooling test. Int Urogynaecol J 4:116.

Hellstrom PA, Tammela TLJ, Kontturi MJ et al. (1991). The bladder cooling test for urodynamic assessment: Analysis of 400 examinations. Br J Urol 67:275.

Hofner K, Kramer AEJL, Tan HK, Krah H, Jonas U (1995). CHESS classification of bladder outflow obstruction. A consequence in the discussion of current concepts. World J Urol 13:59–63.

James ED, Niblett PG, MacNaughton JA, Sheldon C (1987). The vagina as an alternative to the rectum in measuring abdominal pressure during urodynamic investigations. Br J Urol 60:212.

Klevmark B (1974). Motility of the urinary bladder in cats during filling at physiological rates. 1. Intravesical pressure patterns studied by a new method of cystometry. Acta Physiol Scand 90:565–577.

Lim CS, Abrams P (1995). The Abrams-Griffiths nomogram. World J Urol 13:34–39.

Merrill DC (1971). The air cystometer, a new instrument for evaluating bladder function. J Urol 106:865–866.

Reynard J, Lim CS, Abrams P (1995). Pressure flow studies in men: the obstructive effect of a urethral catheter. J Urol in press.

Ryall RL, Marshall VR (1982). The effect of a urethral catheter on the measurement of maximum urinary flow rate. J Urol 128:429–432.

Schäfer W (1990). Basic principles and clinical application of advanced analysis of bladder voiding function. Urol Clin N Am 17:553–566.

Sethia KK, Smith JC (1987). The effect of ph and lignocaine on detrusor instability. Br J Urol 60:516.

Sørensen S, Jonler M, Knudson UB, Djurhuus JC (1989). The influence of a urethral catheter and age on recorded urinary flow rates in healthy women. Scand J Urol Nephrol 23:261–266.

Spangberg A, Terio H, Engberg A, Ask P (1989). Quantification of urethral function based on Griffiths' model of flow through elastic tubes. Neurourol Urodyn 8:29–52.

Thomas DG (1979). Clinical urodynamics in neurogenic bladder dysfunction. Urol Clin N Am 6:237–253.

Torrens MJ (1977). A comparative evaluation of carbon dioxide and water cystometry and sphincterometry. Proc Int Cont Soc Portoroz 7:103–104.

Wein AJ, Hanno PM, Dixon DO, Raezer D, Benson GS (1978). The reproducibility and interpretation of carbon dioxide cystometry. J Urol 120:205–206.

Complex Urodynamic Investigations

Videourodynamics

The advent of cinefluoroscopy of the bladder in the early 1950s was a major stimulus to the development of a better understanding of lower urinary tract function. In the early 1960s pressure studies were synchronised with cystourethrography (Enhorning et al. 1964), providing further information, and this technique has been developed in certain larger urodynamic centres over the last decade as videourodynamics. However in some of these centres it is used as the routine investigation. The author has never agreed with this approach, arguing that videourodynamics should be reserved for more complicated patients where there is a high chance of anatomical abnormality coexisting with bladder and urethral dysfunction. Furthermore it is now necessary to justify each exposure to radiation to minimise an individual's lifetime exposure to X-rays, for patients and staff alike.

Imaging of the urinary tract both at rest and on coughing and straining, during filling and during voiding, allows the following useful information to be obtained:

- *Full, at rest.* Bladder capacity, shape, and outline (e.g., diverticulum, trabeculation). Vesico-ureteric reflux at rest.
- *Strain/cough.* Assessment of degree of bladder base descent and bladder neck competence.
- *Voiding.* Speed and extent of bladder neck opening.
  Calibre and shape of urethra.
  Site of any urethral narrowing/dilatation/diverticula Vesico-ureteric reflux.
- *"Stop test".* Speed and adequacy of voluntary urethral closure mechanism.
  "Milk back" from posterior urethra.
  Trapping of urine in prostatic urethra.
- *Post-voiding.* Residual urine.

For most routine problems conventional urodynamics are sufficient and the additional information given by simultaneous imaging of the urinary tract does not help the patient's management.

Equipment

VUDS requires an image of the urinary tract, given by either a fixed X-ray unit (Fig. 3.69) or an image intensifier (Fig. 3.70). Recently, some units have started to use ultrasound as an alternative, arguing that it gives a better image of the bladder outlet in women and eliminates the risks of irradiation from X-rays. Furthermore, recent data has suggested that the measurement of bladder wall thickness by ultrasound may be a guide to the diagnosis of D): the thicker the wall the more likely there is to be DO. Ultrasound has its limitations:

- Particularly in the male it cannot easily be used to visualise the whole urethra.
- If a vector scanner is used at the introitus in women then there is distortion requiring correction before taking measurements (a linear array scanner cannot be used, because it may alter the vaginal anatomy, by its presence).
- The upper tracts cannot be visualised synchronously.
- Apart from bladder wall thickness, other aspects of bladder wall anatomy are not as well seen.

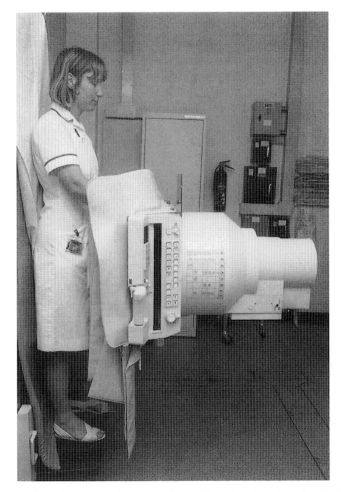

Fig. 3.69 X-ray unit: such apparatus, found only in radiology departments, makes it difficult for a woman to void in "a standing" position. 📖

In view of the limitations of ultrasound, X-ray is still used in most urodynamic departments to image the urinary tract. We have chosen to use our image intensifier system for several reasons:

● We are independent of the X-ray department and can therefore use the system at any time. In most units VUDS is carried out in the X-ray department during set sessions.

● We have been able to create a more friendly and less "hostile" atmosphere than in the more utilitarian X-ray department.

● The patient can sit or stand in a natural position, ensuring the least inhibition to voiding.

However there are disadvantages:

● The image quality is not as high as with fixed X-ray units, particularly if the patient is obese and a lateral view is needed to visualise the bladder neck because it is obscured by anterior vaginal wall descent in the AP (anterio-posterior) view.

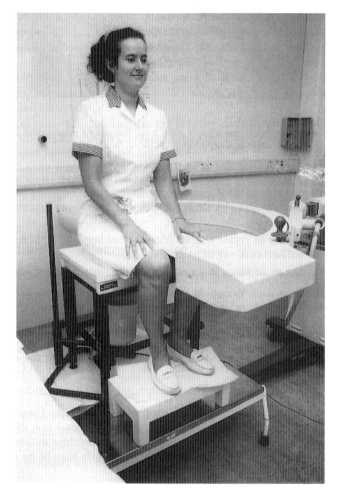

Fig. 3.70 Image intensifier: this apparatus allows a woman to sit normally to void. 📖

● We have to pay to replace the X-ray equipment – a not inconsiderable sum!

Many companies can supply equipment for VUDS. These systems are computerised and convert the analogue urodynamic signals to a digital format; they then mix these with the

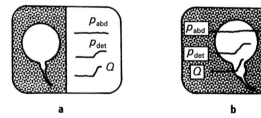

Fig. 3.71 Videourodynamics: **a** screen split with X-ray image and urodynamic data separated; **b** urodynamics superimposed over X-ray image. 📖

digitised X-ray image to produce a combined image on the TV or compluter screen. The presentation of data may be by either of two main methods:

- On a split screen, with the urodynamic traces on one side and the X-ray picture on the other (Fig. 3.71a).
- By superimposition of urodynamic traces over the X-ray image. The traces can be faded so as not to obscure the X-ray image (Fig. 3.71b).

Alterations in Technique During Videourodynamics

- Certain changes in urodynamic technique are necessary to accomodate to the radiological environment. The first is that the contrast medium used for visualising the bladder is of a density different from that of urine. This means that adjustments may have to be made to the flowmeter, which would otherwise record an artefactually high reading because of the greater weight of the voided fluid.
- If it is necessary for women to void in the standing position then a specially shaped funnel system needs to be used to collect the voided urine and pass it to the flowmeter. This may delay further the registration of the flow tracing on the polygraph, relative to the pressure. However, as long as this potential problem is recognised it is unlikely to cause any practical difficulties.
- If the patient is to void in the sitting position some further modification of technique may be required. The simplest way to provide a radiotranslucent commode seat is to construct a thick foam cushion, cut to the shape of a toilet seat, and cover it with a hygienic material. Certain X-ray manufacturers have this equipment available.
- It is useful to be able to visualise the bladder neck in the straight lateral projection. This may mean an increase in the radiation exposure, but is facilitated by the use of special high-density contrast (260 mg I/ml). Such contrast has a higher density and viscosity, though this is less significant if the contrast is heated to 37°C. The effect on flow is not as great as might be expected because the flow is less turbulent.

Interpretation of Videourodynamics

If VUDS is performed with synchronous intraurethral pressure measurement and pelvic floor electromyography then a perfect demonstration of the mechanisms of continence (voiding) can be obtained.

Normal Results. Videourodynamics allows the relationships between anatomical events, for example bladder neck opening, to be related to hydrodynamic recordings. The normal sequence of events on voiding is as follows:

- Bladder base descent, urethral pressure decrease, reduced sphincter EMG activity.
- Bladder neck opening, detrusor pressure increase, EMG silent.
- Flow in progress, detrusor pressure maximal, EMG silent.

- Urethral pressure increased, flow ends, no residual urine, detrusor pressure usually decreases, but may increase (after contraction) EMG transiently increases.

However it should be pointed out that few if any centres in England perform EMG during routine urodynamics. Careful examination of the pressure and flow curves can usually reveal episodes of urethral or pelvic floor overactivity (see "Pressure Flow Studies").

If urine flow is voluntarily interrupted in "mid-stream" (the stop test), then the stream is interrupted at the level of the pelvic floor. The urine in the proximal part of the urethra is "milked back" into the bladder, the bladder base then elevates and the bladder neck closes. When the pelvic floor and urethral sphincter are strong, which often happens with detrusor overactivity, bladder base elevation may appear quite forceful and has been described as a "kick". Under these circumstances the isometric detrusor pressure ($p_{det,iso}$) usually reaches a high level.

During the filling phase of VUDS the bladder neck should be closed, although the bladder neck in up to 50% of continent post-menopausal women opens on coughing. However in younger women and men, if it is seen to open either spontaneously or during stress or postural change, this is abnormal. Such an opening may be due to intrinsic incompetence of the bladder neck or because the bladder neck is being opened in association with an involuntary detrusor contraction. On voiding, the bladder neck should open widely. If it is seen to remain closed this may be because the detrusor is not contracting strongly enough (low p_{det}) or because the bladder neck itself is failing to relax (detrusor-bladder neck dysynergia) and so producing obstruction (high p_{det}). A clue to its existence is the presence of "trapping" of contrast in the posterior urethra, proximal to the distal urethral sphincter mechanism, owing to failure of retrograde emptying of the urethra. Alternatively the failure of the bladder neck to open may be due to fibrosis (bladder neck contraction) or to benign prostatic enlargement "splinting" the bladder neck.

Urethral overactivity during voiding occurs in neuropathic vesico-urethral dysfunction and is characterised by a narrowing at the level of the distal urethral sphincter mechanism, proximal to which the posterior urethra is distended by the force of the detrusor pressure. This subvesical distension may emphasise the bladder neck, which appears as a bar or ring on X-ray or endoscopy. The bladder neck may also appear prominent as part of a global detrusor hypertrophy secondary to detrusor overactivity.

Advantages and Disadvantages of Videourodynamics

VUDS has some advantages over basic urodynamics but there are also disadvantages:

Advantages

- Combining X-ray and urodynamic investigations, VUDS offers the most comprehensive means of assessment. For example radiology is the best way to localise the site of urethral obstruction.
- Videotape recording improves case review sessions, and teaching promotes a greater interest and understanding of urodynamics by allowing clinicians to relate the urodynamic measurements to familiar structural and radiological features.

- Sound recording on the tape adds another dimension to assessment, as well as allowing more spontaneous recording of incidental observations.

Disadvantages

- Not all patients need radiological imaging; in these patients VUDS will lead to unnecessary X-ray exposure. Clinicians should select out such patients.
- Expensive urodynamic equipment may be lying idle in the X-ray department for four days a week unless it is portable and used for basic urodynamics elsewhere.
- The unnatural environment for voiding leads to psychological suppression of micturition in many patients (up to 30% of women). Women especially dislike voiding "in public".
- If VUDS are conducted in the X-ray department the busy atmosphere may mean there is less time for the clinician to spend with the patient in history-taking and discussion. We have found that the overall benefit of assessment depends very much on the time allowed to understand the patient's problem and to set the patient at ease.

Is There a Role for Micturating Cystourethrography (MCUG)?

If VUDS is not readily available in your own hospital or in a nearby centre, then MCUG can be of value. Much information can be acquired by asking the radiologist to take the following films or, even better, record the whole investigation on videotape.

- AP films at rest, on straining and on coughing.
- Lateral film during voiding.

Indications for VUDS

The prime indication for VUDS is when anatomical information is required as well as physiological (urodynamic) data.

- Defining the site of bladder outlet obstruction: VUDS is the best method and is important when the level of obstruction cannot be predicted. In younger men, prostatic obstruction is unlikely and the obstruction may be at the bladder neck or in the urethra, on the other hand, in the older man when the prostate is overwhelmingly likely to be the culprit, VUDS is unnecessary.
- In women the main area of anatomical interest is the bladder base when the clinician is looking for information on bladder neck position, bladder base support and the function of the pelvic floor.
- Patients with neurological disease likely to cause vesico-urethral dysfunction are best investigated by VUDS. In this group of patients there are likely to be both anatomical abnormalities (for example vesicoureteric reflux and bladder diverticula) as well as voiding dysfunction such as detrusor – sphincter dyssynergia.
- Patients with post-operative problems, for example, men with post-prostatectomy incontinence, should be investigated by VUDS to acquire the maximum amount of information prior to further invasive therapy such as artificial sphincter implantation.

Indications for VUDS: Summary

- Suspected bladder outlet obstruction in younger patients.
- Children with abnormal voiding in whom invasive therapy is contemplated.
- Recurrent female stress incontinence if further surgery is planned.
- Neuropathic vesico-urethral dysfunction.
- Postprostatectomy incontinence prior to artificial sphincter implantation.
- Impaired renal function without intrinsic renal disease where urethral over-activity may be a cause.

Ambulatory Urodynamics (AUDS)

In the first edition of this book (1983), AUDS did not appear in the index, and there was only a passing mention of the pioneering work of Douglas James in Exeter. He was considered idiosyncratic in his decision to investigate patients using natural-fill cystometry and to allow the patient to walk around the urodynamic investigation room, something he was able to achieve by using air-filled lines rather than water-filled ones to link the patient to the transducer. The air-filled lines minimised the movement artefacts that prevent fluid-filled lines being used in this situation. Dr James's patients were restricted by the length of the cabling connecting the transducers mounted on a belt around the patient's waist to the urodynamic apparatus.

Little changed until the later 1980s, when workers in Bristol, Maastricht, Newcastle and Oslo developed their own home-made ambulatory systems. Subsequently several companies have developed commercially available systems based on the use of catheter-mounted trans-ducers connected to a microcomputer worn over the shoulder by the patient (Fig. 3.72). This arrangement allows real freedom of movement to the extent that the patient can reproduce the activities that produce incontinence. In principle these systems are the same as those used for conventional UDS and the same basic methodology applies.

Technique of Ambulatory Urodynamics

We record three micturition cycles during AUDS: a resting cycle when the patient sits in a chair; an ambulent cycle when the patient moves around the hospital, and an exercising cycle which should include any specific incontinence-provoking measures, for example walking downstairs or, in a more extreme way, performing an overhead smash in tennis! Once the three cycles are recorded then the information is downloaded onto a desktop computer for analysis. The analysis is relatively time-consuming and requires considerable expertise.

The data acquired during AUDS should include voiding data and information on urine leakage. There are problems associated with both these areas.

Urine Leakage. Because one of the prime indications for AUDS is the detection of inconti-nence, it is important that the episode of leakage is recorded synchronously with the pres-sure data. However recording urine leak has proved problematic: methods have included the

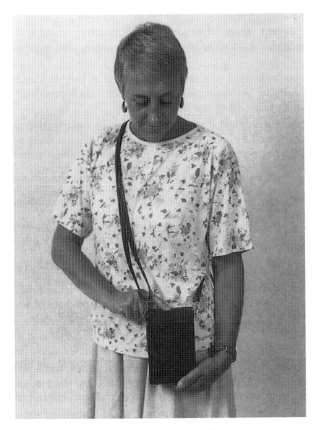

Fig. 3.72 Ambulatory UDS: microcomputer worn over the shoulder. Event marker allows the patient to code events such as urgency or leakage. 📖

Exeter nappy and temperature-sensitive techniques. The Exeter nappy is a body-worn garment in which there is a network of wires in a grid arrangement. A small current is passed through the grid and when leakage occurs, because urine conducts electricity, part of the grid is short circuited. By measuring the resistance of the grid, the occurrence of leakage and to some extent the degree of leakage can be recorded. However, the nappy is rather bulky and somewhat uncomfortable. A temperature-sensitive device has been developed at Bristol in which temperature-sensitive diodes are implanted in a standard incontinence pad, giving a constant reading of perineal temperature of approximately 35°C. When the patient leaks the temperature of the pad is increased because urine is at body temperature (Fig. 3.73). On the other hand, when the patient undresses to void the pad temperature falls (Fig. 3.74) as the pad is taken away from the body.

Voiding Data. The patient unit should allow the connection of a flowmeter so that the urine flow rate can be recorded synchronously with intravesical and abdominal pressure. Unless this is achieved it is difficult to deduce whether or not bladder outlet obstruction exists.

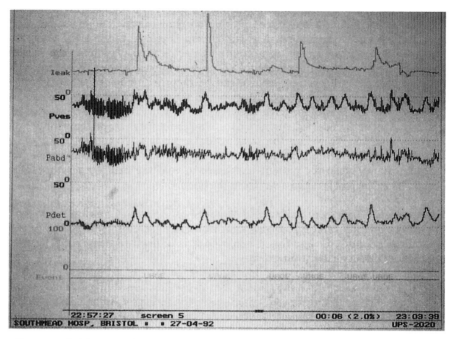

Fig. 3.73 Ambulatory UDS showing on the top trace the temperature rises due to urine leakage. 📖

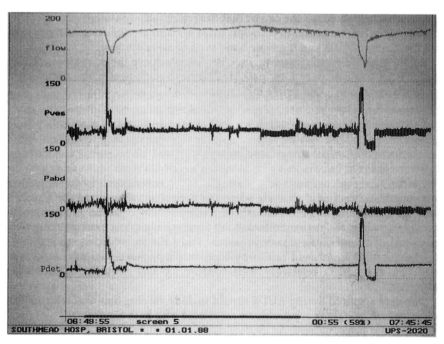

Fig. 3.74 Ambulatory UDS: a normal study; the falls in the temperature trace are due to the pants being removed at normal voids. 📖

As well as measuring p_{abd}, p_{ves}, flow and leakage, the AUDS equipment should have an event-maker which the patient uses in conjunction with a diary to signal sensations such as first sensation of filling, urgency or leakage episodes. In the diary the patient is also asked to record their activities so that leakage episodes can be correlated with physical and other activities.

Interpretation of Ambulatory Urodynamics

As well as providing the evidence for, and the cause of, the patient's incontinence, much additional interesting information is generated by AUDS. Present ideas on detrusor overactivity, compliance and voiding function are being questioned. AUDS on normal individuals have shown a 30% incidence of detrusor overactivity, although this is of no significance to the individual unless accompanied by urgency and urgency incontinence. This provides yet another illustration of the aim of urodynamics "to reproduce and provide a pathophysiological explanation of the patient's symptoms". In a neurologically normal person, without symptoms, the finding of DO is not significant, particularly if a third of normal individuals can be shown to have such findings. Does DO in these circumstances have any positive significance? There are a number of ways in which these findings might be explained:

- All people would have DO if studied long enough.
- DO is an artefact of investigation that results from the presence of an intravesical catheter.
- Thirty percent of normal individuals will develop symptoms of detrusor overactivity in future years.

Klevmark showed that bladder compliance is related to the speed of bladder filling, and AUDS has confirmed this fact. In two groups of patients in whom conventional UDS frequently shows low compliance (namely neurogenic patients and older men with "high-pressure chronic retention"), AUDS has shown that if the bladder is filled naturally then low compliance disappears and is replaced by the finding of phasic detrusor overactivity. Even so, in both groups there are higher filling pressures than seen in patients with simple BOO or neurogenic patients who have DO. (Fig. 3.55).

Voiding pressures during AUDS have been shown to be significantly higher than during conventional UDS (in most females). The explanation may be common to both higher voiding pressures and the apparent uncovering of DO in patients with low compliance on conventional UDS. Fast filling may prevent the detrusor from generating its full contractile force, either because fast fill interferes with the mechanical reorganisation of the muscle or because the biochemical environment of the detrusor is altered. A similar phenomenon can be experienced by any of us if we allow our bladder to overfill with the result that we have hesitancy and poor flow.

Indications for Ambulatory UDS

- To confirm the patient's history of incontinence where conventional UDS has been normal, and
- To determine whether detrusor overactivity or sphincter weakness is the main cause of incontinence if the patient desires further treatment.

AUDS is a valuable method of investigating the lower urinary tract. However the tests are time-consuming and require considerable interpretative skills. AUDS is best used only in the larger units with extensive experience of basic UDS.

Non-Invasive Urodynamics

There has been interest in developing a reliable technique that could avoid the need for pressure-flow studies in some men with suspected bladder outlet obstruction. Efforts have centered on obtaining a measurement of bladder pressure without the need for a catheter passed into the bladder. The technique that appears likely to become available in the near future uses a modified paediatric blood pressure cuff to measure isovolumetric bladder pressure (Blake and Abrams 2004). The cuff is wrapped around the shaft of the penis (Fig 3.75). When the bladder is full, the patient is asked to pass urine. As soon as flow is detected by the flow meter an automatic inflation mechanism inflates the cuff, which increases cuff pressure by 10 cmH$_2$O per second until flow is cut off by the pressure in the cuff. The flow meter detects the cessation of flow and the pressure at that instant has been shown to be close to the true isovolumetric pressure (measured by synchronous conventional urodynamics). Taking the maximum urine flow rate recorded on another occasion and the

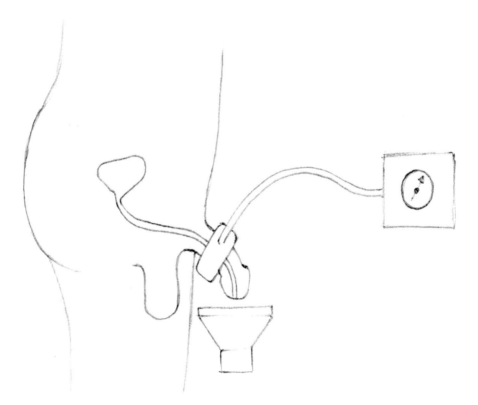

Fig. 3.75 Penile cuff measurement.

isovolumtric bladder pressure from non-invasive urodynamics it will probably be possible to confidently diagnose either bladder outlet obstruction or absence of obstruction in 60% of elderly men with LUTS. This is likely to mean that these men will not need to have PFS. The group who will probably still need to have PFS are those with an intermediate pressure and flow rate.

Urethral Function Studies

As described in the section earlier in this chapter on cystometry, urethral function can be inferred from the findings during filling and voiding. If the patient is continent, urethral function during filling is satisfactory. If voiding is unobstructed then full urethral relaxation can assume to have taken place. However both criteria are met by few patients attending urodynamic clinics, because there is a high likelihood of urethral dysfunction. Urethral function can be more accurately measured in a number of ways:

- Urethral pressure profilometry (UPP)
  - Static
  - Dynamic or stress
  - Voiding
- Urethral electrical conductance
- Fluid bridge test
- Leak point pressure estimation

These tests are clinically used as aids in the diagnosis of incontinence with the exception of voiding UPP, which is used in a few centres to diagnose the presence and site of bladder outlet obstruction. The diagnosis of incontinence is best made by seeing urine leave the external urinary meatus, because this is a *direct* means of diagnosing incontinence. Urethral function studies represent an *indirect* method of diagnosis.

Static Urethral Pressure Profilometry

Definitions

- *The urethral pressure profile (UPP)* indicates the intraluminal pressure along the length of the urethra with the bladder at rest. Appendix 1, Part 5, shows the ICS terminology for urethral pressure measurement. The zero pressure reference point is again taken as the superior edge of the symphysis pubis. When describing the method, it is necessary to specify the catheter type and size, the measurement technique, the rate of infusion (if the Brown and Wickham technique (see later) is used), the rate of catheter withdrawal, the bladder volume and the position of the patient.
- *Maximum urethral pressure* is the maximum pressure of the measured profile.
- *Maximum urethral closure pressure* is the difference between the maximum urethral pressure and the intravesical pressure.
- *Functional profile length* is the length of the urethra along which the urethral pressure exceeds intravesical pressure.

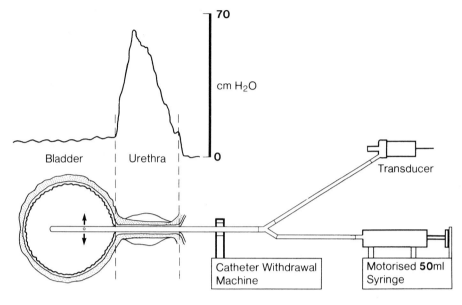

Fig. 3.76 Brown and Wickham technique.

Techniques

Three main methods for urethral pressure measurements are currently used. The Brown and Wickham technique is the best-known method of measuring urethral pressures at rest (Fig. 3.76). However catheter tip transducers may be used, although there is a rotational effect depending on which direction the transducer faces: MUP is highest if it is anterior facing and lowest if posterior facing, so it is suggested that it should be pointed facing laterally. Balloon catheters have previously been used but require frequent recalibration.

Fluid Perfusion Profilometry

The basis of the Brown and Wickham technique is the measurement of the pressure needed to perfuse a catheter at a constant rate. The catheter is passed into the bladder and withdrawn slowly through the urethra. The catheter has eyeholes 5 cm from its tip through which the perfusion fluid escapes into the bladder or urethra. The constant infusion is maintained by a syringe pump. The technique has been shown experimentally to be measuring the occlusive pressure of the urethral walls. Figure 3.76 illustrates the equipment required for urethral closure pressure profile measurement using this technique.

Catheter Size

There is no appreciable difference in pressure measurements provided the catheter is between sizes 4 FG and 10 FG. It seems likely that the sizes above 10 FG may record urethral elasticity as well as urethral closure pressure and therefore give falsely high readings. The comparison of pressure between small and much larger catheters may provide a basis for measuring urethral elasticity.

Catheter Eyeholes

A single end-hole or side-hole is known to be inaccurate, the first because of the lack of adequate mucosal contact and the second owing to differences in pressure measurement due to orientation. A catheter with two opposing side-holes set back from the catheter tip is known to be of adequate accuracy. The presence of more than two holes does not improve the accuracy significantly. If the holes are 5 cm from the tip then catheterisation is facilitated.

Rate of Perfusion

It is desirable that the catheter is perfused at a constant rate. This necessitates the use of a motorised syringe pump *or a very accurate peristaltic pump*. A perfusion rate of between 2 ml/min and 10 ml/min gives an accurate measurement of closure pressure. Perfusion rates of less than 2 ml/min usually fail to record the true urethral pressure unless an extremely slow withdrawal rate is used. The reason for this is outlined below. Perfusion rates in excess of 10 ml/min are likely to lead to falsely high readings, because at such a rate the fluid cannot escape from the catheter eyeholes along the urethra fast enough.

Rate of Catheter Withdrawal

It is most satisfactory to withdraw the catheter mechanically at a constant speed using a motorised system. Speeds of less than 0.7 cm/s are satisfactory when used with perfusion rates of 2 ml/min to 10 ml/min.

Response Time

The technique of UPP requires great attention to detail and illustrates most of the general problems that must be appreciated in order to perform good-quality urodynamics. The issue of response time is important for all urodynamic techniques, particularly now that computerised systems with their limited sampling rates have become the most frequently used systems (see "Cystometry"). The attention to technique is vital and the methods discussed above should allow the investigator to measure pressure profiles accurately. However it is still essential to assess each individual measurement system for its recording accuracy. The response time of the system should be calculated. In a Brown and Wickham system this is most easily done by occluding the eyeholes of the perfused catheter during recording. A graph of pressure against time will be obtained (Fig. 3.77). The slope of the line will give the maximum response at that perfusion rate as centimetres of water per second; for example, if the system has a maximum response at a given perfusion rate of 50 cmH$_2$O per second and the urethral pressure rises by 100 cmH$_2$O in the proximal 2 cm of the urethra then it follows that the catheter must not be withdrawn faster than 1 cm/s at the test infusion

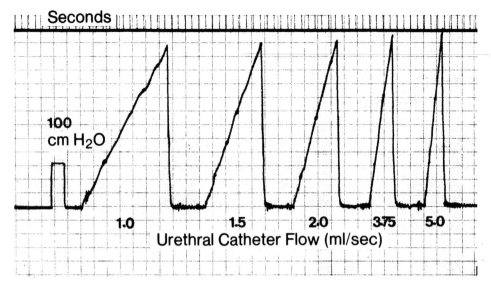

Fig. 3.77 Varying response times for a urethral pressure profile catheter system, showing the pressure response to catheter occlusion at different infusion rates. 📖

rate or the pressure will be underestimated. The response time of the system is determined by three factors: the length and diameter of the tubing from the patient to the external pressure-measuring transducer, the rate of catheter perfusion and the speed of catheter withdrawal. In practice a 100-cm length of manometer tubing is a satisfactory means of connecting the profile catheter to the pressure transducer and to the syringe pump.

By studying the shape of the urethral pressure profile it is relatively easy to decide whether the response time has been adequate to obtain an accurate profile. The tracing we

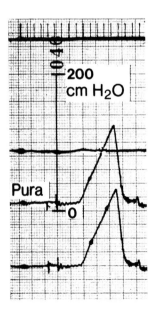

Fig. 3.78 Artefactual "saw tooth" urethral pressure profile, with a straight ascending limb which underestimates the actual urethral pressure. The abbreviations in figures correspond to those suggested by the International Continence Society (Appendix 1, Part 2). 📖

describe as a "sawtooth" profile (Fig. 3.78) is diagnostic of an inaccurately measured maximum urethral pressure. The upstroke of the profile is smooth and straight and looks unphysiological. The downstroke is usually faster than the upstroke and more irregular. If such a profile is recorded then the perfusion rate should be increased or the withdrawal rate decreased. Other factors influencing the response time of the system are air bubbles or fluid leaks.

Reproducibility of the Urethral Pressure Profile

Provided that suitable attention has been paid to detail of technique, the results are highly reproducible. Certain "normal" variations in the urethral pressure profile have been described. The most common reason for pressure fluctuation is voluntary contraction of the urethral or periurethral musculature. It seems likely that most of the maximum urethral pressure of the resting profile is produced by the intramural urethral striated muscle described by Gosling (1979). If the patient is not relaxed during urethral pressure profile measurement, the pelvic floor, which lies in close proximity to the urethra, may by its contraction produce a pressure increment along the urethra. This can be recorded deliberately by asking the patient to contract the pelvic floor voluntarily as if they were holding on when desperate to pass urine. If the urethra is sensitive, it is not uncommon for the first urethral profiles to be of a higher pressure because of the failure of the patient to relax. If reproducible profiles cannot be obtained in any particular case then this is an indication for the performance of a profile which records the maximum urethral pressure with a stationary catheter over a longer period of time. Sometimes vascular pulsations are seen on such recordings; this is not abnormal.

Effect of Posture on the Urethral Pressure Profile

From the technical point of view, it is easier to perform urethral profiles if the patient is supine. Most tests are performed in this position. The posture of the patient does have a considerable influence on urethral muscle tone. The normal response to the assumption of a more upright posture is an increase in the maximum urethral closure pressure of about 23%. In some abnormal patients this increase may not occur, and in others, some neuropathic, the increase in pressure may be excessive (greater than 100%). The absence of an increase in pressure on standing may be a diagnostic test for urodynamic stress incontinence (Tanagho 1979).

The Normal Urethral Pressure Profile

The figures for normal urethral pressures in the available literature are all taken from very small series. The figures in Table 3.4 (*overleaf*) are taken from a large number of our patients who have been assessed and considered to be both clinically and urodynamically normal. The figures are for patients who are in a supine position with the bladder empty. Adequate information on normal pressures in other postures and for other bladder volumes is not available. This does limit the value of urethral pressure profile measurement, because it is the urethral response to bladder filling and postural change which may be most important in diagnosis.

Table 3.4. Values for maximum urethral pressure (cmH$_2$O) in patients in whom no abnormality has been found

	Male		Female	
Age	Mean	Range	Mean	Range
< 25	75	37 to 126	90	55 to 103
25 to 44	79	35 to 113	82	31 to 115
45 to 64	75	40 to 123	74[a]	40 to 100
> 64	71	35 to 105	65[a]	35 to 75

[a] Edwards (1973) quotes figures for normal urethral pressure in the over-45 age groups that are much lower than this, in the range of 20 to 50 cmH$_2$O.

There are certain sex differences. In the male, the maximum urethral pressure does not decline significantly with age, whereas in the female, particularly after the menopause, the maximum urethral pressure is lower. Similarly, in the male, the prostatic length tends to increase with age while in the female the maximum urethral pressure and the functional urethral length tend to decrease (see Figs 3.79 and 3.80).

It is evident that there is a wide overlap between the range for normal urethral parameters and for abnormal situations, e.g. stress incontinence. There is a better correlation between normality and abnormality if an index is used. This is most commonly some estimate of total urethral muscle function such as maximum urethral closure pressure x functional length or, alternatively, a measurement of the area beneath the urethral pressure profile curve.

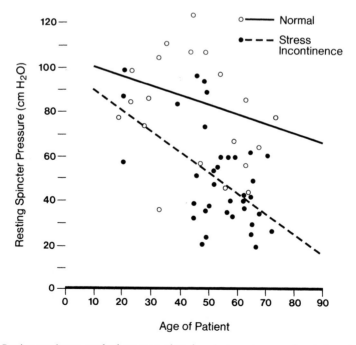

Fig. 3.79 Resting maximum urethral pressure plotted against age in normal and stress-incontinent patients, with regression lines calculated statistically.

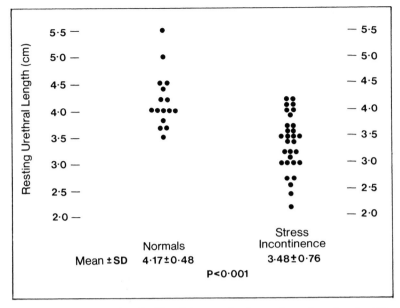

Fig. 3.80 Comparison of urethral length in normal and stress-incontinent females. 📖

The shape of the urethral profile is of diagnostic importance. In the normal male the most important part of the profile, from a functional point of view, is that between the bladder neck and the membranous urethra. The distal bulbar and penile urethra are very variable in length and are not usually described. Certain constant features are seen in male profiles. The

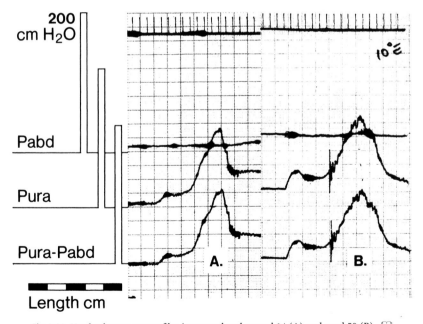

Fig. 3.81 Urethral pressure profiles in normal males aged 14 (A) and aged 50 (B). 📖

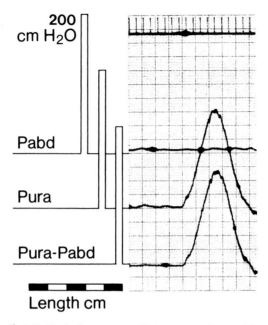

200 cm H$_2$O

Pabd

Pura

Pura-Pabd

Length cm

Fig. 3.82 Urethral pressure profile in a normal female. 📖

presphincteric part of the trace shows, even in boys, a pressure increase due to prostatic tissue (Fig. 3.81). The presphincteric pressure area blends with the pressure zone attributed to the distal urethral sphincter mechanism, which in itself should be more or less symmetrical. As the male patient gets older the length of the presphincteric profile (prostatic length) increases and the pressure within this area may become higher. This is not necessarily abnormal within certain limits.

The normal female urethral pressure profile is symmetrical in shape (Fig. 3.82) and asymmetry is generally due to a faulty measurement technique (e.g., the sawtooth profile).

Classification of Urethral Pressure Profile Abnormalities

Abnormalities may be classified according to the part of the urethra affected and the sex of the patient.

Presphincteric abnormalities are usually seen in male patients with bladder neck or prostatic problems. Commonly, the prostatic plateau may be elevated or elongated. This plateau may be flat or there may be a prostatic peak between the bladder neck and the distal urethral sphincter mechanism (Fig. 3.83). The significance of this peak is uncertain. If it is at the region of the bladder neck then it is sometimes due to bladder neck hypertrophy. A bladder neck peak may also occur on penile erection. A peak in the mid-prostatic region may be related to the meeting of the lateral lobes of a hyperplastic gland. Presphincteric abnormalities in the female are usually produced by surgery where an elongation is related to operations which suspend the bladder neck.

Sphincteric abnormalities are confined to the area of the main urethral pressure peak: mid-urethra in the female and just near the prostatic apex in the male. The pressure here is

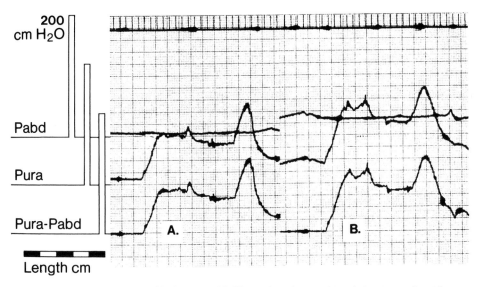

Fig. 3.83 Urethral pressure profile showing a bladder neck and prostatic peak in a man of 60. These peaks are not so prominent in the supine position (A) as they are in the erect position (B). 📖

either too low or too high and may be assessed either at rest or during voluntary contractions, as well as in relation to postural and bladder volume changes. Low pressure is related to damage, atrophy or denervation (Fig. 3.84).

An abnormally high pressure is usually related to involuntary sphincter overactivity or pelvic floor contraction. In the latter case the high pressure is seen only on voluntary

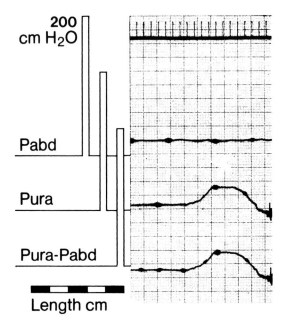

Fig. 3.84 Abnormally low urethral pressure profile in a woman of 84. 📖

contraction when the pressure may reach about 300 cmH$_2$O and this is most commonly encountered while investigating adult enuretics of both sexes with detrusor overactivity. Fowler has recently described a group of younger women with difficulty in voiding due to sphincter overactivity. Many of these patients have abnormally high urethral pressures due to overactivity of the intraurethral striated muscle.

Post-sphincteric abnormalities are less common. Rigid urethral strictures are not well demonstrated by the profile techniques. Adequate demonstration of a stricture depends on the recording catheter being of exactly the same gauge as the stricture, or slightly larger. A small peak, because of meatal stenosis, may be seen in females. Occasionally the urethral pressure from the bulbocavernosus muscle in the male will be greater than that at the region of the distal urethral sphincter mechanism. The significance of this findings and other changes, with age and sexual activity, have not been investigated.

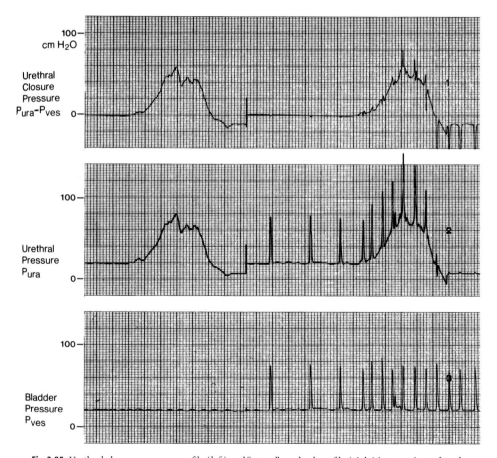

Fig. 3.85 Urethral closure pressure profile (*left*) and "stress" urethral profile (*right*) in a continent female patient. The urethral closure pressure (upper trace) does not become negative until the point of maximum urethral pressure has been passed. ▢

The "Stress" Urethral Profile

This concept of the "stress" profile was introduced by Asmussen and Ulmsten in 1976. Bladder pressure measurement can be made simultaneous with urethral pressure if a suitable dual-lumen catheter is used. For accurate measurement the catheter tip transducer system is recommended. The measuring catheter is withdrawn very slowly through the urethra (1 to 2 mm/s), as described above, with the patient coughing at regular intervals. An alternative method is to hold the measuring catheter stationary at 0.5-cm intervals down the urethra while the patient performs a Valsalva manoeuvre to a predetermined pressure. This method measures the efficiency of pressure transmission to the proximal urethra from the abdominal cavity. It is now well known that decreased conduction of increased abdominal pressure is associated with urodynamic stress incontinence (USI). The transmission may be expressed as the closure pressure, which is the urethral pressure minus the intravesical pressure. If the closure pressure becomes negative on coughing then leakage is likely to occur. Closure pressure may be derived electronically by subtracting intravesical pressure from intraurethral pressure, and this may be displayed on the chart recorder (Fig. 3.85) The best correlation between USI and the findings on stress UPP is found if the test is done with a full bladder and the patient in the erect position. In USI the classical stress UPP shows dips in closure pressure below the 0 cmH$_2$O baseline (Fig. 3.86). Equivocal stress UPPs show dips in the closure pressure trace without reaching the zero line (Fig. 3.87). As with static UPP, there is lack of specificity when normal stress UPPs are analysed against the presence or absence of USI, there being many false negatives where the stress UPP is normal yet the patient on filling cystometry can be demonstrated to have USI. The stress UPP has greater diagnostic specificity when it is abnormal or equivocal, when most patients will be found to have USI.

There is probably little role for stress UPP unless it is carried out in the erect patient with a full bladder: the easiest position in which to demonstrate USI. However the erect position is more difficult from the technical point of view; for example, the withdrawal device must be held vertically and the catheter tends to fall out unless carefully supported. The stress UPP is rarely used now, however it illustrates the basic mechanism that maintains continence when abdominal pressure rises.

Urethral Electrical Conductance (UEC)

This is an electrical fluid bridge test and can be measured either at the bladder neck (BNEC) or in the distal female urethra (DUEC). The DUEC can distinguish between the shortlived increase in conductance seen in USI and the more lengthy increase seen when incontinence is secondary to DO. The principle of both methods is that the resistance to the current flow between the two electrodes on the catheter will reduce, resulting in an increase in current, if there is urine in the area between the two electrodes (Fig. 3.88).

The UEC has little place in diagnostics but has been used in two particular circumstances:

- In needle suspension surgery for USI the BNEC can be used to determine how tightly the sutures must be tied in order to achieve bladder neck closure.

In patients with urgency without DO, the BNEC has been used as part of a biofeedback technique to teach patients how to voluntarily close the bladder neck and abolish the symptom of urgency.

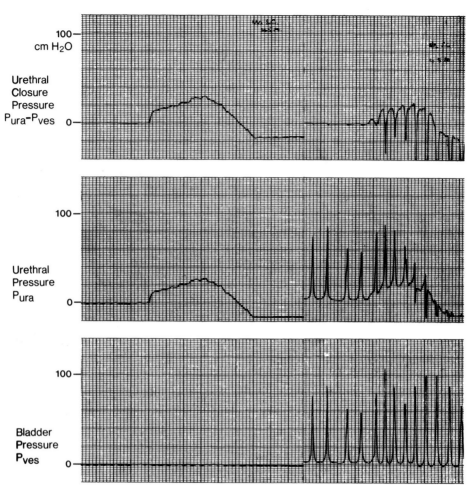

Fig. 3.86 Urethral closure pressure profile (left) and "stress" urethral profile (right) in a patient with a low urethral closure pressure, and poor transmission of cough pressure to the urethra. The urethral closure pressure becomes negative on coughing. 📖

Urethral Leak Point Pressure Measurement

This technique was described by McGuire and seeks to define overall urethral function in terms of the intravesical pressure, or the detrusor pressure, at which urine starts to leak from the urethra. The abdominal leak point pressure (also known as the Valsalva leak point pressure, VLPP) is defined as the intravesical pressure at which urine leakage occurs due to increased abdominal pressure in the absence of a detrusor contraction. The Valsalva manoeuvre (expiration against the closed glottis) is the easiest and most controlled way of achieving a graded increase in intravesical pressure. The technique is based on the assumption that the urethral catheter present during the test does not significantly alter the seal of the urethra. It also assumes that straining does not produce urethral distortion, which might

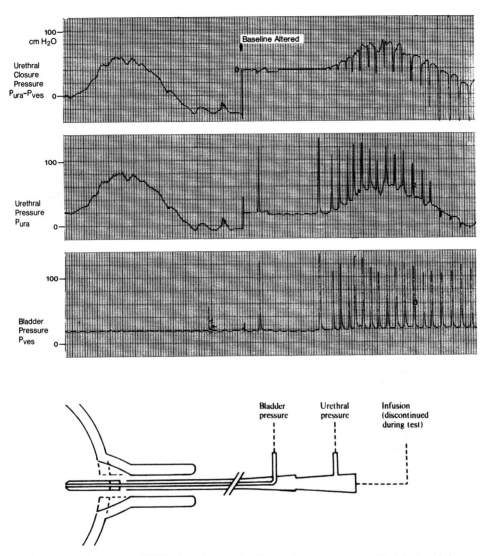

Fig. 3.87 "Equivocal stress UPP", where the negative dips on the upper trace reach but don't go below the 0 baseline. The patient has an acceptable static maximum urethral closure pressure of 60 cmH$_2$O.

falsely raise the VLPP. The third assumption is that there is no pelvic floor relaxation or contraction during the test. While the technique has not been examined as closely from the technical point of view, as urethral pressure profilometry, it is clear that there is an association between poor urethral function and a low VLPP.

The Valsalva LPP has been used to identify those women with USI who have intrinsic urethral failure (intrinsic sphincter deficiency) rather than urethral hypermobility as the cause of their incontinence.

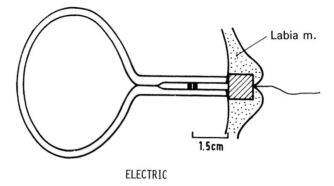

ELECTRIC

Fig. 3.88 Distal urethral electrical conductance test.

The detrusor LPP is defined as the lowest detrusor pressure at which leakage occurs in the absence of either a detrusor contraction or increased abdominal pressure. It is used to predict which meningomyelocele children will develop upper tract dilatation secondary to obstructed voiding due to well-preserved sphincter function (detrusor LPP; see Chapter 5).

Indications for Urethral Function Testing

Specific indications for testing have been discussed in the sections on urethral electrical conductance and leak point pressure measurement. In view of the poor specificity of stress UPP, its use has declined significantly. The measurement of static UPP has several uses:

- In postprostatectomy incontinence there is a close association between sphincter damage and reduction in maximum urethral closure pressure (MUCP).
- In women with USI there is some evidence that a preoperative MUCP of less than 20 cmH$_2$O is associated with poor outcome. If further research bears this out then UPP measurement may define a group of women who require "obstructive" surgery in order to become continent.
- In women with unexplained incontinence measurement of MUCP for a period of minutes may (Fig. 3.89) suggest inappropriate urethral relaxation incontinence.
- In patents being considered for undiversion the MUCP gives a good indication as to whether implantation of an artificial sphincter or bladder neck suspension is necessary. If the MUCP is greater than 50 cmH$_2$O then the patient will be continent if a good-volume, low-pressure reservoir is created.
- Fowler Syndrome: Idiopathic voiding dysfunction or idiopathic urinary retention is a condition of younger adult women and associated with polycystic ovary syndrome. Treatment is by intermittent self catheterisation, suprapubic catheterisation, or more recently, by sacral neuromodulation. Urodynamics are characterised by a high MUCP,

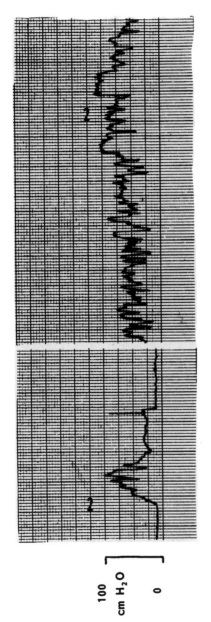

M.U.C.P.

Fig. 3.89 Urethral Pressure fluctuations. The left-hand trace shows static urethral pressure profilometry with normal maximum urethral closure pressure (MUCP) but an irregular shape. The right-hand trace is recorded by positioning the catheter at the MUCP: marked dips in pressure were recorded suggesting the diagnosis of urethral relaxation incontinence. ▯

usually greater than 100 cmH$_2$O, a normal bladder on filling and no observed voiding contraction.

Neurophysiological Testing

There are no urodynamic centres using routine neurophysiological assessment in Great Britain. Some centres in North America, Continental Europe and Japan do use these techniques more frequently. There is no doubt that neurophysiological testing has been, is and will be most important in developing a better understanding of lower urinary tract function. The question is, "What additional information do these tests give that helps patient investigation and management?"

There are two situations where testing may influence diagnosis or help in management:

- In women who have voiding difficulty or who are in retention. By using bipolar urethral sphincter electromyography, Fowler has shown a high percentage to have electrically bizarre sphincter activity, including complex repetitive discharges and decelerating bursts, as the likely cause.
- In children with dysfunctional voiding, perineal skin surface patch electrodes can be used, as part of biofeedback, to train the child to properly relax the pelvic floor muscles during voiding.

One of the reasons why many urodynamicists believe there is little role for these tests in clinical practice is that, with the exceptions above, almost all tests are only found to be abnormal in the presence of a clinically detectable neurological deficit. Hence careful physical examination coupled with a detailed analysis of the urodynamic traces can provide the same answers that neurophysiological tests can give.

The 1988 ICS collated report includes definitions and descriptions of the neurophysiological tests that can be used. The ICS report gives some idea of the complexity of neurophysiological testing. These tests require specific skills and are best carried out separately from urodynamic studies in an appropriately staffed and equipped neurophysiological laboratory.

References

Videourodynamics

Enhorning G, Miller ER, Hinman F (1964). Urethral closure studied with cineroentgenography and simultaneous bladder-urethra pressure recording. Surg Gynaecol Obstet 118:507–516.
Norlen LJ, Blaivas JG (1986). Unsuspected proximal urethral obstruction in young and middle aged men. J Urol 135:972.
Perkash I, Friendland GW (1985). Real-time gray-scale transrectal linear array ultrasonography in urodynamic evaluation. Semin Urol 3:49–59.
Versi E, Cardozo L, Studd JWW, Brincat M, O'Dowd TM, Cooper DJ (1986). Internal urinary sphincter in maintenance of female continence. Br Med J 292:166.
Webster GD, Older RA (1980). Videourodynamics. Urology 16:106.

Ambulatory Urodynamics

Blake C, Abrams P (2004). Nonivasive techniques for the measurement of isovolumetric bladder pressure. J Urol 171:12-19.

Griffiths CJ, Assi MS, Styles RA, Neal DE (1987). Ambulatory long-term monitoring of bladder and detrusor pressure. Neurourol Urodyn 6:161-162.

James D. Continuous monitoring. (1979) Urol clin N Am 6: 125-135.

Kulseng-Hanssen S, Klevmark B (1988). Ambulatory urethro-cysto-rectometry. A new technique. Neurourol Urodyn 7:119-130.

Kulseng-Hanssen S, Klevmark B (1996). Ambulatory urodynamic monitoring of women. Scand J Urol Nephrol 30 suppl 179 pp 27-37.

Paseini-Glazel G. Cisternino A, Artibani W, Pagano F (1992). Ambulatory urodynamics. Preliminary experience with vesico urethral holter in children. Scand J Urol Nephrol suppl 141:87-92.

Robertson AS, Griffiths C, Neal DE (1996). Conventional urodynamics and ambulatory monitoring in the definition and management of bladder outflow obstruction J Urol 155:506-511.

Swithinbank LV, James M, Shepherd A, Abrams P (1999). Role of ambulatory urodynamic monitoring in clinical urological practice. Neurourol Urodyn 18:215-22.

Van Waalwijk van Doorn ESC, Remmers A, Janknegt RA (1992). Conventional and extramural ambulatory urodyamic testing of the lower urinary tract in female volunteers. J Urol 147:1319-1326.

Webb RJ, Ramsden PD, Neal DE (1991). Ambulatory monitoring and electronic measurement of urinary leakage in the diagnosis of detrusor instability and incontinence. Br J Urol 146:336-337.

Pad Testing

Jørgensen L, Lose F, Andersen JT (1987). One hour pad-weighing test for objective assessment of female urinary incontinence. Obstet Gynaecol 69:39.

Gosling JA (1979) The structure of the bladder and the urethra in relation to function. Urol Clin N Am 6:31-38.

Lose G, Versi E (1992). Pad-weighing tests in the diagnosis and quantification of incontinence. Int Urogynecol J 3:324.

Versi E, Orrego G, Hardy E, Seddon G, Smith P, Anand D (1996). Evaluation of the home pad test in the investigation of female urinary incontinence. Br J Obstet Gynaecol 103:162-167.

Urethral Function Studies

Abrams P, Torrens MJ (1977). Urethral closure pressure profiles in the male. Urol Int 32:137-145.

Asmussen M, Ulmsten U (1976). Simultaneous urethrocystometry with a new technique. Scand J Urol Nephrol 10:7-11.

Brown M, Wickham JEA (1969). The urethral pressure profile. Br J Urol 41:211-217.

Bump RC, Elser DM, Theofrastous JP, McClish DK (1995). The continence program for women research group. Am J Obstet Gynaecol 173/2:551-7.

Edwards LE (1973). Investigation and management of incontinence in women. Ann Roy Coll Surg 52:69-85.

Hilton P (1983). The urethral pressure profile under stress: a comparison of profiles on coughing and straining. Neurourol Urodyn 2:55.

Kulseng-Hanssen S, Stien R, Fønstelien E (1987). Urethral pressure variations in women with neurological symptoms. In relationship to urethral and pelvic floor striated muscle. Neurourol Urodyn 6:71-78.

Kulseng-Hanssen S (1983). Prevalence and pattern of unstable urethral pressure in 174 gynaecologic patients referred for urodynamic investigation. Am J Obstet Gynaecol 146:895

Lose G (1992). Simultaneous recording of pressure and cross-sectional area in the female urethra: a study of urethral closure function in healthy and stress incontinent women. Neurourol Urodyn 11:55-89.

McGuire EJ, Fitzpatrick CC, Wan J et al. (1993). Clinical assessment of urethral sphincter function. J Urol 150:1452-1454.

Tanagho EA (1979). Urodynamics of female urinary incontinence with emphasis on stress incontinence. J Urol 122:200-204.

Thind P, Lose G, Jørgensen L et al. (1991). Urethral pressure increment preceding and following bladder pressure elevation during stress episodes in healthy and stress incontinent women. Neurourol Urodyn 10:177.

Ulmsten U, Henriksson L, Iosif S (1982). The unstable female urethra. Am J Obstet Gynaecol 144:93.

Neurophysiological Testing

Fowler CJ, Christmas TJ, Chapple CR, Parkhouse HF, Kirby RS, Jacobs HS (1988). Abnormal electro-myographic activity of the urethral sphincter, voiding dysfunction, and polycystic ovaries: A new syndrome? Br Med J 297:1436–1438.
Siroky MB (1996). Electromyography of the perineal floor. Urol Clin N Am I 23:299–307.
Vodusek DB (1996). Evoked potential testing. Urol Clin N Am II 23:427–447.

Chapter 4

Patient Assessment

Introduction

The vast majority of patients with lower urinary tract dysfunction present with symptoms. An occasional patient will present "silently", with a palpable mass in the lower abdomen, due to an enlarged bladder, or perhaps the symptoms of uraemia. Despite our extensive experience of assessing patients with voiding disorders, we remain impressed by the unreliability of symptoms, even when taken by a urodynamically trained and experienced clinician. This is one of the reasons for the use of urodynamic testing. We commend any approach that lends objectivity to diagnosis, and in particular the use of frequency-volume charts (urinary diaries). The frequency-volume chart forms the basis for the interview during which the clinician attempts to reach a diagnosis, evaluate the patient's most troublesome symptoms, judge the severity of these symptoms, assess the impact of the symptoms on the patient's life and judge the patient's expectations in terms of treatment.

During discussion of the patient's presenting complaints, the clinician should seek information on both the storage and the voiding phases of the micturition cycle. In our unit, history-taking is based on the completion of a proforma (Appendix 3) which leads the interviewer through the phases of bladder function: the storage phase, premicturition symptoms, voiding symptoms and post-micturition symptoms. If the symptoms are interpreted in the context of the normal function of the lower urinary tract, then it may be possible to produce a provisional symptomatic diagnosis. Urodynamics and other investigations then become tests of a clinical hypothesis. If these steps are taken consciously then there is feedback from functional urodynamic information which helps to improve symptomatic diagnosis. Although symptoms have been considered individually in this section, they may be grouped together in symptom complexes, which have more diagnostic significance.

Frequency-Volume Charts

The ICS describes three types of charts (ICS 2002)

- *Micturition time chart:* This records only the times of micturition, day and night, for at least 24 hours.
- *Frequency-volume chart:* This records the volumes voided as well as the time of each micturition, day and night, for at least 24 hours.
- *Bladder diary:* This records the times of micturition, voided volumes, incontinence episodes, pad usage, and other information, such as fluid intake, the degree of urgency, and the degree of incontinence.

The clinician has to deal with a range of urinary symptoms, many of which are variable in nature. It may be unnecessary to proceed with urodynamic investigation, because the basic abnormality in many patients may be related not to detrusor or urethral dysfunction, but rather to alterations in renal excretion, circadian rhythms or the psychological control of micturition. In addition, minor abnormalities of bladder dysfunction may be exacerbated by alterations in renal function, and it is important to identify such alterations before instituting major surgical treatment. Over a period of more than thirty years we have obtained considerable experience in the use of frequency-volume charts completed by the patient. We have found these an essential method of investigating the function of the male and female lower urinary tracts. The charts were developed originally as part of a research project evaluating the response to treatment (Torrens 1974). While Fig. 4.1 represents our normal chart,

Name _____   Date of appointment 14 : 1 : 92

DAY	time / volume (mls.)	DAY-TIME							NIGHT-TIME			Number of pads used in 24 hour period
1	↑a.n. 08.30 09.30 200 50 50	17.30 200	15.00 W	17.30 200	22.30 250				00.30 05.00 50 200			3
2	08.00 08.30 10.00 150 50 100	11.30 100	18.20 W	17.30 —	18.10 100	22.30 150			01.00 05.30 100 200			2
3	08.00 09.00 10.30 100 W W	12.00 100	14.30 200	18.00 W	21.00 200	22.30 100			00.15 01.30 05.15 200 200 200			4
4	07.45 09.00 10.15 100 100 100	11.30 100	12.00 250	17.45 250	22.00 250				04.00 07.10 150 100			2
5	08.00 09.15 10.30 100 100 100	13.45 100	16.00 W	17.15 100	22.30 250				01.30 04.45 200 200			3
6	07.10 08.15 09.30 100 50 50	10.45 W	12.00 W	14.30 200	16.00 100	18.15 100	22.30 200		01.45 04.10 07.00 200 200 100			4
7	08.00 09.15 10.00 100 100 100	13.00 200	13.45 W	16.00 100	17.45 150	19.45 W	23.00 100		02.15 06.30 250 200			4

Fig. 4.1 Standard frequency-volume chart. The time of voiding and the volume voided are recorded for each micturition. Incontinence episodes are recorded as "W", pad usage is recorded in the right-hand column and the fluid intake is estimated.

RECORD DATE, TIME, VOLUME, URGENCY, LEAKAGE AND NUMBER OF PADS USED AS SHOWN IN THE EXAMPLE BELOW

DATE	DAY-TIME (from time out of bed to time to bed)							NIGHT-TIME (in bed)			NO OF PADS
Example 15 Febr	9.00 175 1, +	11.30 150 1, ++	1.00 175 2, +	3.30 200 1, +	5.00 175 2,	7.15 175 2, ++	9.30 125 1, ++	12.30 175 1, +	3.00 150 2, +	5.50 125 1, ++	1 + 1 + 1 or = 3
MARCH 27	7.30 250 1	8.30 50 1	11.00 — 1	2.00p— 1	400 150 1	6.30 100 2+	7.45 300 1	9.45 100 2	10.15 1	3.00a— 5.00 2	1
28	6.30 100 1	8.30 100 1	11.30 100 1	1.00p— 150 2	3.15 300 1	5.15 400 2+	8.00 200 1	1000 200 2+	10.30 100 1	3.30 450 2+	1
29	8.45 150 1	1.45p— 100 2+	4 150 1	5.45 150 +1	7.00 200 1	8.15 100 2++	10.30 350			—	2
30	7.30 900 2+	9.30 —	11.00 —	12.45 —	2.15 —	4.30 —	8.00 —	1000 —	11.p—	3.15 500 2	1
31	9.00 300 1	10.45 100 1	12.30 150 1	1.30 150 2	5.00 300 2+	6.50 150 1	8.00 300 2+	9.00 100 1	11.45 200 2++	—	2
APRIL 1	8.30 400 1	10.00 50 1	1.00p— 150 1	1.45 100 2+	4.00 300 1	4.30 300 1	6.15 100 1	8.45 150 1	1.00o 11.00o 250 280 2 1	—	2
2	8.00 500 2	11.00 —	1.00 100 2+	400 150 1	5.45 200 2	7.00 250 2++	8.00 350 2	9.30 250 1	11.00 1.50	—	2

1 = No urgency   2 = Urgency   + = a little/wet pants   ++ = a lot/wet clothes or pads

Fig. 4.2 Frequency-volume chart also recording urgency (1 or 2) and degree of leakage (+ or ++).

it is possible to use more complex charts if more information is required, for example, when evaluating a new treatment (Fig. 4.2, *above*).

For a period of seven days prior to an outpatient appointment, the patient is asked to record, as accurately as possible, the time and volume of each micturition. In addition, the chart is used to record episodes of urinary incontinence and can be used to record the degree of urgency at each micturition, as well as the use of incontinence aids, such as pads. The patient is not instructed to "hold on" until the bladder is very full, as suggested by some authorities (Turner Warwick et al. 1979), but told to void as normal. No effort is made to make a precise assessment of the patient's fluid intake, because this makes the chart too complex. However, the patient is asked to estimate how much he or she drinks per day, in cups. More accurate estimates of intake are difficult, not only because socially it would appear strange to be measuring the volumes of fluids imbibed but also because food is a significant source of fluid. Patients eating large amounts of fruit and vegetables are often mystified by their high urine output when they appear to be drinking relatively little.

We have found that these charts are well accepted, even by elderly patients and, in the majority of cases, are completed with accuracy and enthusiasm. Even when enthusiasm outstrips ability, the patient still provides useful information. The chart facilitates history-taking and avoids exaggeration or minimisation of the patient's symptoms. By examination of the chart the clinician is able to obtain accurate information as to the exact frequency and nocturia, together with the maximum and average volumes of urine passed at each episode of voiding. This method is the only way of obtaining a value for the average voided volume, a parameter which is important when deciding what volume a patient's bladder should be filled to during cystometry.

From the frequency-volume charts, abnormalities in the circadian rhythm of urine production may be detected, and psychogenic voiding patterns are often identified. In addition, it has been shown that certain patterns suggest particular types of bladder or urethral pathology. Abrams and Klevmark (1996) has classified frequency-volume charts into six basic patterns:

1. Normal volumes, normal frequency: as seen in normal patients with a normal 24-hour urine volume.

2. Normal volumes, increased frequency: such patients have an increased 24 hour urine production (polyuria), indicative of increased fluid intake. Most frequently this is high fluid intake by choice, but occasionally will indicate a significant pathology such as diabetes insipidus or uncontrolled diabetes mellitus.

3a. Reduced *fixed* volumes, day and night; this pattern is suggestive of an intravesical pathology, such as "interstitial cystitis" or carcinoma *in situ*.

3b. Reduced *variable* volumes, day and night. This pattern is often indicative of detrusor overactivity.

We would also add further types.

4. Normal early morning void, reduced variable day volumes. This pattern usually indicates a psychosomatic cause for frequency. The patient sleeps well and voids a normal or even increased volume on rising but passes small, variable amounts during the day.

5. Nocturnal polyuria: these patients void with normal frequency and normal volumes by day, but with increased frequency at night, with more than 33% of the 24-hour urine production being passed during the 8 hours of rest. This pattern is the classical one of nocturnal polyuria which may be due to congestive cardiac failure or abnormalities of antidiuretic hormone or atrial natriuretic hormone secretion, but is often idiopathic.

Alterations in Fluid Excretion

The normal daily fluid output from the kidneys varies between 1 litre and 3 litres every 24 hours. It is worth remembering in the context of deciding what filling rate to use during urodynamics that a urine output of 1.4 litres in 24 hours represents a renal excretion of 1 ml of urine per minute. Approximately 80% of this volume is excreted during the waking hours, and therefore in the normal condition it is not necessary to empty the bladder at night. Abnormalities of renal excretion may be induced by sudden increase in the volume of fluid ingested, or by an alteration in the normal circadian rhythm.

Alterations in the quantity of fluid imbibed may occur at times of stress and during periods of social change, for example, at times of redundancy or retirement. An example is shown in Fig. 4.3 (*overleaf*), where a sudden change in lifestyle has resulted in a dramatic increase in the patient's fluid intake, leading to frequency and nocturia, with large volumes voided on each occasion: the subject had become the teaboy in a prison! Abnormalities of the normal circadian rhythm may be induced primarily by disease itself, such as renal failure or heart failure, or be secondary to drugs used in the treatment of such conditions, for example, diuretic therapy. It is important to identify abnormalities such as a renal cause at an early stage, as they may exacerbate minor abnormalities of bladder function. Nocturnal polyuria in elderly men appears to be secondary to subclinical cardiac failure which results in increased production by the right atrium of the heart of atrial natriuretic

DAY	time / volume (mls)			DAY–TIME						NIGHT-TIME		
1	10·30 / 500	11·09 / 400	2·17 / 375	4·37 / 400	8·15 / 450	9·43 / 300				12·40 / 400	5·00 / 450·	
2	6·00 / 200	9·17 / 350	11·05 / 450	1·57 / 350	4·24 / 350	6·31 / 400	8·14 / 200	9·41 / 350		12·00 / 300	5·11 / 450	
3	9·00 / 250	11·34 / 325	2·26 / 400	4·02 / 300	6·08 / 350	7·59 / 450	9·36 / 300	11·00 / 500	4·50 / 200	6·15 / 150		
4	9·14 / 325	11·00 / 400	2·15 / 300	4·00 / 350	6·51 / 400	9·23 / 400	10·11 / 300		1·00 / 400	4·23 / 200	5·45 / 1·50	
5	10·45 / 300	12·25 / 250	1·40 / 250	2·21 / 350	4·34 / 400	16·40 / 350	9·25 / 300·		1·15 / 200	4·05 / 300	5·45 / 250	
6	10·30 / 350	11·26 / 375	12·33 / 300	1·22 / 400	3·13 / 700	4·56 / 350	9·04 / 400		1·12 / 300	4·00 / 200		
7	6·00 / 200	10·37 / 400	12·27 / 350	4·22 / 400	6·09 / 350	8·23 / 350	9·32 / 350	10·30 / 250	3·04 / 400	5·25 / 300		

AVERAGE DAILY FLUID INTAKE (in cups) = ___12___

Fig. 4.3 The recording chart for frequency-volume assessment showing an alteration in frequency due to excessive intake. 📖

peptide (ANP), the powerful natural diuretic, which causes urine production to be increased. ANP provides the essential mechanism by which excess fluid is excreted at night. Lastly, alterations in circadian rhythms may be due to a primary defect in posterior pituitary function. Although such abnormalities are easily identified by examination of the frequency-volume charts, they may be resistant to treatment. Antidiuretic hormone (DDAVP) administration may be helpful but must be used with care.

Psychogenic Voiding Patterns

The bladder has often been referred to as "the mirror of the mind", and it is common for psychological problems to manifest themselves initially as urological symptoms. Such psychogenic voiding patterns are often "diagnoses of exclusion" following persistently negative urological studies. However, the frequency-volume chart may identify such abnormalities at an early stage. Such alterations in voiding patterns are those of frequency and sometimes nocturia, occurring at times of social and mental stress. In Fig. 4.4 it is shown that frequency is occurring during periods at work, but disappears at the weekend. We have also found that patients may be able to interpret these findings themselves and make a self-assessment of their condition if they are given the opportunity to complete a frequency-volume chart. Another characteristic of the psychogenic voiding pattern is the absence of nocturia despite quite marked frequency during the day (Klevmark's type 4; see above).

Intravesical Pathology

Although serious bladder pathology (e.g., infiltrating carcinoma or carcinoma *in situ*) is usually associated with other symptoms including haematuria, such individuals may present with the symptoms of frequency and nocturia. These patients' frequency-volume

Name _____   Date of appointment **4.6.50**

DAY	time / volume (mls) DAY-TIME								NIGHT-TIME		
1	7.30/200	9.45/110	10.45/110	12.30/150	2.30/110	5.15/100	7.0/80	10.00/100	2.0/150		Mon
2	6.30/180	9.15/110	2.0/100	5.0/100	7.45/100	10.0/100			12.30/100	3.0/150	Tues
3	6.30/200	9.30/100	11.0/110	2.0/110	3.15/–	5.30/100	7.45/100	10.0/150	1.0/150	3.15/150	Wed
4	6.0/180	9.0/110	10.30/–	12.30/100	3.15/100	6.30/100	10.0/110		3.30/190	5.15/150	Thurs
5	7.45/150	9.15/100	10.45/180	12.15/100	130/100	3.30/100	6.45/150 / 9.30/50 / 11.30/100		2.30/200	5.0/150	Fri
6	8.0/100	11.0/125	3.30/110	6.45/100	10.30/100						Sat
7	8.45/200	10.15/100	2.15/150	5.0/130	10.30/100				1.30/150		Sun

AVERAGE DAILY FLUID INTAKE (in cups) = **6**

Fig. 4.4 Frequency-volume chart showing excessive frequency during periods at work. At the weekend daytime frequency becomes normal and nocturia reduces markedly. 📖

charts frequently demonstrate "fixed" voided volumes with relentless frequency and nocturia. For example, Fig. 4.5 (*below*) is from a patient who exhibited such characteristics and was subsequently shown to have bladder carcinoma. The finding of such a pattern on a frequency-volume chart should indicate the need for further investigations, including urgent cystoscopy.

Name _____   Date of appointment **20.8.80**

DAY	time / volume (mls) DAY-TIME									NIGHT-TIME					
1	11.30 AM/100	12.00/100	12.30/100	12.55/100	1.20/100	2.00/100	2.55/100	3.50/50	4.45/50						
✶	6.45/50	7.45/75	8.45/25	9.45/25	10.15/25					12.30/50	2.55/25	2.10/25	2.40/25	3.45/25	4.40/25
2✶	6.30/50	7.20/50	8.00/25	8.50/100	9.25/50	10.10/50	11.10/50	11.45/50	12.80/50						
✶	3.15/50	4.20/25	6.00/25	6.50/25	7.30/25	8.30/50	9.10/25			9.50/25	12.20/25	1.00/25	1.50/25	4.10/25	5.40/25
3✶	5.50/25	6.30/25	7.50/25												
✶															
✶															

AVERAGE DAILY FLUID INTAKE (in cups) = **4**

Fig. 4.5 Frequency-volume chart, showing frequency due to fixed bladder capacity in a patient with bladder carcinoma. 📖

Overactive Bladder and Detrusor Overactivity

Overactive bladder (OB) is defined as urgency with or without urge incontinence, usually with frequency and nocturia. OAB symptoms are presumed to be due to involuntary detrusor contractions characteristic of detrusor overactivity.

Following the exclusion of the abnormalities described above, there remain a group of patients in whom the basic pathology remains unclear. From the clinician's point of view the most important factor is to consider whether the patient's symptoms are related to bladder outlet obstruction or to an abnormality of detrusor function such as detrusor overactivity.

Patients with detrusor overactivity often show reduced but variable volumes of urine during the day. Their night-time volumes and the first void on waking in the morning are often of larger quantity.

Bladder Outlet Obstruction

We are not aware of any clear pattern on a frequency-volume chart that will allow the diagnosis of bladder outlet obstruction to be made.

Analysis of Symptoms

In this section each symptom is defined and explained in functional terms. The object, as ever, is to provide a pathophysiological understanding of the patient's complaints. Such an approach requires some conceptual thinking, but allows the clinician to develop a hypothesis as to the patient's underlying condition as the history is taken.

The interpretation of a patient's symptoms is modified by many factors, not least by the time the clinician is able to spend with the patient. The limits of normality are not adequately defined, and in an individual case may be what the patient, rather than the doctor, considers to be normal. The adequacy of communication is important, as are many preconceived ideas held by the medical staff. For this reason, for each symptom, a specific wording of the question to the patient about that symptom is suggested.

In the analysis of each individual symptom it is important not only to assess the presence or absence of any symptom, but also to define its frequency and severity; as Fig. 4.6 shows, patient-completed questionnaires now attempt to grade each of the symptoms in terms of frequency and/or severity, and bother.. Lower urinary tract symptoms (LUTS) should be divided into the phases of micturition: storage, voiding, post-micturition and others.

Storage Symptoms

Frequency of Micturition

Increased daytime frequency is defined as the complaint by the patient who considers that he or she voids too often by day.

> Question: "How often do you pass urine (your water) from the time you wake in the morning until the time you go to sleep at night?"

21. HESITANCY

1 = none
2 = only on full bladder
3 = occasional
4 = usually
5 = always strains to void urine
6 = cannot void urine
X = unknown

if 1, 5, 6 or X in 21 go to 22

FREQUENCY (of hesitancy)

1 = more than x 1/day
2 = x 1/day
3 = more than x 1/week
4 = x 1/week
5 = less than x 1/week
X = unknown

Fig. 4.6 Urodynamic questionnaire: an example of the question format with the presence/absence of the symptom followed by a supplementary question as to its frequency.

Abnormality of urinary frequency is a change from that to which any particular patient is accustomed. There is surprisingly little objective data on frequency in the normal population, however three excellent papers by Larsson and Victor (1988), Swithinbank and Abrams (2001) and Carter et al. (1992) give us information on women and men respectively. We would consider normal diurnal frequency to be between 3 and 7 voids per day.

Increased urinary frequency is seldom the patient's only complaint; it is usually associated with other symptoms – most frequently, urgency of micturition. Frequency of up to 10 to 12 times per day may be tolerated by many patients; above this it is usually socially embarrassing. However this statement must be modified according to the patient's occupation, and if the patient works on a factory production line, or is a long-distance lorry driver, then it becomes essential that they can hold urine for at least two hours. Patients are notoriously inaccurate in their assessment of urinary frequency, and for this reason an objective means of assessing frequency, such as the frequency-volume chart, is essential.

Mechanisms of Increased Urinary Frequency. It is useful in understanding the mechanisms of frequency if the causes are categorised according to the voided volume.

1. *Normal voided volume.* We consider the normal voided volume to be 300 ml to 600 ml in the adult. A child's expected voided volume can be calculated on the basis of 30 ml plus 30 ml for each year of life, so that a child of three can be expected to void 120 ml at a time. In this group, with normal voiding volumes increased frequency must be due to an increased intake, resulting in increased output. This may be secondary to:

   ● Polydypsia, which may occasionally be psychotic, but is more usually because the patient enjoys a favourite beverage, be it tea, water or beer.

   ● An osmotic diuresis (e.g., diabetes mellitus).

   ● An abnormality of anti-diuretic hormone production, e.g. in diabetes insipidus.

2. *Reduced voided volumes.* This term implies that the bladder capacity under general or regional anaesthetic would be normal, but the voided volumes are consistently small – less than 300 ml. The causes of reduced voided volumes include the following:

● Detrusor overactivity.

● A significant residual urine resulting either from bladder outlet obstruction, detrusor underactivity or a combination of the two.

● Non-inflammatory causes of increased bladder sensation, for example, anxiety or the idiopathic hypersensitive bladder.

● Inflammatory bladder conditions (e.g., acute cystitis, carcinoma *in situ* or bladder stone).

● A fear of urinary retention, especially in older male patients who experience increasing hesitancy as the bladder becomes full, and who compensate by voiding frequently.

● Fear of incontinence. Some patients, both with urodynamic stress incontinence and/or with detrusor overactivity, have increased frequency in order to keep their bladder volumes low, and minimise the risk of leakage.

3. *Reduced structural bladder capacity.* In this case the bladder capacity is smaller than normal under regional or deep general anaesthesia, resulting in consistently small voided volumes. The reduction in capacity may be due to:

● Post-infective fibrosis (e.g., tuberculosis).

● Non-infective cystitis (e.g., interstitial cystitis (Hunner's ulceration)).

● Post-pelvic irradiation fibrosis (e.g., after radiotherapy for bladder or cervical cancer).

● After surgery (e.g., partial cystectomy).

Mechanism of Decreased Urinary Frequency. Infrequent voids of large volumes of urine usually provoke admiration rather than complaints. Decreased frequency may be due to the profession of the patient, for example, "check-out girls" working in supermarkets may develop the ability to hold their urine for long periods of time. Similarly lorry drivers working on the motorways may void infrequently. Reduced detrusor contractility and impaired bladder sensation may be factors that can lead to decreased frequency, or indeed may result from the habit of holding large volumes.

When faced with patients, usually women, with recurrent urinary infections, it is important to ask the patient's voiding habits between infections, because quite often they can be discovered to be "infrequent voiders". Part of their management then consists of advising them to void at least four-hourly.

Nocturia

Nocturia is the complaint that the individual has to wake one or more times to void.

> Question: *"How many times, on average, are you woken from your sleep because you need to pass urine?"*

Unless the clinician's definition of nocturia is made clear, the patient may include a void before going to sleep, or the first void in the morning. Furthermore the frequency of nocturnal voiding, in relation to age, needs to be considered when judging the significance of the symptom.

This complaint is dependent on age in both sexes. We have defined nocturia as being woken from sleep each night by the need to urinate. It is usual for men over 65 and women over 75 to awaken once at night in this way.

Other patients will attempt to include all voids during the hours of darkness, giving the paradox of increased nocturia during the winter, compared with during the summer. It is also important to ask whether the patient sleeps well, and whether he or she drinks during the night. Some patients sleep poorly for no apparent reason, and some because of a restless partner or chronic painful conditions such as arthritis. These patients, once awake, are often unable to settle until they have emptied their bladders, thus producing apparent nocturia. However most such patients have no increase in daytime frequency.

Mechanisms of Nocturia

Most causes of nocturia are the same as those described for increased diurnal frequency. However, in addition, nocturnal production of urine may increase (nocturnal polyuria). Often this is due to the reabsorption of oedema fluid in patients with mild congestive cardiac failure: it is therefore important to examine the ankles and sacrum of all elderly patients for oedema fluid. However increased nocturnal urine production is often seen in the absence of demonstrable oedema, although oedema does not become clinically detectable until there is at least 1 litre of fluid lying in the interstitium. When the patient goes to bed, oedema fluid is reabsorbed into the circulation and the venous pressure increases. In the right atrium an increase in venous pressure results in the secretion of atrial naturetic peptide. Nocturia may also be due to loss or reduction of antidiuretic hormone production at night: a reversal of the diurnal pituitary rhythm. If there is diurnal frequency and urgency then nocturia is most likely to be due to detrusor overactivity. Other causes of nocturia include habitual poor sleep patterns, a partner who disturbs the patient, pain for any reason (e.g., arthritis), and sleep apnea (van Kerrebroeck et al. 2002)

Urgency

Urgency is the complaint of a sudden compelling desire to pass urine which is difficult to defer (because of fear of leakage)

> Question: "When you get the feeling of wanting to pass your water, can you hold on or do you have to go immediately?"

If the patient appears to have urgency then the following two supplementary questions may be useful:

> "If you are watching your favourite TV programme, and get the feeling of wanting to pass urine, can you delay it until the programme has finished, or do you have to leave the room more or less immediately?"

> "How much time does your bladder give you from the time you first feel you want to go until you think you are desperate and likely to leak – five minutes, ten minutes, half an hour?"

Mechanisms of Urgency

Urgency is usually due to detrusor overactivity, when urgency frequently results in *urgency* incontinence. Urgency is felt lower down than either bladder pain or a normal strong desire to void, as felt when voiding is delayed.

Bladder Pain

> Question: *"When your bladder fills do you have any pain in your bladder?"*

Bladder pain is felt suprapubically and increases slowly and gradually with bladder filling. The pain leads to frequency, not because of fear of incontinence, but due to increasing discomfort and fear of pain. Bladder pain, although often relieved by micturition, may persist after voiding, most classically in interstitial cystitis.

Mechanisms of Bladder Pain

Bladder pain may be due to:

- Inflammatory conditions of the bladder, e.g. acute cystitis or interstitial cystitis.
- Increased bladder sensation without inflammation but due to irritation by intravesical pathology such as bladder carcinoma ("malignant cystitis") or bladder stone.

Urinary Incontinence

Urinary Incontinence is the complaint of any involuntary leakage of urine.

> Question: *"Do you ever leak urine or wet yourself?"*

The original ICS definition, "incontinence is a condition in which involuntary loss of urine is a social or hygienic problem, and is objectively demonstrated" remains useful as it encompasses the concept of quality of life (Appendix 1, Part 5). Loss of urine through channels other than the urethra is defined as extraurethral incontinence, for example when due to a vesico-vaginal fistula. Strenuous effort should be made on history-taking to decide which type of incontinence is suffered by the patient.

It is unwise to ask patients if they are incontinent, because they will often answer "no", either through embarrassment or because they imagine that incontinence means being wet all the time.

Stress Incontinence

Stress urinary incontinence is the complaint of involuntary leakage on effort or exertion, or on sneezing or coughing.

> Question: *"Do you ever leak urine when you cough, sneeze, exercise, lift heavy objects or walk on rough ground or down hill?"*

Stress incontinence denotes a symptom, a sign or a condition. The symptom of stress incontinence indicates the patient's statement of involuntary urine loss during physical exertion. The sign of stress incontinence denotes the observation of urine loss from the urethra, synchronous with a physical exertion such as coughing. The condition "urodynamic stress incontinence" has been defined by the ICS as" the involuntary loss of urine occurring when, in the absence of a detrusor contraction, the intravesical pressure exceeds the maximum urethral pressure". Clearly, it is important that abdominal pressure is measured during urodynamic studies in order to satisfy the needs of this definition.

Mechanisms of Stress Incontinence. The first line of continence is normal closure of the bladder neck throughout filling. The second line is a competent distal urethral sphincter mechanism. It follows that stress incontinence must involve a degree of inadequacy of both these mechanisms. The physiology of urethral incompetence has been discussed in Chapter 2.

The clinical situations in which bladder neck and urethral incompetence occur include:

- A weakened pelvic floor, especially in the obese and multiparous.
- A paralysed pelvic floor in lower motor-neurone lesions.
- Abnormally high pressures in a distended bladder where distension tends to open the bladder neck.
- Iatrogenic damage to the sphincter mechanisms, for example, following transurethral resection of the prostate.
- Congenital short urethra.

One important differential diagnosis is between urodynamic stress incontinence and stress-induced detrusor overactivity (see Chapter 3). It is important to ask the patient whether they have any sensation of urgency prior to leakage which occurs when detrusor overactivity follows coughing or change of posture.

Urgency Incontinence

Whilst deliberating the new ICS definition, and later when discussing the difficulties of measuring the symptom urgency, a semantic discussion arose over the meanings of the words "urge" and "urgency". "Urge", in the English language denotes 'wish' or need". On the other hand urgency is defined by Webster's as "immediate action, insistent", as in the ICS definition of urgency: a sudden compelling desire to pass urine which is difficult to defer. Perhaps the phrase, "because of fear of leakage" should have been added to the definition. Given this discussion it would be more consistent to call "urge incontinence", urgency incontinence. Unfortunately this thought never occurred to the terminology committee when they met through 2000 and 2001: it was suggested by Michael Craggs.

Urgency incontinence is defined as "the complaint of involuntary leakage accompanied by or immediately preceeded by urgency

> Question: "When you want to pass urine, do you ever leak before you can get to
> the toilet because you can't hang on long enough?"

Most frequently there is no specific trigger for urgency incontinence, but some patients do report certain provoking factors such as hand washing, answering the telephone or putting the key in the front door when returning home.

Mechanisms of Urgency Incontinence. Urgency incontinence may, as in the case of urgency, be associated with

- Detrusor overactivity, when it is known as detrusor overactivity incontinence.
- Urethral relaxation incontinence, which is defined as leakage due to urethral relaxation in the absence of raised abdominal pressure or detrusor overactivity. It is an unusual cause of urgency incontinence.

Giggle Incontinence

This type of incontinence is usually a complaint of younger women. The history is clear and usually not associated with other urinary disturbance. Because of the problem of reproducing this symptom in the urodynamic laboratory the mechanism is not clearly understood. The definition is implicit in the name. Suggested mechanisms for giggle incontinence include urethral relaxation, detrusor overactivity and congenital urethral weakness.

Nocturnal Enuresis

> Question: *"Do you ever wet the bed or your pyjamas (nightgown) when you are asleep, either at night or during the day?"*

Strictly speaking, enuresis can refer to any incontinence, day or night. However the term is most often used to mean a normal act of micturition occurring during sleep, that is nocturnal enuresis. Enuresis may be divided into primary, when the patient has never been dry at night, and secondary, when enuresis follows a period of nighttime continence. Nocturnal enuresis is often a significant factor in the past history of young adults with nocturia. A family history should be sought and the presence or absence of concurrent diurnal symptoms noted. When talking to children it is useful to assess diurnal symptoms by asking the questions, *"Do you have to leave the classroom in the middle of a lesson in order to pass urine?"* and *"Do you have to get up to pass urine when you are watching your favourite TV programme?"*

Mechanisms of Enuresis. Enuresis is fundamentally a disturbance of brain function whereby bladder distension, for one reason or another, does not elicit normal cortical arousal. Various other factors may contribute to the situation, including:

- Increased nocturnal secretion of urine due to an inappropriately low level of ADH secretion at night.
- Reduced bladder or urethral sensation, such as in neuropathic patients.
- Detrusor overactivity.
- Inappropriate cerebral sedation, for example, by drugs or alcohol.
- Reduced bladder capacity.

It is very common to hear from parents that the enuretic child sleeps much more deeply than all the other children.

Incontinence Without Obvious Cause

Incontinence in the absence of sensation, without an associated desire to micturate and in the absence of raised abdominal pressure, is seen only in patients with neurogenic bladder.

Continuous Incontinence

Patients not infrequently complain of being "continuously incontinent". However, true continuous incontinence can only be due either to a fistula between the ureter, bladder or urethra above the distal sphincter mechanism, and the vagina, or to an ectopic ureter entering into the urethra below the distal mechanism or into the vagina in the female. Patients with severe sphincter weakness may be more or less continuously incontinent during the day, but when they lie down in bed they are usually dry for considerable periods of time.

When assessing incontinence it is essential to document the frequency and severity of incontinence. Figure 4.7 shows how we ask about severity and the measures the patient takes to cope with leakage. In addition, if the patient uses pads then the type of pad, the proportion which are wet and the degree of wetness all need to be ascertained.

Incontinence During Sexual Intercourse

Incontinence may be related specifically to sexual activity. Penetration may precipitate involuntary detrusor contractions. Leakage during intercourse may also occur in women

27. DEGREE OF INCONTINENCE

1 = drops, wets underclothes
2 = 'floods', wets outer clothes
3 = 'floods', on floor
X = not known

28. MANAGEMENT OF INCONTINENCE

1 = no protective measures, no clothes change
2 = changes underwear/clothes
3 = pads for safety
4 = pads for necessity
5 = appliance
6 = catheter
7 = urinary diversion
8 = other
X = unknown

complete ONLY if 3 or 4 in 28

PADS PER DAY

PADS PER NIGHT

Fig. 4.7 Urodynamic questionnaire: the section enquiring as to the degree of incontinence and the measures taken to control leakage. 📖

with stress incontinence. Leakage at orgasm in the woman may be secondary either to urethral sphincter weakness, or perhaps to inappropriate urethral relaxation. In the man, occasional ejaculation of urine with semen may occur, and this is most frequently seen in patients with a neurological disease such as spina bifida.

It must also be recognised that incontinence can have a profound effect on the sexual activity of patients and may be a cause of marital disharmony. Because of the considerable psychological repercussions this can have, it is particularly important that the sexual history is taken in detail so that proper practical advice can be given. As patients are often embarassed it is important to ask directly about leakage during intercourse.

Voiding Symptoms

Hesitancy

Question: "After you have had the feeling that you want to pass water, and you are in the toilet and ready to urinate, does your urine come immediately or do you have to wait?"

If the patient has hesitancy ask a supplementary question:

"How long do you have to wait, 10 seconds, 30 seconds, 1 minute or more than 1 minute?"

This symptom is defined as difficulty in initiating micturition resulting in a delay in the onset of voiding after the patient is ready to pass urine. The complaint of hesitancy should be assessed in terms of the volume voided. It may be normal for any individual to have hesitancy when trying to void with less than 100 ml in the bladder. Conversely, a patient may complain of hesitancy only with a full bladder; this is often taken as a sign of impending urinary retention. However, even a normal person may have problems initiating voiding if the bladder gets exceptionally full.

Mechanisms of Hesitancy. Hesitancy may be due to:

- Bladder outlet obstruction. Here the patient has to wait for the detrusor contraction to generate sufficient pressure to overcome increased outlet pressure
- Detrusor factors. These include detrusor underactivity, and either over- or underdistension of the bladder.
- Urethral factors. For neurological reasons, or in some instances without obvious cause, the urethra may fail to relax, as in detrusor-sphincter dys-synergia (see p. **00**). In neurologically normal patients it is difficult to know whether failure of urethral relaxation is the primary problem rather than an inability to initiate a detrusor contraction.
- "Psychological" factors. Many normal male patients are unable to void except when alone. Two patients spring to mind. The first was a man who could only void when locked in his toilet at home, having made sure that there was nobody else in the house. This man was impossible to investigate! The second man had sea fishing, as his hobby, which involved many hours at sea in an open boat. All his colleagues were able to micturate over the side of the boat, but he went into urinary retention, as he was too inhibited to "perform".

● Penile erection is an unusual but frustrating problem for some elderly men who, woken from their sleep, find that they have an erection due to a full bladder, and are then unable to void until the erection dies away.

Decreased Urinary Stream

Slow stream is reported by the individual as his or her perception of reduced urine flow, usually compared to previous performance or in comparison to others.

Question: "When you pass urine, does the flow come out in front of you in a good flow, or does it drop to your feet?" (Brian Peeling's diagram is a useful way for the patient to visualise this question (Fig. 4.8).)

Urine flow rate depends on the volume voided, and therefore the patient should be asked about the quantities he voids, although this information should have been available from the frequency-volume chart. In addition to the question already mentioned, the patient should be asked about the characteristics of the stream. For example, is it thin and forceful, as would be seen in a patient who had a meatal stenosis? A patient with meatal stenosis might also notice that during micturition the penis enlarges because the penile urethra becomes distended by urine.

Mechanisms of Decreased Urinary Stream. A reduced urine flow may be due to:

● Any cause that reduces the voided volume is usually associated with frequency.

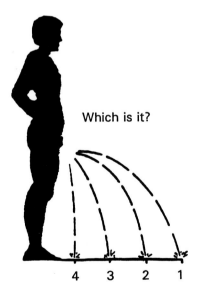

Which is it?

4   3   2   1

Fig. 4.8 Brian Peeling's figure to allow the patient to indicate his stream.

- Bladder outlet obstruction at any level from the bladder neck to the external meatus. Bladder outlet obstruction may be mechanical or functional. The commonest mechanical obstruction is benign prostatic enlargement and the functional obstructions that may be noted are dysfunctional voiding, detrusor sphincter dyssynergia and non-relaxing urethral sphincter obstruction.
- Decreased detrusor contractility, which may be either neurogenic or myopathic. Myopathic abnormalities may be any primary disturbance of bladder muscle, any toxic influence upon bladder muscle, or secondary to overstretching. There are a variety of neurogenic causes affecting both the upper and the lower motor neurones. Most classically, detrusor underactivity would be associated with lower motor neurone damage as, for example, after abdominal perineal resection of the rectum.

Intermittency

Intermittency is the term used when the individual describes urine flow, which stops and starts, on one or more occasions, during micturition.

Question: "Is your urine flow continuous or does it stop and start?"

Figure 3.20 shows intermittency, which has in common many of the same causes as a variable stream when the stream is of varying strength without actual interruption.

Mechanisms of Intermittency. An interrupted or variable flow may be due to:

- *Urethral overactivity.* Actual closure or narrowing of the urethra during voiding usually occurs at the level of the pelvic floor and is termed *dysfunctional voiding* in the neurologically intact and *detrusor sphincter dyssynergia* in those with a neurological disease such as multiple sclerosis.
- *Detrusor underactivity.* A poorly sustained, wave-like detrusor contraction produces a variable or interrupted trace. Similar patterns are produced if the patient has an acontractile detrusor and has to strain to pass urine.
- *Straining during voiding.*

Straining

Straining to void describes the muscular effort used to initiate, maintain, or improve the urinary stream.

Question: "Do you strain either to start your stream or to keep it going?"

Patients may strain through habit or necessity. If the bladder contains little urine it often helps to strain a little to initiate a detrusor contraction. Patients without outlet obstruction can increase their flow by straining, although men with BPO cannot. Patients with detrusor underactivity and/or urethral obstruction may rely on straining to achieve adequate bladder emptying.

Pain on Voiding

Question: "Does it hurt when you pass urine?"

The term dysuria can be confusing: some clinicians, particularly in Europe, use "dysuria" to mean difficulty in voiding. The term "dysuria" has also been used for the urethral pain typically felt in acute cystourethritis. It is better to describe the type and site of pain for example "burning urethral pain" usually indicative of urethritis, prostatitis or cystitis. Some patients with increased bladder sensation, without infection, for example, hyper-sensitive cases and those with the urethral pain syndrome, may also report bladder or urethral pain.

Terminal Dribble

Question: "Does your urine flow end quickly or do you have a dribble before you finish?"

If the patient says there is a dribble they should be asked how long it lasts. Terminal dribble, can be defined as a prolongation of the final part of micturition, when the flow slows to a trickle/dribble: this may last 30 s to 60 s or more. Terminal dribble is due to a failing detrusor contraction associated with bladder outlet obstruction and must be distinguished from post-micturition dribble.

Post-Micturition Symptoms

Post-Micturition Dribble

Question: "After you have passed urine, dressed and left the toilet, do you leak in the next few minutes?"

It is important to distinguish between terminal dribble and post-micturition dribble. Terminal dribble is continuous with the main flow of urine, whereas post-micturition dribble is defined as the involuntary loss of urine after the individual has finished passing urine, usually after leaving the toilet in men, or rising from the toilet in women. Post-micturition dribble is seldom associated with any demonstrable abnormality. This type of leakage is most commonly seen in men.

Mechanisms of Post-Micturition Dribble. This symptom may be due to:

- Failure of the bulbo-cavernosus and bulbo-spongiosus muscles to empty the penile urethra after micturition has ended.
- Failure of the normal "milk-back" mechanism whereby the urine lying between the distal urethral sphincter mechanism and the bladder neck, at the end of micturition, is returned to the bladder: leakage may occur later if the distal sphincter relaxes and the urine passes distally.

- In women, post-micturition dribble is due to urine being deflected by the external genitalia into the vagina, so that when the woman stands the urine drips from the vaginal lumen.

Feeling of Incomplete Emptying

> Question: "After you have passed your water, does the feeling of wanting to urinate go away, or do you feel that the bladder is still not empty."

The normal patient, after micturition, completely loses any awareness of the bladder. Persistence of symptoms is usually felt as incomplete emptying or sometimes as a continued desire to void. These symptoms may often be misleading, as the patient may be shown to have emptied the bladder completely.

Mechanisms of Sensation of Incomplete Emptying. The reasons include:

- Increased sensation, e.g. acute cystitis, interstitial cystitis, urethritis and prostatitis.
- Persistent detrusor contraction (after-contraction), in which the bladder contracts after it is empty, producing high post-micturition pressure. This phenomenon is not related to detrusor overactivity, and is not always felt, so that its significance is unknown. However on occasions it does give rise to a persistent desire to void or to a feeling of incomplete emptying after micturition.
- Residual urine; many patients are unaware of the fact that they fail to empty their bladder, but others do have a feeling of incomplete emptying in this situation.

Post-Micturition Bladder or Urethral Pain

Pain may also be felt after micturition, and this is often indicative of intravesical or intra-urethral pathology and is frequently an indication for further investigation.

Strangury. Strangury describes a very unpleasant powerful feeling low in the pelvis, penis or urethra after voiding. It is usually indicative of an intravesical pathology such as a bladder stone or acute cystitis.

Other Symptoms

Haematuria

In almost every instance this symptom is an indication for further urological investigation and should never be ignored. Investigation of haematuria will usually take precedence over the investigation of other lower urinary tract dysfunction.

Loin Pain

It is unusual for the complaint of loin pain to be directly related to lower urinary dysfunction, although it can be secondary to vesico-ureteric reflux, or have an infective origin (pyelonephritis), and these conditions may occur in association with lower urinary tract dysfunction. Similarly calculus obstruction of the lower end of the ureter may present with a combination of upper and lower urinary tract symptoms. In a patient with lower urinary tract symptoms, loin pain is an indication for further investigation, most frequently an intravenous pyelogram or ultrasound.

Urinary Infections

It is appropriate to note here that there is a need for accuracy in the diagnosis of urinary infection. The condition is often diagnosed from symptoms or an inadequately taken "midstream specimen of urine" (MSU). If there is need for a midstream specimen then it should be properly supervised. If there is any doubt about the validity of an MSU, then either a suprapubic aspiration or a catheter specimen of urine may be taken. A catheter specimen should be sent to the laboratory at the commencement of urodynamic investigations. Alternatively a "Stix" test for nitrites, leukocytes, protein and blood, has been shown to be an excellent and cost-effective alternative to the MSU.

Retention of Urine

The patient should be asked whether they have had any retention episodes. The most common causes of urinary retention are benign prostatic obstruction, pelvic surgery, childbirth, the commencement of drug therapy with agents having effects on the bladder or urethra (see Appendix 4), and acute neurological conditions such as prolapsed intervertebral disc. Hence a history of previous urinary retention should alert the clinician to the possibility of detrusor underactivity, asymptomatic bladder outlet obstruction or an underlying neurological cause.

Sexual History

Sexual function and lower urinary tract function are subserved by similar innervation and therefore sexual function should be discussed with most patients. Men should be asked whether erection is present or absent, whether ejaculation if present is forceful and clonic, or if emission is weak. In addition patients should be asked whether or not they have orgasm and questioned as to its character and acuity.

In the absence of previous surgical intervention, for example, surgery of the rectum, psychogenic factors are the most common cause of impotence. However these symptoms in the male patient may be due to demonstrable neurological disease, for example, after spinal cord injury or in multiple sclerosis. They may also be the first indication of a peripheral neuropathy, as in diabetes mellitus or alcoholism. Each of these pathological processes may also lead to lower urinary tract dysfunction.

Erection may occur as a reflex and is mediated by the sacral roots via the pelvic nerves, whereas a psychogenic erection requires intact cholinergic and sympathetic nerve fibres in the pelvic and hypogastric nerves. Ejaculation depends on the co-ordinated action of the striated musculature of the pelvic floor which is innervated by the pudendal nerves. Orgasmic sensation is a combined afferent bombardment through the sympathetic hypogastric and somatic pudendal nerves.

A sexual history should also be taken from female patients asking about orgasm and any associated urine symptoms such as incontinence.

Bowel Function

Bowel function is similarly closely related to lower urinary tract function, and patients should be asked about their frequency of bowel action as well as the mechanics of defecation, that is, do they relax or do they need to strain, or is it essential that they use some artificial means such as manual evacuation, suppositories or enemas to empty their bowel. They should also be asked about their control of bowel function, that is, whether or not they ever soil or have an accident. Faecal incontinence may be passive (equivalent to stress urinary incontinence) or related to urgency (equivalent to urgency urinary incontinence), and patients may be incontinent with respect to gas, loose faeces or solid faeces. In patients both with and without neurological disease, correction of bowel problems may produce a significant improvement in lower urinary tract symptoms.

Medical History

Obstetric History

The incidence of stress incontinence increases with the number of pregnancies and the difficulties of parturition. Electromyography has shown evidence of pelvic floor denervation that is associated with stress incontinence. This denervation is worsened by factors which affect the pelvic floor: the number of pregnancies, the length of labour, the size of the baby, any episiotomies or tears and the use of forceps during delivery. The use of post-partum exercises designed to improve pelvic floor tone may help to prevent stress incontinence.

Gynaecological History

The relationship between the lower urinary tract and the hormonal status of the woman is often significant; for example, patients with urodynamic stress incontinence frequently report that their symptoms are worse in the week before their period begins: this is probably due to increased progesterone levels and relative tissue laxity. Therefore it is important to inquire about not only the patient's menstrual cycle but also her menopausal status. Operations on the uterus may interfere with the innervation of the bladder or may lead to distortion of the lower urinary tract. Denervation, more properly termed decentralisation, is most likely after radical hysterectomy for neoplasia, and may act at both the bladder and urethral levels. Any history of vaginal or suprapubic procedures for prolapse or incontinence may be relevant, because such procedures can produce urethral or bladder neck distortion, scarring or narrowing.

Urological History

The significance of urological symptoms has already been discussed. The patient should be asked about his or her previous urological operations, as such operations have their complications, of which recurrent or persistent obstruction and sphincter damage after prostatectomy are the most common.

Surgical History

The operations most relevant to lower urinary tract function are those on the lower large bowel, where dissection at the side wall of the pelvis may result in nerve damage, especially during abdominal-perineal resection of the rectum.

Trauma History

Trauma to the urethra resulting in stricture formation and obstruction, or trauma to the spinal cord leading to an upper or lower motor neurone lesion, are the accidents most relevant to the lower urinary tract. Trauma to the urethra may be severe and obvious, as in a fractured pelvis with disruption of the pubic symphysis, but problems may follow an apparently trivial perineal injury from which the patient appears to recover in minutes or hours, only to develop a urethral stricture years later.

Other Significant Conditions

Systemic disease processes which influence the lower urinary tract may do so by affecting the innervation. Diabetes mellitus and multiple sclerosis are two such common conditions. Infections such as tuberculosis and schistosomiasis must be remembered. Degenerative disease of the cervical and lumbar spine, spinal tumours and many cerebral conditions may also present as incontinence. Pelvic radiotherapy may produce a post-irradiation cystitis with limitation of the bladder capacity, together with increased frequency and sometimes bladder pain. Mucosal telangectasia following radiotherapy may occasionally cause haematuria.

Drug Therapy

Enquiries should be made as to any drugs the patient is or has been taking, and whether these drugs have any effect on bladder function or produce side-effects. Drugs may be taken intentionally to modify urinary function, or urinary symptoms may be a side effect of a drug taken for another purpose. All drugs with enhancement or blocking effects on cholinergic, alpha-adrenergic or beta-adrenergic receptors and all drugs with calcium channel effects have a potential effect on lower urinary tract function. Most of these drugs are listed in Appendix 4.

Drugs Enhancing Bladder Emptying

Bladder emptying may be improved by giving drugs either to increase contractility or to decrease bladder outlet resistance. In theory, cholinergic drugs increase detrusor contractility and may produce frequency, whilst alpha-adrenergic blockers decrease outlet resistance, and may precipitate or exaggerate stress incontinence. Whilst alpha-blockers are thought to be effective, most clinicians have little faith in cholinergic medication designed to improve detrusor contractility.

Drugs Enhancing Bladder Storage

Bladder storage may be improved by increasing functional bladder capacity or by increasing bladder outlet resistance.

Antimuscarinic drugs, in patients with detrusor overactivity help to achieve continence and increase bladder capacity. Whilst antimuscarinic drugs are felt to be helpful in patients with detrusor overactivity during storage, their effectiveness is limited by side-effects: it is ironic that the most troublesome of these is dry mouth, which encourages the patient to drink more! Alpha-adrenergic stimulating drugs are used to increase bladder outlet resistance, although they have only a marginal effect.

Other Drugs

Other drugs of significance include *diuretics*, which increase urinary frequency in a variable way. The action of diuretics varies in accordance with the patient's age in particular, and the onset of the resulting increased urine output may also vary according to the gastrointestinal absorptive function. *Anti-depressants*, such as the tricyclic drugs, of which amityptyline is an example, often have effects on lower urinary tract function: these drugs have anti-cholinergic actions which tend to increase storage and decrease voiding efficiency. *Oestrogen* therapy may improve lower urinary tract symptoms, decreasing urinary frequency and improving the symptoms of urethral pain/discomfort and urgency.

Full discussion of the actions of drugs on the lower urinary tract is beyond the scope of this book. Some further information is provided in the chapter on anatomy and physiology, or the reader is referred to the excellent chapter edited by, Karl-Eric Andersson in the books from the International Consultations on Incontinence, and the writings of Alan Wein. It is suggested that if the patient is on a drug prescribed to them to influence lower urinary tract function, or on a drug with urinary side-effects, then the investigator should interpret the urodynamic findings in the light of the known drug effects. In certain circumstances the clinician may prefer to withdraw the relevant drug two weeks before urodynamic testing, or before completion of a frequency-volume chart.

General Patient Assessment

Whilst discussing the presenting symptoms with the patient, the clinician will have made a subjective assessment of the patient. It is clear that there is a considerable interaction between the patient's personality and mood on the one hand, and the urinary symptoms on the other. It is a common experience that anxiety leads to urinary frequency and even urgency. Such factors as age, degree of stoicism, degree of neuroticism and mood should be assessed. Some patients are extremely tolerant of symptoms that other patients would refuse to accept, and the presence of nocturia is a good example. Whilst the factors mentioned above cannot be quantified easily, they remain important when the clinician comes to interpret the patient's symptoms and urodynamic findings, particularly with respect to proposals for treatment. It will be necessary occasionally to seek a psychiatric or psychological opinion where the clinician is uneasy about the patient's mental state, but cannot define the abnormality in its relation to urinary symptoms.

In addition to the mental state, the mobility and dexterity of patients can have a profound influence on management. Are they well motivated? Could they manage a urinary appliance? Would they be continent if more mobile and able to reach a toilet? Will they co-operate with follow-up or take drugs reliably? Often the fact that these aspects of assessment are overlooked prevents the subsequent urodynamic diagnosis and efforts at management from achieving the optimal result. The reader is referred to the Scientific Committee report from the 3rd International Consultation on Incontinence (2005) for further details.

Physical Examination

It is assumed that a general examination of the patient has been undertaken already. This section will discuss only aspects of examination that are of special relevance to the lower urinary tract.

Abdominal Examination

It is appropriate that the lower abdomen should be palpated and percussed in an attempt to demonstrate the bladder. In an adult, only a bladder containing in excess of 300 ml is likely to be palpable or can be percussed above the pubic symphysis. Even though a patient is in urinary retention the bladder may be difficult to palpate, although it should be demonstrated readily by percussion. Other enlarged bladders reveal a clearly palpable outline. The poorly defined ("floppy") bladder is associated with lower intravesical pressures and normal upper tracts, whilst the firm and tense bladder is often associated with high intravesical pressures and upper tract dilatation. In most cases seen in the urodynamic laboratory the patient is unaware of their bladder distension. However, pressing on the suprapubic region, and asking if the patient feels a need to void, if positive, is a good indication of a full or enlarged bladder. Suprapubic examination also reveals the degree of sensitivity of the bladder in some cases where bladder pain is a symptom. The degree of obesity of the patient should be noted.

Examination of the External Genitalia

In the female, abnormalities such as meatal stenosis or fusion of the labia are found occasionally. In male patients, phimosis should be excluded, and the fore-skin retracted to reveal the external meatus which should be examined carefully for stenosis. The urethra should be felt for fibrous thickening, which may indicate inflammation or stricture in either sex.

Vaginal Examination

Initially the introitus should be viewed with the patient lying on her back with the legs flexed and abducted.

- Part the labia and inspect the introitus: the position and appearance of the meatus should be noted. The clinician should look to see whether there is evidence of wetness at the introitus, whether the introital mucosa is well oestrogenised, showing a pink, moist and healthy appearance or whether there are signs of oestrogen deficiency when the mucosa appears thin, red and atrophic. If the mucosa is red and there is an offensive discharge it is likely that the patient is suffering an infective vaginitis. The patient should be asked to contract her pelvic floor (as if "holding on") and the perineum should be seen to lift.
- Test for urine leaking by firstly asking the patient to cough repeatedly and secondly by asking the patient to bear down (strain), observing the meatus for urine leakage.
- Assess prolapse: prolapse can be divided into three categories: I, where the prolapse does not reach the introitus; II, where the prolapse reaches the introitus; III, where the prolapse is through the introitus. The presence and degree of anterior vaginal wall descent and posterior vaginal wall descent should be assessed. Uterine descent and/or enterocele will often be missed in this position.
- Assess vaginal capacity and mobility. This has particular significance in choosing the type of surgery in patients with urodynamic stress incontinence. In order to perform a repositioning procedure (e.g., a colposuspension), it is necessary to evaluate the vagina on both sides of the urethra, and place it in contact with the back of the symphysis pubis. The Bonney test, whereby a finger is put either side of the bladder neck, will successfully assess vaginal mobility, but should not be relied on as a test of continence as the elevating fingers may well compress the bladder neck and urethra.

The woman should now be asked to turn onto the left lateral position and examined using the Sim's speculum to systematically assess the three possible elements of prolapse: (anterior, posterior and middle compartments). Detailed measurements should be made in research studies and prior to prolapse surgery, to be repeated after operation. The details of the methodology can be found in Appendix 1, Part 2.

- Use a Sim's speculum to retract the posterior vaginal wall, and assess the resting position of the bladder neck/bladder base and the degree of descent of the anterior vaginal wall on straining. It may be easier to demonstrate incontinence on coughing in this position. Any vaginal scarring should be noted.
- Assess posterior vaginal wall by using the Sim's speculum to retract the anterior vaginal wall (the second blade of the speculum passes over the anterior abdominal wall).

- Assessment of uterine descent or vault prolapse (after hysterectomy) can be achieved by retracting both anterior and posterior vaginal wall either using the Sim's speculum plus a long forceps or by using Cuscow's speculum. Cuscow's speculum cannot be used to assess anterior or posterior vaginal wall prolapse.
- The vaginal examination is an excellent opportunity to assess the voluntary contractile ability of the patient's perivaginal muscles. These muscles are part of the pelvic floor and the ability to contract them forms the basis of the pelvic floor exercises. The left and right pelvic floor muscles should be palpated in the lateral vaginal walls and their strength assessed (Oxford scale).

Rectal Examination

Rectal examination should also be systematic.

- *Inspection.* Does the anus appear normal? If a hand is placed on the perineal skin either side of the anus and lateral traction exerted then in patients with poor anal function the anus will begin to open.
- *Perineal sensation.* Because the dermatones S_2, S_3 and S_4 serve the perianal and perineal region, intact sensation is likely to mean that the innervation of the bladder and urethra, and indeed the rectum and anal canal is intact.
- *Anal reflex.* If the perineal skin is scratched the anus should "wink" at the investigator. This is best seen in patients with upper motor neurone lesions, for example, high spinal cord injury.
- *Anal tone.* As the examining finger passes into the anal canal the tone of the anal sphincter can be assessed. In lesions such as meningomyelocele anal tone may initially appear good, but after removal of the examining finger the anus may remain open.
- *Voluntary squeeze.* Patients should be able to increase anal sphincter pressure by voluntarily contracting the levator ani. If a woman has been unable to contract the perivaginal muscles during vaginal examination then the rectal examination may provide more stimulation, allowing her to appreciate which muscles need to be exercised as part of pelvic floor rehabilitation.
- *Faecal impaction.* If the rectum is impacted the subsequent urodynamics will be affected both because of the difficulty of inserting and monitoring the position of a rectal catheter but also because rectal distension inhibits detrusor contraction.
- *Prostate evaluation.* In men the prostate gland should be assessed for size, shape, consistency and abnormal tenderness.

Neurological Examination

All patients must have a simple neurological examination, including a gross assessment of sensation, reflexes and muscle function in the legs. In particular, special attention should be paid to the sensory sacral dermatomes, the motor divisions of which supply the bladder (S_2 S_3 S_4). In patients found to have, or known to have, neurological abnormalities, a full neurological examination should be performed. In injuries to the spinal cord, the level of the lesion and whether or not the lesion is complete should be documented.

Certain reflex responses are described in the assessment of sacral function. The anal reflexes are listed by pricking the perianal skin and watching to see if the anal sphincter contracts reflexly. This is quite easy to do at the time of rectal examination. The second reflex is the bulbo-cavernosus reflex, and this involves digital squeezing of the glans penis (or clitoris) and the observation of contraction in the anal sphincter or bulbo-cavernosus muscle. In the neurologically intact patient this procedure may provoke a certain amount of discontent and perhaps encourage them to be less co-operative. In any case a positive response is present only in 70% of normal people. If the reflex is considered to be important then it should be demonstrated electrophysiologically.

As a result of neurological examination the patients can be crudely grouped into four:

- Normal.
- Lower motor neurone: with decreased muscle tone, decreased power, decreased reflexes and absent sensation. This picture occurs in low spinal cord injury patients, affecting the conus medullaris.
- Upper motor neurone: upgoing Babinsky responses, increased muscle tone, increased reflexes, muscle spasms and absent sensation. This is typically seen in a high spinal cord injury patient
- Mixed: lower motor neurone and upper motor neurone such as in spina bifida.

Investigations

Urinalysis

A catheter specimen of urine should be obtained at each urodynamic investigation. If the urine is obviously infected then urodynamics should not be performed because of the risk of provoking bacteria or septicaemia. It is sensible, in patients who have a past history of infection, to cover the urodynamic investigations by antibiotics. If investigation is essential in a patient who has an infection and has not been treated, then an adequate dose of the correct antibiotic should be given intravenously in order to ensure an adequate blood level at the time of investigation. The urine specimen should be routinely tested. We now routinely use "Stix" testing to detect leucocytes, nitrites, blood and protein. If "Stix" testing is abnormal, the urine should be sent for microscopy and culture.

Cytology

Cytological studies of urine, vagina or cervix may be indicated. Patients with widespread *in situ* bladder carcinoma, which carries a poor prognosis, may present with the symptoms of cystitis or bladder hypersensitivity. In these patients the urine specimen often shows white cells or red cells, and urine for cytology is likely to show malignant cells. In female patients with lower urinary tract symptoms the hormonal status of the patient may be assessed by lateral vaginal wall cytological smear. It has been shown that the urinary symptoms of patients whose vaginal cells show oestrogen deficiency often improve with oestrogen therapy.

Radiology

Non-contrast Radiology

A plain X-ray of the abdomen and pelvis can be useful. The X-ray should be critically examined to look at soft tissue abnormalities such as an enlarged bladder, bony abnormalities such as spondylosis, spina bifida or metastasis, and for opacities such as bladder or ureteric stones. In patients with straightforward LUTS, X-ray is very unlikely to show any abnormality.

Intravenous Urography

Traditionally many patients with lower urinary tract symptoms had an intravenous urogram (IVU) performed, but there is no evidence to show that in patients with lower urinary tract symptoms the IVU gives any useful information. This is because static films give very little idea of function: bladder shape may alter during contraction and diverticula may appear; the evaluation of residual urine is also notoriously inaccurate. Equally the absence of residual urine or of a basal prostatic filling defect does not exclude significant bladder outlet obstruction.

An IVU and/or ultrasound is indicated however, if the patient has blood in the urine or an abnormal plain x-ray. Similarly if the patient reports haematuria or has localised upper tract symptoms imaging is essential. It should also be carried out in patients who have undiagnosed continuous incontinence, as it may reveal a duplex kidney, suggesting an ectopic ureter. In patients with a proteus urinary tract infection, imaging may show an infected "matrix" renal calculus which can be difficult to see on a plain film.

Micturating Cystourethrography

The conventional micturating cystourethrogram (MCUG) consists of visualisation by a radiologist of abnormally fast filling, followed by emptying of the bladder: a number of spot films are taken at appropriate (or inappropriate) occasions. However, this can be a valuable assessment of lower urinary tract structure, because changes may be seen during the micturition cycle. It is appropriate to make the most of the investigation and to provide the maximum amount of clinical information to the radiologist. In order to do this the whole investigation should be recorded on videotape. The MCUG is a "second best" investigation to videourodynamics. However if videourodynamics is not available then MCUG should be performed (see "Videourodynamics" in Chapter 3).

Endoscopy

Endoscopy is not indicated in the assessment of lower urinary tract functions unless there are specific symptoms or signs. Endoscopy is indicated if the patient complains of bladder pain or haematuria or if there is an abnormal MSU or abnormal radiology. Occasionally clinical "desperation" may be an indication for endoscopy.

Endoscopy should always consist of urethroscopy followed by cystoscopy. It is particularly important that urethral inspection is not omitted, as it may give information as to the site of obstruction in patients with obstructed voiding. However, if the obstruction is functional rather than structural, for example, detrusor-bladder-neck dyssynergia or detrusor-sphincter dyssynergia, then the site of obstruction will not be demonstrated by endoscopy. Bladder neck and/or bladder wall hypertrophy does not indicate obstruction, nor does trabeculation of the bladder: these features are more strongly associated with detrusor overactivity. If urethroscopy is normal and the urodynamic assessment has shown obstructed voiding, videourodynamics is the investigation of choice to determine the site of obstruction. The correlation between endoscopy and urodynamic findings is discussed Chapter 5 under "Urodynamics in Men".

Ultrasound

Considerable progress has been made in the level of sophistication in ultrasound technology. In assessing patients with lower urinary tract problems, ultrasound can be used in several ways:

- As basic screening test in place of the plain abdominal X-ray.
- To assess bladder emptying. Simple hand-held machines are now available which can be used during urodynamics, in the outpatient clinic, on the ward and even in the patient's home (Fig. 3.24).
- To exclude upper tract problems. It is useful to be able to scan the kidneys as in some situations vesico-urethral dysfunction can result in upper tract dilatation (see "Neuropathic Bladders" in Chapter 5). However renal ultrasound is probably best left to the radiologists.
- Vaginal ultrasound. Ultrasound can be used as an alternative to X-rays in videourodynamics (see Chapter 3). A vector scanner placed at the introitus is preferred as an intravaginal probe may distort lower urinary tract anatomy.
- Rectal ultrasound: this can be used to visualise the prostate in men, and the lower urinary tract in both men and women.

References

Abrams P, Klevmark B (1996). Frequency volume charts: An indispensable part of lower urinary tract assessment. Scand J Urol Nephrol 30 suppl 179.

Bailey R, Shepherd A, Tribe B (1990). How much information can be obtained from frequency/volume charts? Neurourol Urodyn 9:382–385 (abst).

Caine M (1984). The pharmacoloogy of the urinary tract. London: Springer-Verlag.

Carter P (1992). The role of nocturnal polyuria in nocturnal urinary symptoms in the healthy elderly male. MD Thesis University of Bristol.

Donovan JL, Abrams P, Peters TJ, Kay HE, Reynard J, Chapple C, de la Rosette JJMCH, Kondon A (1996). The ICS-'BPH' study: the psychometric validity and reliability of the ICS male questionnaire. Br J Urol 77:554–562.

Jackson S, Donovan J, Brookes S, Eckford S, Swithinbank L, Abrams P (1996). The Bristol female lower urinary tract symptoms questionnaire: development and psychometric testing. Br J Urol 77:805–812.

Klevmark B (1989). Objective assessment of urinary incontinence. The use of pad-weighing and frequency-volume charts. Dan Med Bull Special Supplement Series 8:28–30.

Larsson G, Victor A (1988). Micturition patterns in a healthy female population, studied with a frequency-volume chart. Scand J Urol Nephrol supp. 4:53–57.

Larsson G, Abrams P, Victor A (1991). The frequency/volume chart in detrusor instability. Neurourol Urodyn 10:533–543.

Larsson G, Victor A (1992). The frequency/volume chart in genuine stress incontinent women. Neurourol Urodyn 11:23–31.

Nørgaard JP (1991). Pathophysiology of nocturnal enuresis. Scand J Urol Nephrol suppl. 140.

Reynard JM, Lim C, Peters TJ, Abrams P (1996). The significant of terminal dribbling in men with lower urinary tract symptoms. Br J Urol 77:701–710.

Reynard JM, Peters TJ, Lamond E, Abrams P (1995). The significance of abdominal straining in men with lower urinary tract symptoms. Br J Urol 75:148–153.

Robinson D, McClish DK, Wyman JF, Bump RC, Fantl JA (1996). Comparison between urinary diaries completed with an without intensive patient instructions. Neurourol Urodyn 15:143–148.

Swthinbank L, Abrams P (2001). Lower urinary tract symptoms in community-dwelling women: defining diurnal and nocturnal frequence and the "incontinence case". Br J Urol 88(Suppl2):49–50.

The Third Edition of Incontinence (2005). Eds. Abrams P, Cardozo L, Khoury S, Wein A. Health Publications Ltd. Editions 21-76, rue de la Pompe, 75116 Paris (+33 1 45 03 31 96; FAX: +33 1 45 72 89; e-mail: progress.urologie @wanadoo-fr. Also available through www. amazon.com.

Torrens MJ (1974). The effect of selective sacral nerve blocks on vesical and urethral function. J Urol 112:204–205.

Turner Warwick R, Milroy E (1979). A reappraisal of the value of routine urological procedures in the assessment of urodynamic function. Urol Clin N Am 6:63–70.

Van Kerrebroeck P, Abrams P, Chaikin D, et al. (2002). The standardization of terminology in nocturia: report from the standardization subcommittee of the International Continence Society. Br J Urol 88(Suppl 3):11–15.

Chapter 5
Urodynamics in Clinical Practice

Introduction

The principles of urodynamics having been discussed and the reader provided with a proper understanding of urodynamic techniques, it is important to place urodynamic studies in a proper clinical context. The purpose of this chapter is to show the clinician the four main ways in which urodynamic tests can improve diagnosis and treatment.

- The investigations may assist in the evaluation of an individual case, providing objective evidence on which to base decisions.
- The analysis of groups of patients may, over a time, improve both the understanding of pathophysiology and the selection of patients for treatment.
- Urodynamics may provide objective information before and after therapeutic intervention, allowing the clinician to monitor the results of treatment more accurately.
- The tests assist the continuing education of clinicians themselves.

As clinicians become more experienced in the urodynamic investigation of patients, their confidence in their diagnostic ability as to the significance of symptomatic complaints increases. This increase in confidence is only partially justified. We shall refer to the study in which the diagnostic ability of the urodynamic investigations was tested. The computer proforma (Appendix 3 Part 1) contains a question that is asked of the investigator at the end of the symptomatic enquiry, (i.e., they are asked to predict the urodynamic findings from the symptomatic complaints). Even for the experienced investigator the results are salutary!

The urodynamic diagnosis is used by us as the "arbiter of truth". This statement assumes that the explanation for the patient's symptomatic complaints will unfold as the urodynamic investigations proceed. If the symptomatic history and the urodynamic investigations are at variance then the studies should be repeated or extended.

In 1995 we investigated 3578 patients in our unit. By far the most common investigation was urine flow studies with the ultrasound estimation of residual urine. Table 5.1 shows the

Table 5.1. 1995 urodynamic workload (children are defined as = 16 years old)

	Children	Female	Male	Total
Ambulatory UDS	1	79	3	83
Pad test	0	61	0	61
Routine UDS	5	809	418	1232
Uroflowmetry	27	133	1589	1749
Video UDS	48	190	175	413
Total	81	1312	2185	3578

proportions of children, men and women investigated and the investigations these patients had. The median age of women investigated was 52 years and that of men 66 years.

Urodynamics in Children

Three main groups of children are considered for urodynamic studies (UDS):

- Children with neurological disease and possible vesicourethral dysfunction.
- Children with lower urinary tract symptoms and/or dysfunction.
- Children with non-neurological congenital abnormalities and possible vesicourethral dysfunction.

Children with Neurological Disorders

These are most commonly related to dysgenesis of the spine and the associated nervous system. The neurological deficit is frequently more complicated than that in acquired neurological problems, and this makes the interpretation of bladder dysfunction more difficult.

The largest group of children with neuropathic bladders are those with myelodysplasia. It is important to recognise that the level of the neurological lesion does not correlate with the functional classification of the bladder. This is true in many types of neurological disease, but is particularly evident in these children, most of whom have spina bifida in addition to their neurological lesion. The role of urodynamics is to make the crucial functional distinctions between a high-pressure bladder (unsafe) and a low-pressure one (safe), the former being associated with the worse prognosis. Blaivas et al. (1977) emphasised that there was no statistical correlation between the pressure generated in the bladder and the level of the neurological lesion. They noted that detrusor-urethral dyssynergia can occur in both "high-" and "low-pressure" bladders. The timing of UDS in these children is much debated. McGuire has been the protagonist for early UDS, within the first few months of life. Using leak point pressure measurements he advocates the early use of clean intermittent catheterisation to prevent upper tract drainage being compromised. It had our habit to investigate these children later when continence would normally be expected to develop, at around 5 years of age. However, we now perform VUDS in the first year of life. Figure 5.1 describes our protocol.

VUDS will have to be repeated if an interventional therapy such as ileocystoplasty or artificial sphincter implantation is planned. VUDS are used in these children in view of the relatively high incidence of abnormalities such as vesicoureteric reflux and sphincteric obstruction during voiding.

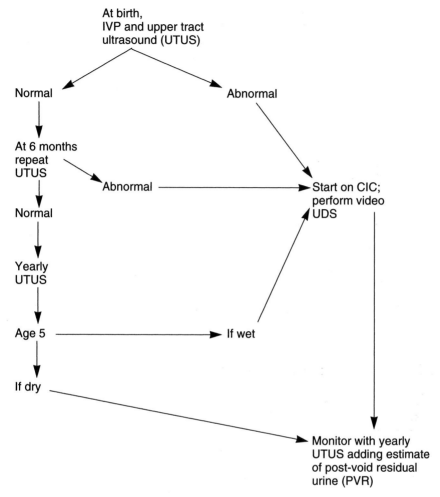

Fig. 5.1 Algorhythm for the investigation of children with neuropathic vesico-urethral dysfunction based on upper tract ultrasound (UTUS) and the use of clean intermittent catheterisation (CIC). 📖

With the reducing incidence of meningomyelocele births many born now have minimal defects and develop normal bladder and bowel function. The principles of management of these children are similar to that of the adult neuropathic patient and are discussed later.

Children Born with Non-Neurological Defects

There are two main groups in this category:

● *Urethral valves.* Boys born with urethral valves have often been diagnosed prenatally and are treated very early in life. However there are often long-term sequelae to valves, with poor bladder compliance and upper tract dilatation. These boys need to be followed in a similar fashion to the meningomyelocele children with early urodynamics if there is upper tract dilatation.

- *Ano-rectal abnormalities.* The frequency of voiding dysfunction in these children depends on the extent of the abnormality and the presence of associated sacral bony defects: the higher the lesion the more likely the child is to have disturbed voiding due to an associated neurological deficit. Urodynamic studies before and after pelvic surgery, aimed at restoring bowel continuity to the anus, give useful information, although it is unclear whether or not UDS are essential in management or whether the "watch and wait" policy outlined above is adequate.

Normal Children with Vesico-Urethral Dysfunction

These children have no physical abnormality and fall into several main groups, but present chiefly with enuresis and daytime incontinence or recurrent urinary infections. On urodynamic investigation the main abnormalities found in children are detrusor overactivity, dysfunctional voiding and vesico-ureteric reflux, and these may occur alone or in combination.

- *Detrusor overactivity.* The toddler's bladder goes from the reflex organ of the infant to the adult bladder by the age of five in most individuals. Between, there is a stage at which children have partial control over bladder activity. All those who have brought up children are familiar with the techniques children use to control involuntary detrusor contractions: boys pinch the end of their penis, and girls squat, pushing the heel into the perineum. In performing these manoeuvres both boys and girls are probably using the bulbo-cavernosus reflex to inhibit an unwanted contraction. In this period toddlers often make mistakes whilst playing a favourite game, delaying too long and wetting themselves. However by the age of 5, 90% of children are reliably dry, day and night, although the remaining 10% continue to have problems. Parents and some children understandably become distressed by continued poor bladder control with the wet beds and embarrassing daytime incidents that result. There is considerable pressure on the health care professionals to "do something". However we know that 90% of those wet at 5 will become dry by adulthood and therefore resist the pressure for any interventional treatments.

  *Enuresis may or may not be associated with detrusor overactivity and it has to be remembered that enuresis is a phenomenon with a number of possible causes in addition to detrusor overactivity: low bladder capacity, reduced bladder sensation, failure of arousal from sleep and overproduction of urine at night are the most important. For those readers interested in this topic, the work of the Aarhus group in Denmark has been most important. They have shown that a proportion of children have deficient production of antidiuretic hormone at night and therefore fail to concentrate their night-time urine and produce higher volumes. Such children are better treated by synthetic antidiuretic hormone (DDAVP) than by an antimuscarinic drug.

  Management involves a presumptive diagnosis followed by empiric treatment, although in our view children should be screened by urine flow studies (UFS) and ultrasound estimates of residual urine, as UFS show that a small proportion of enuretic children exhibit disordered voiding, that is, dysfunctional voiding.

- *Dysfunctional voiding.* This term is reserved for those children unable to micturate with a continuous flow because of pelvic floor overactivity during voiding. The cause of the overactivity is not understood, although such children may also have bowel problems (chronic constipation) and often exhibit behavioural difficulties. The pelvic floor overactivity produces an interrupted flow pattern that looks very similar to detrusor-sphincter dyssynergia. As far as we know dysfunctional voiding is not seen commonly in asymptomatic children. An effect of stream interruption is to lead to detrusor inhibition before the bladder is emptied, resulting in an increasing residual urine. Voiding occurs against a partially closed sphincter, and that may be the reason that most children have detrusor overactivity during filling. This combination may produce detrusor hypertrophy, resulting in reduced bladder compliance with upper tract dilatation as well as incontinence, enuresis, infections and vesicoureteric reflux.

This condition was first described by Himan in 1956 and later by Allen in 1977. They used the term "non-neurogenic neurogenic bladder", which is confusing in many senses – the term "dysfunctional voiding" is to be preferred.

- *Children with vesico-ureteric reflux (VUR)*. VUR is likely to be discovered after a child has presented with urinary tract infection often complicated by secondary enuresis. If screening studies, flow rates and ultrasound estimates of residual urine, together with upper tract ultrasound, are normal then urodynamics is not indicated. If reflux and upper tract dilatation coexists then urodynamics is indicated. However the interpretation of bladder compliance in the presence of gross reflux, or indeed a diverticulum, is very difficult because the refluxing ureter and kidney increase bladder compliance. In such children any change in compliance should be regarded as dangerous to the upper tract and renal function.

Modifications of Urodynamic Technique in Children

In children there may be specific problems in using conventional techniques for two main reasons, namely the small size of the child or lack of co-operation from the child.

The small size of children requires obvious alteration in techniques such as reducing the speed of bladder filling: Nijman recommends that the bladder should be filled at 10% of the expected bladder volume per minute. Expected bladder volume can be calculated by the formula 30 ml + (30 ml times age), giving a 3-year-old a capacity of 120 ml (i.e. 30 + (3 × 30)). In children with compromised neurology resulting in reduced urethral sensation, or who have been taught to do clean intermittent catheterisation, a urethral catheter can be used for pressure measurement and the 6 Fr dual-channel catheter works well. The combination of an epidural catheter for pressure recording and a 6 Fr catheter for filling can be used although the dual channel catheter is preferred because it facilitates doing two full-void cycles. It is wise to record two fill and void sequences in children, as recommended by Griffiths and Scholtmeyer, because this allows the child to become used to the strange environment of the urodynamic room: a more relaxed micturition is often seen on the second void.

If the child is likely to be upset by urethral catheterisation, and this will apply to most neurologically normal small children not doing intermittent self-catheterisation (ISC), there are two choices: perform urodynamics under sedation, or prior to urodynamics put in suprapubic catheters under anaesthetic. Urodynamics works well for infants and toddlers under one year. They are admitted to the paediatric ward, where they receive an appropriate dose of a sedative such as Vallergan. The baby comes with its mother to the laboratory and can be breast-fed, given a bottle or given a dummy or comforter if they cry. In older children sedation is not so satisfactory and the child becomes very difficult to pacify if roused;

we would prefer to use suprapubic catheters (two epidural catheters, one for filling and one for the measurement of p_{ves}, or a single dual-channel 6 Fr catheter). The suprapubic route allows the fill-and-void cycle to be repeated.

Passage of the rectal catheter for p_{abd} measurement can be a problem in children who are fearful of rectal examination. Most children over 5 can be calmed, provided the atmosphere is relaxed and the child is not pressurised. We once advocated the exclusion of parents from the urodynamic room, but this is now socially unacceptable and even the parent who adds to the child's anxiety has to be accepted. Our urodynamic laboratory has a plentiful supply of children's books and videos which have proved an excellent distraction: the child is invited to bring their favourite video.

Who Should Do Paediatric Urodynamics?

Paediatric UDS should only be performed in centres with an active urodynamic unit with staff expert in dealing with children and where there is active collaboration with the paediatricians and paediatric urologist (see Chapter 7).

Indications for Urodynamic Investigation in Children

Because these studies are often upsetting for children we only use UDS if:

● The results will affect management.
● Empirical treatment has failed and invasive therapy is contemplated requiring confirmation of the presumptive diagnosis.
● Screening tests have been shown to be abnormal.

We are still asked to do urodynamics in children with enuresis who have failed to respond to bladder training, enuretic alarm and anticholinergics. We refuse, but offer to do screening flow studies and offer to become involved in their management as their medical therapy may not have been aggressive enough. Only if invasive therapy such as ileocystoplasty is being contemplated would we agree to do full urodynamics in the non-neurogenic child.

Urodynamics in Women

UDS in women should be set in a therapeutic context. Incontinence in women forms a large part of the workload of any urodynamics unit; two-thirds of the women referred to the Bristol unit fall into this category. Stress incontinence is almost entirely a female problem which may occur alone or be associated, to a variable extent, with urgency. Leakage associated only with urgency (urgency incontinence) is also a common problem. The overactive bladder symptom complex allows an index of suspicion about the nature of the functional disorder, but it is not entirely reliable. One of the principal roles for urodynamics is the identification of the main cause of incontinence, detrusor or urethral, in any particular case.

Table 5.2 shows the distribution of the different types of incontinence among patients referred to our unit; 64% complain of either stress or urgency incontinence. The reason why

Table 5.2. Different types of female incontinence categorised by symptoms

Incontinence (types)	%
None	22.3
Stress	19.0
Stress/urge	25.1
Urge	14.4
Urge/enuresis	5.1
Enuresis	2.9
Post-micturition dribble	0.8
Continuous	6.4
Other	4.0

Table 5.3. Percentage of female patients presenting with incontinence according to age

Age	Stress	Stress/Urge	Urge
20–30	14%	15%	15%
40–50	30%	34%	16%
60–70	12%	32%	20%

female incontinence is more frequent, and more troublesome, than in males is that the predisposing factors work together to compound the problem. While there is a natural tendency for the bladder to become overactive with advancing age, there is also a tendency for the urethra to become less competent in women. The pattern of presentation therefore varies with age (Table 5.3) and the overall prevalence increases with age.

As incontinence occurs with a high prevalence in the community, it is unrealistic and indeed unnecessary for all women to have urodynamic studies to confirm a diagnosis. Treatment should begin in the community and only if this is unsatisfactory or fails should urodynamic referral be made (see Chapter 6). Management is detailed in the algorithms produced by the International Consultations on Incontinence.

Symptom Presentation in Women

There are several common types of presentation:

- Stress incontinence
- Overactive bladder symptoms
- Frequency
- Mixed urge and stress incontinence
- Urinary infections

Urodynamics has a role in further defining the underlying vesico-urethral disorders when empirical treatment has failed.

Stress Urinary Incontinence

In the first edition of this book we stated that if the patient had pure stress incontinence then UDS were not indicated. Our attitudes have changed some-what and there are several advantages to performing UDS on all women before invasive surgery:

- Confirmation of incontinence and its cause.
- Definition of detrusor activity during filling.
- Assessment of detrusor voiding function.
- Assessment of degree of sphincter weakness.
- Assessment of pelvic floor function.

Both the confirmation of incontinence and the definition of its cause is highly desirable. Twelve percent of women with apparently pure stress incontinence can be shown to have detrusor overactivity rather than USI as the cause of their symptoms. Very careful physical examination is a reputable way of making a clear diagnosis of stress incontinence if leakage is synchronous with the first cough, but only in a minority of women with USI can this be shown. The reason for this is clear on video, when many women will leak after the third or fourth cough as the bladder neck is progressively opened by successive coughs (Fig. 5.2). Even if the woman leaks on the first cough and a diagnosis of USI is certain, UDS do give further information on other aspects of urethral and detrusor function. These other pieces of information allow the surgeon to counsel the woman on the likely outcome of surgery. If the detrusor is underactive or acontractile on voiding then it is reasonable to warn the patient that spontaneous voiding may be delayed and that it might be necessary for her to go home with a catheter for a period of time. In some patients with apparently pure stress incontinence, detrusor overactivity (DO) may be found. In recent reports on the findings of ambulatory urodynamics in USI patients it has been suggested that asymptomatic DO preoperative becomes symptomatic after USI surgery. Certainly if DO is found preoperatively then the patient should be told that USI surgery is for stress incontinence and cannot be guaranteed to cure DO. UDS also allows the assessment of urethral and pelvic floor function. If despite USI the patient has reasonable urethral function as judged by the maximum urethral closure pressure (MUCP) and can effectively interrupt voiding using her pelvic floor then the outcome of USI surgery is likely to be excellent. If however the MUCP is low

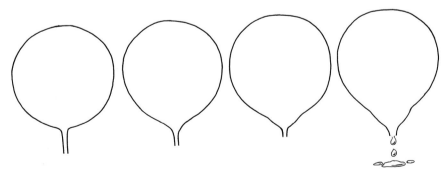

Fig. 5.2 Diagram of the video appearance of the bladder neck changing with successive coughs: leakage occurs after four coughs. 📖

(below 20 cmH$_2$O) then there is evidence that the outcome for a repositioning procedure such as Burch colposuspension is less successful.

The Diagnosis of Urodynamic Stress Incontinence (USI)

USI is the involuntary leakaged urine during increased abdominal pressure in the absence of a detrusor contraction during filling cystometry. Much nonsense has been talked about videourodynamics being the "gold standard" test for the diagnosis of USI. In fact, the "gold standard" is seeing urine leak from the external meatus when the patient raises her intra-abdominal pressure in the absence of a detrusor contraction. Videourodynamics is *not* necessary for the routine diagnosis of USI, and indeed it is easy to miss the loss of a few drops of urine if the urodynamicist watches the TV monitor rather than the patient. Urodynamics is always an embarrassing investigation for patients, and much effort must be made to put the woman at her ease, so that she will tolerate the investigator "staring" at her perineum. To demonstrate USI the patient should be seated as in all female UDS. If USI is not demonstrated then it is useful to ask the patient to flex and abduct one thigh to open the introitus: this reduces the support offered by the pelvic floor and may allow the demonstration of USI (Fig. 3.56).

Other urodynamic tests such as urethral profilometry may provide interesting and useful information but cannot be used to diagnose USI if it is not seen during filling cystometry. Figure 3.78 shows how the maximum urethral pressure, whilst significantly lower in USI patients, has inadequate specificity to be used for diagnostic purposes. If despite carrying out UDS as described above USI is not demonstrated in patients with the symptom of stress incontinence, and if surgery is being contemplated then ambulatory urodynamics (AUDS) is the test of choice. If after AUDS no incontinence can be demonstrated then the patient should be told that surgery would not be wise when the cause of incontinence remains to be defined.

The Overactive Bladder

The overactive bladder (OAB) is urgency, with or without urgency incontinence, usually with frequency and nocturia. OAB is presumed to be due to detrusor overactivity (DO). In OAB due to DO, frequency and urgency may precede the onset of urgency incontinence. In the nulliparous woman the pelvic floor has significantly better function than after childbirth and the patient can often use her pelvic floor to retain continence until the involuntary contraction fades. In DO, bladder sensation is usually normal with the exception that the desire to void becomes accentuated.

Symptoms are not always adequate to distinguish the cause of OAB and if a definitive diagnosis is required then UDS are essential. The correlation of OAB with DO is best for both men and women when all OAB symptoms are present and there are no other LUTS. OAB has been divided into "OAB wet" (includes urgency incontinence) and "OAB dry" (without incontinence).

In OAB "wet", most urgency incontinence follows urgency and is due to an involuntary detrusor contraction. Some patients have incontinence owing to increasing pain. Hence some women with bacterial cystitis will have incontinence because bladder wall inflammation makes it more desirable to be a little wet rather than suffer extreme pain as the bladder fills: this type of leakage is not urgency incontinence Evidence from ambulatory urody-namics is increasingly showing that in women with urgency incontinence without any stress incontinence symptoms the cause of incontinence is almost always DO, whereas conven-tional urodynamics show that only two-thirds have DO. Because the association of urgency incontinence and DO in this group of women appears so strong, UDS are not needed except in the research setting, for example trials of new drugs, and if invasive therapy is being contemplated after conservative and drug therapy have failed.

If all investigations fail to show DO in patients with urgency incontinence then an alter-native mechanism needs to be proposed. In DO incontinence occurs either because the increased bladder pressure overcomes the combined resistance of the intrinsic urethral muscle plus help from the pelvic floor or because the urethra relaxes as part of a premature micturition reflex. *Urgency incontinence* in the absence of a detrusor contraction can only happen if urethral relaxation occurs. Here there exists an overlap and some confusion with the previously used term "urethral instability", which was defined as a fall in urethral pres-sure of greater than 20 cm H_2O recorded when measuring the maximum urethral closure pressure, during bladder filling or at capacity. However it is very unusual to witness urethral relaxation leading to incontinence whilst doing UDS, and we believe it to be an very unusual single cause of incontinence. Nevertheless we have seen the occasional woman who has flooding incontinence without any prior warning, such as the feeling of urgency. In such patients, if conventional UDS fail to show a cause for incontinence then it is helpful to record urethral pressures over a 5 to 10 minute period, at capacity, to see if the MUCP fluctuates (see Fig. 3.89, page 117). In other women, for example, those with urodynamic stress incon-tinence, urethral pressure fluctuations might make incontinence worse if the fall in urethral pressure corresponds to an increase in abdominal pressure due to coughing or straining.

In "OAB dry" the situation is less clear. Firstly, if the patient has never been wet (leaked urine), it is difficult to be sure he or she has ever experienced true urgency (for fear of leakage). OAB dry would also be termed the "frequency-urgency" syndrome and needs to be distinguished from bladder hypersensitivity and painful bladder syndrome. (see below)

"Bladder Hypersensitivity"

Bladder hypersensitivity is a urodynamic diagnosis made not infrequently in our unit. We use this term for individuals with increase bladder sensation characterised by an early first sensation of filling and an early first desire to void which persists into a normal and a strong desire without a break. In most individuals there will be absence of sensation between first sensation and normal desire to void. In bladder hypersensitivity the bladder capacity is less than 250 mls. The frequency-volume chart may show a larger voided volume on rising in the morning but will show voided volumes, consistently less than 250 mls throughout the day. By taking a careful history and determining that the patient's frequency is not due to urgency for fear of leakage, it is possible to suspect the subsequent urodynamic diagnosis.

Painful Bladder Syndrome

The ICS has recommended this term and has defined it as the complaint of suprapubic pain related to bladder filling, accompanied by other symptoms such as increased daytime and nighttime frequency, in the absence of urinary infection or other obvious pathology. The ICS believes that it is unhelpful to put all such patients into the category of "interstitial cystitis" because of the assumption that this is a single disease, when it seems likely that several disease processes will ultimately be shown to contribute to the spectrum of painful bladder syndrome. Bladder pain is a symptom that warrants further insert investigations including urine microscopy, cytology and cystoscopy.

Mixed Urgency and Stress Incontinence

This combination is experienced by the largest group of women referred for UDS. Initial treatment is conservative (see therapy for LUTD, p. 173) but if this fails then UDS are required to direct future management. The assessment of mixed incontinence should be both symptomatic and urodynamic, and the key questions are:

- Is urgency or stress incontinence most frequent?
- Is urgency or stress incontinence most troublesome?
- Are both USI and DO seen on UDS?
- Do the symptoms and the urodynamic findings correlate?

Because DO can be regarded as the premature activation of the micturition reflex, urgency incontinence usually involves a larger loss which occurs more rapidly and which may be too much for any incontinence pad the woman is wearing, as compared to the typical urine leak in stress incontinence. Hence even though incontinence secondary to DO may occur less frequently in a woman with mixed incontinence, it is often judged more troublesome.

When assessing DO during filling cystometry it should be remembered that the pattern of DO is dependant on urethral function. It is easy to underestimate the severity of DO in a woman with poor urethral function: if the MUCP is 20 cmH$_2$O and the pelvic floor function poor, when the intravesical pressure rises to 20 or 30 cmH$_2$O due to an involuntary contraction, incontinence will occur. However after surgery, which improves overall urethral function the DO may appears much more spectacular on UDS, with high pressures during filling: this is particularly true after implantation of an artificial sphincter. When judging DO in a woman with poor urethral function the degree of symptoms and frequency of involuntary contraction are good guides to the problems she may face after USI surgery. DO can be more accurately assessed in women with poor urethral function if a Foley balloon catheter is used for filling and the balloon is pulled down to occlude the bladder neck (Fig. 5.3). This manoeuvre should only be used after conventional studies have demonstrated DO because the presence of a balloon catheter has been shown to increase the incidence of DO in older men.

In our unit 45% of women with symptomatic mixed incontinence are found to have both USI and DO. However a high proportion of those women with USI who complain of urgency incontinence do not have DO demonstrated on conventional UDS. There has been no large study to investigate such women by ambulatory UDS which might confirm the diagnosis of DO. It remains a clinical impression that women with symptoms suggestive of DO but without DO on UDS, do better from USI surgery. The symptoms of urgency and urgency incontinence in these patients may reflect the fact that the woman is well aware that, as the bladder fills towards capacity, she is more likely to leak and it therefore becomes a matter of "urgency" to empty the bladder in these circumstances.

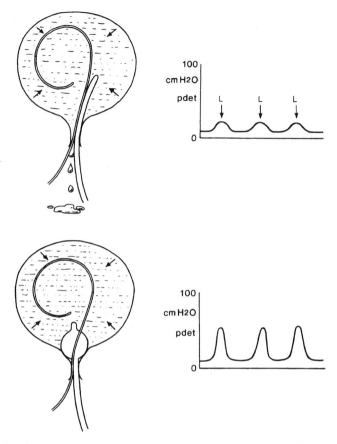

Fig. 5.3 Technique for assessing detrusor overactivity in women with poor urethral function (L signifies leakage). 📖

Urinary Infections

These are common in women and are not usually associated with voiding dysfunction except in the elderly. Poor bladder emptying due to bladder outlet obstruction (BOO) is rare in women. BOO has a variety of structural causes: meatal strictures, urethral distortion secondary to genito-urinary prolapse, urethral obstruction secondary to prolapsed uretero-coele, urethral cancer or stricture after surgery, but may also be functional (see "Dysfunctional voiding", pp. 80–81). Detrusor underactivity (DUA) as a cause of poor bladder emptying is more common. Although DUA may be secondary to drugs (tricyclic antidepressants), surgery (for example after hysterectomy (Wertheims most classically), or rectal operations), injury (spinal cord trauma) or spinal disease, it is most commonly idiopathic and seen in elderly women.

Urinary infections are the most common presentation of voiding dysfunction, because few women complain of poor stream and hesitancy. UDS have little part to play, although we use urine flow studies and ultrasound estimates of residual urine to screen older women with recurrent infections. Flow patterns will usually give an indication if BOO is present, because the maximum flow rate will be consistently reduced. If poor emptying is due to DUA then the flow pattern will often show that reasonable flows can be achieved, often with the help of abdominal straining, but ultrasound shows that the bladder does not empty. We often catheterise the patient in outpatients to exclude any significant mechanical obstruction to flow, to obtain a urine specimen for microscopy and culture, and to accurately measure post-void residual.

Urodynamics in Men

In men, lower urinary tract symptoms (LUTS) are generally due to three main causes of lower urinary tract dysfunction (LUTD):

- Detrusor overactivity (DO)
- Bladder outlet obstruction (BOO)
- Detrusor underactivity (DUA)

Detrusor Overactivity

This may persist from childhood or develop in middle or old age, when it may or may not occur in the presence of BOO. Because urodynamic stress incontinence does not occur in normal men, the confusion of symptoms that occur between stress and urgency incontinence is rarely a problem. Hence a man with urgency and urgency incontinence almost always has DO as the cause and UDS are only indicated if invasive therapy is being contemplated after conservative treatment has failed.

Bladder Outlet Obstruction

The suspicion of BOO is the usual reason for performing UDS in men. All men should be screened by urine flow studies (UFS) and the ultrasound estimate of post-void residual (PVR). In older men the prostate gland has been traditionally held responsible for many of the symptomatic complaints of male patients, and there has been a tendency to use prostatectomy as a panacea for lower urinary tract symptoms. The need for objective evaluation of these symptoms was answered by the introduction of pressure-flow analysis of micturition. Urodynamic studies have provided alternative explanations for certain symptoms and they have contributed to our understanding of some of the common disorders. However, they have not in any way *superseded* the importance of a careful and methodical clinical assessment. The history and clinical examination, followed by the routine urine and appropriate radiological investigations, remain the basis for urological management.

The correlations between symptoms and urodynamic diagnosis are poor, and the only symptom with a reasonable urodynamics correlation is urgency incontinence with DO. Symptoms have been found to be neither sex nor age specific. For these reasons the term "prostatism" has been abandoned in favour of the term "LUTS", divided into "storage" and "voiding" symptoms, and not the old terms "irritative" and "obstructive" symptoms (Table 5.4). The terms referring to prostate histology (benign prostatic hyperplasia: BPH), prostatic size (benign prostatic enlargement: BPE) and the coexistence of BPE and BOO (benign

Table 5.4. LUTS

Storage Symptoms	Voiding Symptoms
Frequency	Hesitancy
Nocturia	Straining to void
Urgency	Poor stream
Urgency incontinence	Intermittent stream
Stress incontinence	*Dysuria*
Enuresis	Feeling of incomplete emptying
Bladder pain	Terminal dribble

prostatic obstruction: BPO) should be used appropriately and consistently so that clinicians and urodynamicists can communicate clearly about both individual patients and groups of patients. As Fig. 5.4 shows, the presence of BPH or BPE may have no impact on voiding but BPO does, producing the classic urodynamic finding of low flow rate and high voiding pressure. If the terms LUTS, BPH, BPE, BPO and BOO are used then misleading terms such as "clinical BPH", "symptoms of BPH", "symptomatic BPH" and "prostatism" can be abandoned.

Should all older men with LUTS have pressure-flow studies (PFS)? The answer depends on the treatment intentions of the patient and clinician. If conservative treatment is planned then basic urological tests should be performed after a routine physical examination and an analysis of symptoms, but unless there are definite indications for surgery then no urodynamic tests are needed at this stage (see treatment of LUTD). If conservative treatment has failed and the patient remains symptomatic to the extent that he wishes to consider surgery then urine flow studies (UFS) and the ultrasound estimate of PVR should be carried out. If the maximum flow rate (Q_{max}) is below 10 ml/s then the chance of the patient having BOO is 90%; 38% of our patients would fit into this category. However if the Q_{max} is 10 ml/s to 15 ml/s then the incidence of BOO falls to 71% or less (Table.5.5). Because 29% of these patients will not be shown to have BOO, we believe that *all patients with a Q_{max} of 10 ml/s or more should have PFS before invasive therapy.*

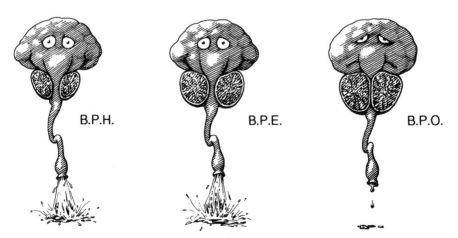

B.P.H.   B.P.E.   B.P.O.

Fig. 5.4 Diagrammatic representation of benign prostatic hyperplasia (BPH), benign prostatic enlargement (BPE) and benign prostatic obstruction (BPO) when BPH leads to BPE, which in turn results in bladder outlet obstruction. 📖

Table 5.5. Predictive ability of first flow rate for a voided volume of 150 ml or more

Flow rate ml/s	Number	Pressure Flows	
		Obstructed	Not obstructed
< 10	135 (38%)	119 (89%)	16 (12%)
10 to 15	130 (37%)	92 (71%)	38 (29%)
> 15	91 (26%)	44 (48%)	47 (52%)
Total	356 (100%)	255 (71%)	101 (28%)

How is the diagnosis of BOO made? In some men either flow is very low (< 10 ml/s) or voiding pressure is so high ($p_{det}, Q_{max} > 100$ cm H_2O) that BOO is highly likely. However for most patients the diagnosis of BOO is made by plotting the maximum flow rate (Q_{max}) against detrusor pressure at Q_{max} (p_{det}, Q_{max}) into the ICS nomogram which is derived from the Abrams-Griffiths, LPURR and URA nomograms. If the clinician wishes to describe the degree of obstruction then the Bladder Outlet Obstruction Index (BOOI) can be calculated and BOO diagnosed without reference to the nomogram from the simple equation:

$$BOOI = p_{det}, Q_{max} - 2Q_{max}$$

If the BOOI is greater than 40 then BOO exists; if it is below 40 then no definite BOO exists. By further analysing the urodynamic trace it is possible to categorise those patients with a BOOI of less than 40. To do this the minimum detrusor pressure during voiding ($p_{det\,min,\,void}$) must be read from the trace: usually this is seen at the end of voiding. If both the p_{det}

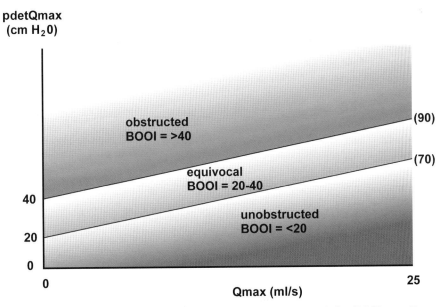

Fig. 5.5 The ICS pressure-flow nomogram using bladder outlet obstruction index ($BOOI = p_{det}, Q_{max} - 2Q_{max}$).

Q_{max}/Q_{max} point and the point of $P_{det\ min,\ void}$ are plotted then the LPURR (linear passive urethral resistance ratio) is obtained. The $P_{det,\ min\ void}$ point is where the flow-pressure curve reaches the pressure axis. For a BOOI of less than 40, BOO exists if:

- The $p_{det\ min,\ void}$ is 40 cmH$_2$O or more.
- The slope of the LPURR line is greater than 2 cmH$_2$O/ml/s. The slope of the LPURR line is calculated in cmH$_2$O/ml/s simply by the following equation:

$$slope = (p_{det,\ Qmax} - p_{det\ min,\ void})/Q_{max}$$

Many clinicians had been baffled by the various methods for diagnosis and grading BOO, but the degree of agreement in the diagnosis of obstruction was very high (95%), so now only the ICS nomogram is recommended. Research on more complex methods continues but in our view is unlikely to offer large patient benefits

Conventional, Video or Ambulatory UDS?. The older the man, the less likely that there will be a functional disorder producing BOO. However in younger men with poor flow there is a higher likelihood of either bladder neck obstruction (BNO) or detrusor underactivity (DUA) being the cause, and therefore video UDS are the investigation of choice as VUDS allows identification of the site of any obstruction. Whilst ambulatory UDS are more physiological and give interesting results they are unnecessarily complex for routine use in the male patient. In fact there are few instances when AUDS are indicated in men. Hence for the majority of male patients, that is the group of older men with LUTS suggestive of BOO, basic (conventional) UDS are the investigation of choice. Non-invasive urodynamics may partly replace conventional UDS (pressure-flow studies) in the future.

Detrusor Underactivity (DUA)

This is responsible for the symptoms of a significant minority of patients. As defined earlier, DUA either results in a significant post-void residual urine or results in the bladder being emptied more slowly than normal. DUA cannot be diagnosed with certainty from the flow trace, although an irregular flow curve with Q_{max} occurring in mid-trace is highly suggestive. DUA is a diagnosis made after pressure-flow studies (PFS): 10 to 20% of men with low flows have a degree of DUA. On the PFS trace, DUA can appear as a low sustained contraction or as a wavelike contraction. If urethral relaxation is normal during voiding then the flow trace will reflect the detrusor pressure changes. However the patient with DUA will often use straining to assist micturition and the PFS curves can look confusing as a result.

What are the interrelationships between DO, BOO and DUA? These three common urodynamic diagnoses are not exclusive of each other, and commonly DO and BOO are found together (in up to 40% of patients). In fact the largest sub-group of older men, whose lower tract function has been defined by UDS, have both DO and BOO. DUA can exist with prostatic obstruction, but it is likely that most men with DUA and severe BOO will develop urinary retention early on. DUA and DO together are uncommon in the neurological intact male patient. Whilst DUA seems to occur with a similar prevalence in most age groups, the prevalence of DO rises with age, so that 50% of asymptomatic men of 70 can be shown to have DO on UDS, although DO may not give the patient troublesome symptoms and may be interpreted as a *normal* desire to void.

Urodynamics in the Younger Man

Video UDS are the investigation of choice after screening flow studies. Bladder neck obstruction and inadequate urethral relaxation are observed in younger men. Such abnormalities appear to be functional rather than structural abnormalities. Younger men are less phlegmatic than older men when investigated and require more careful handling. Fainting (syncope) is most common in this group and if the patient goes quiet, looks worried and pale and starts to sweat, lie him down! It is wise to stop the filling and allow the patient at least 20 minutes to recover. Usually the patient can then stand and the UDS can be continued. If the patient is very inhibited by the investigation then it may be necessary to leave him to void alone, in which case the video part of the study may have to be abandoned.

It should be reiterated that all patients should be screened by flow studies and the flow study results compared with the flow recording from the PFS: if they are not similar the PFS should be repeated. This rule should apply to all patients investigated by urodynamics.

Postprostatectomy Problems

Patients with postprostatectomy problems present as three main symptomatic groups:

- Persistent OAB symptoms suggestive of detrusor overactivity.
- Persistent symptoms suggestive of obstruction.
- Incontinence.

Therefore, several symptom complexes are seen which may suggest a single disorder or, as in the non-operated patient, a combination of symptoms suggesting, for example, detrusor overactivity and obstruction. The symptoms of frequency, nocturia, urgency, urgency incontinence and bladder discomfort are suggestive of persistent DO: the symptom of slow stream, is suggestive of persistent BOO. The symptom of incontinence is likely to be regarded even more seriously by the patient after surgery than before operation. The patient should be asked the frequency and severity of his incontinence and whether or not he suffers social restriction or has to take protective measures to safeguard his clothes. It is also important to establish whether or not the incontinence was present before operation and then to determine what kind of leakage the patient suffers. The incidence of postprostatectomy incontinence has been estimated at 1 to 3% after TURP, but higher after radical prostatectomy. Video-urodynamic studies (VUDS) are the investigation of choice and urethral pressure profilometry can be very useful. Post prostatectomy incontinence is now being seen more frequently because radical prostatectomy for localised prostrate cancer is being performed more often.

Persistent Symptoms Suggestive of Detrusor Overactivity

Those patients with persistent symptoms suggestive of detrusor overactivity are shown by the cystometric findings to have a high incidence of DO. The symptoms of DO are known to improve after prostatectomy and 62% of overactive detrusors revert to normal on post-operative cystometry (Abrams 1978). However, 19% of patients continue to show DO after an adequate prostatectomy. Price et al. (1980) have shown that those patients with the symptoms of urgency and urgency incontinence, and with demonstrable severe DO before operation, are most likely to have persistent problems after operation. The reason for the conversion of DO to normal detrusor behaviour on cystometry is unclear. It has been suggested that lower voiding pressures after prostatectomy, or the denervation of the bladder neck and posterior urethra resulting from surgery, may be important factors.

Persistent Symptoms Suggestive of Obstruction

The postoperative complaints of slow stream and hesitancy have in the past led to repeated transurethral resections with the increased likelihood of damage to the intrinsic urethral sphincter mechanism. The urodynamic results of this group of patients show clearly that the minority of such patients with reduced flow have persistent outlet obstruction. A higher proportion of patients have a slow stream due to an underactive or acontractile detrusor. If urethral pressure profilometry shows no residual prostatic tissue (Fig. 5.6) then a second prostatectomy will not help the patient. However, should profilometry show the presence of residual prostatic tissue (Fig. 5.7) then transurethral resection of the remaining prostatic tissue may be expected to improve voiding, even when the detrusor is underactive.

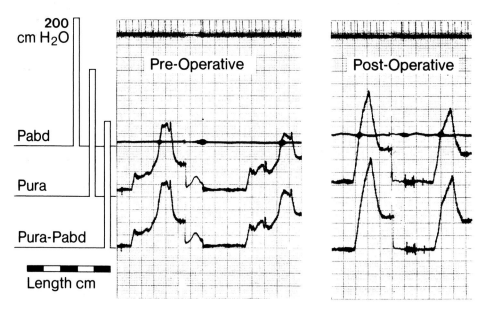

Fig. 5.6 Two Urethral pressure profiles before and after prostatectomy. There is no residual prostatic pressure area post-operatively. 📖

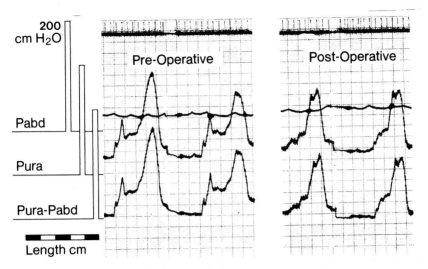

Fig. 5.7 Two Urethral pressure profiles before and after prostatectomy. In this case enough prostatic tissue remains to produce a presphincteric pressure rise. 📖

When assessing postprostatectomy problems a reasonable time interval following the operation should be allowed for the gradual improvement of symptoms, which can be expected to occur for six months following surgery. The appearance of new complaints after surgery suggests that a change has occurred in the lower urinary tract. Symptoms of over-activity may be due to a urinary tract infection and those of obstruction to a developing stricture. If a patient complains of urgency incontinence following prostatectomy then he will usually have had the symptoms of urgency and possible urgency incontinence prior to operation. Because these symptoms may fail to improve after operation, patients with urgency prior to operation should be counselled, explaining that although an improvement in urine flow rate is anticipated, one cannot be similarly confident about the symptoms of DO, which may persist.

Incontinence

Incontinence following prostatectomy is either urgency incontinence, stress inconti-nence or very occasionally a mixture of the two types. The symptom of stress inconti-nence in neurologically normal male patients does not occur in the unoperated case. Therefore, the appearance of this symptom following surgery implies per-operative damage to the distal urethral sphincteric mechanism, or possibly the weakening of the pelvic floor support to the sphincter mechanism by removal of a large adenoma at open operation. In urological practice it is relatively common to see transient stress inconti-nence following open prostatectomy for benign disease, but more commonly after radical prostatectomy for cancer. Persistence of stress incontinence, in our view, indicates per-operative sphincteric damage. In male patients, stress incontinence is effectively treated by implantation of an artificial sphincter (see "Treatment of Lower Urinary Tract Dysfunction," in Chapter 6).

Urodynamics in the Elderly

Many patients we investigate are elderly, and we like to distinguish the *frail elderly* from other patients. If an old person is clearly in the last few years of life, then our approach to urodynamic investigations will be different because the therapeutic options will be limited. For example, if a frail old man has failed to respond to antimuscarinic treatment for urgency incontinence that persists after prostatectomy then there is little point in confirming that DO is the cause as he will never be considered for ileocystoplasty. However this will not be the case if the man is 70 years of age and walks or exercises daily. Our use of urodynamics is governed by an assessment of the patient's *biological and not chronological age*.

The prevalence of DO increases with age and if there is mental impairment then DO is almost inevitable. Urodynamics on patients who are confused is often upsetting for the patient and difficult for the urodynamic staff. Whilst we are always prepared to do studies if they will help the management of patients, the value of UDS is limited in the frail elderly. However urine flow studies and the estimation of post-void residual (PVR) is often helpful in excluding significant BOO or DUA. If a significant PVR is seen then it may be beneficial to treat this by catheterisation and thereby improve the quality of the patient's life. Many of the very elderly may be troubled by recurrent infections made worse by a failure to achieve proper bladder emptying: knowledge of the PVR in these patients will aid treatment.

Urodynamics in the Neurological Patient

A number of neurological conditions commonly lead to lower urinary tract dysfunction. In patients with these conditions, urodynamics are often a vital part of the investigation and management process. These conditions may be congenital, for example meningomyelocele or sacral agenesis, or else acquired, including multiple sclerosis, cerebrovascular accidents, spinal cord trauma and Parkinson's disease.

In the neurological patient symptoms may be altered or absent even though marked vesico-urethral dysfunction exists. For example in spinal cord trauma or meningomyelocele there can be changes in bladder behaviour that threaten kidney function even though the patient notices little change in symptoms. Therefore in the neurogenic patient, urodynamics have a surveillance role in several conditions such as those mentioned above: spinal cord trauma and meningomyelocele. Neurological disease produces two important dysfunctions:

- *Neurogenic Detrusor Overactivity (NDO)* is the term often given to DO in the neurogenic patient. There are no real differences in urodynamic appearances between NDO and idiopathic DO.

- *Functional bladder outlet obstruction* secondary to urethral overactivity occurs classically in spinal cord injury, meningomyelocele and multiple sclerosis (MS). The functional obstruction is due to either intermittent urethral overactivity, as in spinal cord injury or MS when it is known as *detrusor-sphincter dyssynergia*. Meningomyelocele patients may have a continuous obstruction to voiding known as *nonrelaxing sphincter obstruction*. The effect of urethral overactivity is to produce a reduced interrupted flow rate and incomplete bladder emptying: in non-relaxing urethral sphincter obstruction, the interrupted flow is due to the patient needing to strain to overcome the functional obstruction.

In the neurological patient, bladder behaviour is difficult to predict from the neurological signs, although broad principles apply in complete lesions. If there is damage to the lower motor neurones, for example after an injury to the lower part of the lumbar spine, then:

- Bladder sensation is lost.
- Detrusor contractility is absent.
- Bladder compliance may be reduced.
- Sphincter function is reduced.
- Voiding is by straining.

If the upper motor neurone is damaged within the central nervous system, for example by a high spinal cord injury:

- Bladder sensation is lost.
- Detrusor overactivity is likely.
- Bladder compliance may be reduced.
- Sphincter function is normal during filling but may be overactive during voiding. (DSD)
- Voiding is reflex.

In conditions like MS and meningomyelocele the neurological lesions are more complex and the pattern is less constant because the lesions are incomplete.

Urodynamic Technique in the Neurogenic Patient

For reasons that are poorly understood the neurogenic bladder is particularly sensitive to the speed at which it is filled. Hence fast filling tends to produce artefactual low compliance. In neurogenic patients the bladder should *not* be emptied at the start off UDS unless the patient is on intermittent self-catheterisation and it is their normal time to catheterise. It is better to fill slowly on top of the residual.

Filling Rate. A flexible approach needs to be taken. From the patient's frequency-volume chart and knowledge of the patient's residual urine (usually from ultrasound estimates) a policy for that patient can be defined. Generally filling should start at 10 ml/min. If there is no rise in the detrusor pressure this can be increased to 20 ml/min or 30 ml/min. However if pressure begins to rise then filling should be stopped for 5 min to 10 min until the pressure has settled, and then restarted at 10 ml/min. In the neuropathic child the filling rate should be slower, 2 ml/min to 5 ml/min.

Patient Position. Many male neuropathic patients will not be able to stand or even sit, either to be filled or to void. In neurological disease bladder behaviour is less dependent on patient position and if the patient has to lie down throughout filling and voiding this is likely to give appropriate information. Patients with paraplegia have to be investigated lying, because few can manage to sit for UDS. With the patient lying the voiding phase presents problems but in male patients urine can be voided so that it flows down a tube (a piece of builder's drainpipe) to the flowmeter; (after a considerable delay) the flow is eventually registered by the flowmeter.

Which tests? In the neuropathic patient video UDS are the investigation of choice in view of the higher incidence of anatomical abnormalities, such as vesico-ureteric reflux and prostatic duct reflux. VUDS also make it easier to study any abnormalities of co-ordination between the detrusor and the urethra, for example, detrusor-sphincter dyssynergia. As VUDS are required, if the patient needs to be investigated lying, the couch has to be suitable for X-ray investigation (Fig. 5.8) Special problems exist in the neurogenic patient, such as muscle spasms and autonomic dysreflexia which produce particular difficulties during VUDS. Leg spasms in spinal injury patients may make it difficult to pass the catheters, but usually spasms settle during the investigations. *Autonomic dysreflexia* tends to occur in patients with high spinal cord injury. It is a dangerous syndrome where stimuli such as bladder filling or urinary infection lead to dramatic increase in blood pressure, increased pulse rate and sweating. If this occurs during VUDS the bladder should be emptied immediately and the situation will resolve.

Occult Neuropathy. Neurological disease may present with lower urinary tract dysfunction (LUTD) before the onset of neurological signs: MS regularly presents to the urodynamicist, who may be the first to suspect the diagnosis. The sudden onset of LUTD in a younger person, and the occurrence of voiding difficulties in patients with back or neck pain, are two relatively common indications that an underlying neurological disease may be present.

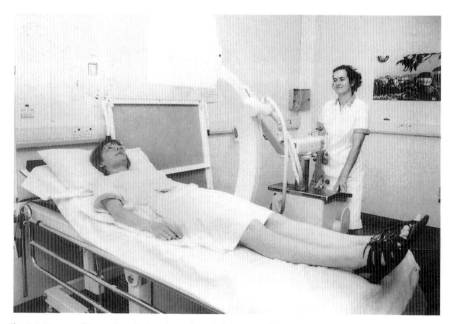

Fig. 5.8 Neuropathic patient being investigated lying on the examination couch with the image intensifier in position over the lower abdomen.

References

Abrams P (1978) Urodynamic changes following prostatectomy. Urol Int 33:181–186.

Abrams P (1994). New words for old. Lower urinary tract symptoms for 'prostatism'. Br Med J 308:929–930.

Abrams P (1999). Bladder outlet obstruction index, bladder contractility index and bladder voiding efficiency: three simple indices to define bladder voiding function. Br J Urol 84:14-15.

Allen T (1977). The non-neurogenic bladder. J Urol 177:232–238.

Andersen JT, Bradley WE (1976). Abnormalities of detrusor and sphincter function in multiple sclerosis. Br J Urol 48:193–198.

Andersen JT (1988). Urodynamics terminology and normal values in children, females and males. Scand J Urol Nephrol suppl 114.

Bhatia NN, Bergman A (1986). Urodynamic appraisal of vaginal pressure versus rectal pressure recording as indication of intraabdominal pressure changes. Urology 27:482.

Blaivas J, Labib KL, Bauer SB, Retik AB (1977). Changing concepts in urodynamic evaluation of children. J Urol 117:778–781.

Byrne DJ, Hamilton Stewart PA, Gray BK (1987). The role of urodynamics in female urinary stress incontinence. Br J Urol 59:228–229.

Chancellor MB (1993). Urodynamic evaluation after spinal cord injury. Physical medicine and rehabilitation clinics of North America 4:273–298.

Gierup J (1970). Micturition studies in infants and children. Scand J Nephrol 5:12 suppl.

Griffiths DJ, Scholtmeijer RJ (1982). Precise urodynamic assessment of meatal and distal urethral stenosis in girls. Neurourol Urodyn 1:89.

Houle A, Gilmour R, Churchill B et al. (1993). What volume can a child normally store in the bladder at a safe pressure. J Urol 149:561.

Koff S (1982). Estimating bladder capacity in children. Urology 21:248.

Lim CS, Abrams P (1995). The Abrams-Griffiths Nomogram. World J Urol 13:34–39.

Mayo ME, Chetner MP (1992). Lower urinary tract dysfunction in multiple sclerosis. Urology 39:67–70.

McGuire EJ (1994). Idiopathic detrusor instability. In Kursh ED, McGuire EJ (eds): female urology. Philadelphia: Lipincott p 95.

Nijman R (1994). Course on paediatric urodynamics. Utrecht.

Philp T, Read DJ, Higson RH (1981). The urodynamic characteristics of multiple sclerosis. Br J Urol 53:672–675.

Price DA, Ramsden PD, Stobbart D (1980) The unstable bladder and prostatectomy. Br J Urol 52:529–531.

Poulsen A, Schou J, Puggaard L, Torp-Pedersen S, Nordling J (1994). Prostatic enlargement symptomatology and pressure/flow evaluation: interrelations in patients with symptomatic BPH. Scand J Urol Nephrol suppl 157:67–73.

Shepherd AM, Powell PH, Ball AJ (1982). The place of urodynamic studies in the investigation and treatment of female urinary tract symptoms. J Obstet Gynaecol 3:123–125.

Chapter 6
Management of Lower Urinary Tract Dysfunction

Urodynamic data provides the basis for sound management of lower urinary tract dysfunction (LUTD). However as explained in Chapter 4, UDS follow a proper evaluation of the patient by symptom analysis, physical examination, urine microscopy and abdominal X-ray or ultrasound. This assessment may provide the basis for an initial period of empiric treatment, because precise diagnosis by UDS in every woman with incontinence and every older man with LUTS is not practical in most areas of the world. This chapter is intended to provide no more than the principles involved in treatment and their relationship with urodynamic investigation at different levels. The principles of treatment are common to all patient groups, although some treatments are not applicable initially; for example, bladder training for detrusor overactivity cannot be used, in the accepted sense, in patients without bladder sensation.

The books from the International Consultations on Incontinence the third of which was published in 2005 provide detailed evaluation of the techniques used for the management of LUTD.

Storage Phase Problems

The principal patterns of the storage phase are detrusor overactivity and urethral sphincter incompetence.

Detrusor Overactivity

Idiopathic or Neurogenic Detrusor Overactivity (IDO or NDO) and reduced bladder compliance may lead to problems in two main ways:

- Overactive bladder symptoms, with or without urgency incontinence, which in neurogenic patients can be difficult to categorise.

- Upper tract dilatation leading to renal impairment.

Treatments for detrusor overactivity can be divided into three main groups: conservative, medical, and surgical.

Conservative Treatments

These consist of:

- *Advice on fluid and food intake* including the twenty-four hour total and the timing and type of fluid and food intake, for example:
  - Don't drink before going out.
  - Don't drink before going to bed or during the night.
  - Maintain an adequate fluid output: one to two litres.
  - Avoid fluids that produce symptoms, for example containing caffeine or alcohol.
  - Water containing foods (fruit, salads, vegetables, rice and pasta) should be treated as if they are fluids, and the quantity and timing should be adjusted as necessary
- *Bladder training.* The use of the voiding diary to encourage the voiding of increasing volumes at increasing intervals.
- *Pelvic floor exercises.* Increasing pelvic floor strength may work by reflex inhibition of the detrusor or by aiding urethral closure until the involuntary contraction has passed and the detrusor has relaxed.
- *Other treatments* such as biofeedback, in which the patient is given information on bladder activity so that when the detrusor pressure rises they can see an increasing number of lights illuminated, hear a louder sound or see the pressure tracing change.

Medical Management

For detrusor overactivity this is confined to drugs with an antimuscarinic action such as oxybutynin propiverine, tolterodine and trospium. Two new drugs with apparent relative selectivity for the M3 receptor, darifenacin and solifenacin, have recently been licensed (2004/2005). These anti-muscarinic drugs all have some activity in blocking the five muscarinic receptors, M1 to M5. In vitro, their effects are different, but this does not necessarily translate to differences in clinical efficacy or tolerability. In addition some drugs are better started at a low dosage and titrated up, whilst others are started at a standard dose and increased or decreased as necessary. Oxybutynin and tolterodine are available, in some countries, in two formulations immediate-release and extended-release. It is useful to have the immediate-release formulations available as they allow for occasional use, for example, when going to the cinema or theater, and they enable greater flexibility of dosage. It is not unusual to use both the immediate and the extended release formulations of a drug simultaneously to provide a higher dose at specific times of the day. It is ironic that their principal side-affect is dry mouth, which encourages the patient to drink more. Other side-effects include difficulty in visual accommodation, due to effects on the ciliary muscle of the eye, indigestion and constipation. Of particular concern are possible central nervous system side-effects such as dizziness, confusion and memory loss. However there is little published evidence on the prevalence of such side-effects although there is cognitive testing research ongoing which should define the problem, if one exists.

Many theoretical mechanisms could be exploited in "new possibilities" for medical therapy of DO, but at the time of writing none of these drugs has undergone a clinical trial beyond phase II.

Intravesical Medical Management

Intravesical oxybutynin has been used for many years in patients who catheterise regularly and require anti-muscarinic medication for detrusor overactivity. This form of oxybutynin therapy is used when oral oxybutynin is unacceptable because of side-effects. Oxybutynin is absorbed through the bladder wall and passes into the general circulation avoiding the liver where the first pass effect metabolises a high proportion of oxybutynin absorbed by the gut after an oral dose: the metabolites of oxybutynin are responsible for many of its side-effects.

Intravesical capsacacin and, more recently, resinaferatoxin have been used in neurogenic DO. These drugs work by a different mechanism, being vallinoid receptor antagonists active on C-fibre afferents. The way in which C-fibre afferents are reactivated, having been previously active in early childhood, is not fully understood. Whether these compounds are active in idiopathic DO remains to be determined. Obviously it is a disadvantage that these compounds can only be given by catheter and this is likely to limit their use.

Botulinum toxin A is the latest intravesical therapy for DO. At the time of writing there is reasonable evidence of efficacy in neurogenic DO and some evidence in idiopathic DO. It is hoped that good quality clinical trials will soon define its role in the therapeutic armamentarium against DO. The substance is diluted and injected, at multiple sites into the bladder wall and blocks nerve transmission to muscle cells for 6 to 12 months: hence treatments usually require repeating.

Neuromodulation

Sacral nerve stimulation is now an established treatment for bothersome DO that has failed conservative and medical treatment. The most recent technique involves the percutaneous insertion of an electrode through one S3 foramen with the patient lying on his or her front. The procedure is under local anaesthetic and the electrode is adjusted so that when stimulated, the best anal contraction (perineal lift) is obtained. The electrode lead is tunnelled to emerge from the skin above the iliac cest on the same side. A temporary connection is made to an external stimulator and a period of test stimulation begins. If after several days there has been significant (defined variously as 50% or better improvement), then the electrode lead will be connected to a permanent battery driven stimulator which is implanted beneath the skin of the lower back. Neuromodulation had been used successfully in idiopathic DO but not yet in neurogenic DO.

Surgical Management

Until the new techniques mentioned above, there were no effective managements between conservative and medical treatments on the one hand and major surgery on the other. Bladder augmentation or substitution is the most effective procedure for the symptomatic relief of detrusor overactivity (DO low bladder compliance). Augmentation cystoplasty can be achieved in a variety of ways by using ileum (ileocystoplasty), colon (colocystoplasty) or stomach (gastrocystoplasty); ureter (ureterocystoplasty) is used when the kidney is being removed for non-function and a widely dilated ureter is available).

In all these procedures the bladder is first split either side to side (coronally) or front to back (sagitally). The bowel segment (15 cm-30 cm long) is also split along its length, on the antemesenteric border, and sewn into the bladder defect. The ureters are left undisturbed unless there is reflux, when the surgeon may wish to reimplant them. Bladder substitution is used if the bladder wall is excessively thick or diseased. For substitution cystoplasty similar techniques are used, although ileum and/or colon would be the tissues of choice and up to 45 cm may be needed: the ureters may require reimplantation although the trigone is usually preserved. Cystoplasty carries significant morbidity and the patient must be counselled in detail on the main complications, namely:

- *Intermittent self-catheterisation (ISC)*. Owing to intentional weakening of the detrusor, Incomplete bladder emptying often occurs in up to 50% of patients. Because the resulting need for ISC is so frequent it is unwise for patients to undergo bladder augmentation until they have demonstrated their ability to perform ISC.
- *Mucus production from the bowel segment*. This can cause blockage, making ISC more difficult.
- *Urinary tract infections*. These are likely to occur with increased frequency after cystoplasty, probably due to mucus production and more difficult bladder emptying.
- *Tumour formation*. With time this may occur in the neobladder, but probably not for ten to twenty years. However the possibility necessitates regular check cystoscopies.
- *Metabolic complications* may occur due to reduced Vit. B12 absorption or from the acidosis that occurs that may lead to calcium loss from bone.

Detrusor myectomy (autoaugmentation) is a newer procedure and involves removing the detrusor muscle, leaving the urothelial layers intact, from the upper half of the bladder. It is inferior to bowel cystoplasty in producing symptom relief, but is a more minor procedure without most of the longer-term risks of cystoplasty although, with time, many patients need to self-catheterise. If detrusor myectomy produces inadequate symptomatic effect then bowel cystoplasty can be performed.

Urethral Sphincter Incompetence

This can result in the symptom of stress incontinence and may be managed conservatively, medically, or surgically.

Conservative Therapy

This should be used in all patients who are suspected of having or who have been demonstrated to have urodynamic stress incontinence (USI). Such therapy includes:

- *General advice* on:
  - Fluid intake (see above)
  - Weight loss: losing weight reduces abdominal pressure and therefore increases the urethral closure pressure, resulting in reduced leakage.

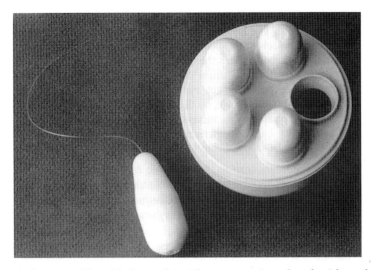

Fig. 6.1 Vaginal cones used for pelvic floor training. The cones contain graduated weights and are used for progressively longer periods at increased weight. 📖

- *Pelvic floor exercises (PFE)*. In order to be effective, these should be performed repetitively, using the $10 \times 10 \times 10 \times 10$ rule. The woman is asked to increase her PFE until she does ten 10-second contractions, ten times a day (roughly hourly) for ten weeks. Most women cannot sustain a pelvic floor contraction for 10 seconds initially and a contraction held for 5 seconds with 5 to 10 seconds between contractions is more realistic at first.

  If the patient is unable to contract her pelvic floor then it may be necessary to use "aids" such as perineometry, vaginal cones (Fig. 6.1) or electrical stimulation to help re-educate the muscles. Faradism is a technique which uses electrical stimulation as therapy rather than to re-educate the pelvic floor muscles.

- *Continence aids*. These have increased in number and variety and both intravaginal and intraurethral devices have been developed. *Intravaginal devices* (Fig. 6.2, *overleaf*) are designed to support the bladder neck and also to prevent anterior vaginal wall descent. Intraurethral devices (Fig. 6.3, *overleaf*) aim to prevent urine leakage by obstructing the urethra: voiding occurs either by a pressure-activated valve mechanism or by removing the device. A third type of device is stuck by adhesive hydrogel onto the external urethral meatus and removed for micturition (Fig. 6.4, *overleaf*). Most of these devices are no longer available, or failed to reach clinical use. In general, intraurethral devices are uncomfortable and poorly tolerated.

Medical Therapy

Historically, medical therapy for stress incontinence has been of disappointing efficiency, although a few patients benefit from alpha-adrenergic agonists such as phenylpropanolamine. These drugs are not generally used except in patients with sphincter weakness associated with neuropathic vesico-urethral dysfunction.

A new drug, duloxetine, a dual serotonin and noradrenaline reuptake inhibitor appears effective in reducing the number of stress incontinence episodes. The drug appears to act

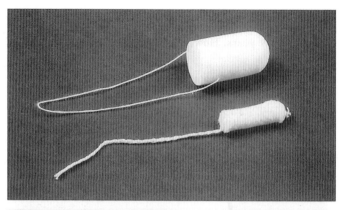

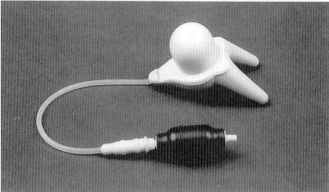

Fig. 6.2 Intravaginal devices designed to prevent stress incontinence: a large tampon for use during exercise compared with a standard tampon, and an inflatable prosthesis shown with the pump connected and the balloon inflated to press on the urethra. 📖

centrally on Onuf's nucleus in the anterior horn of the spinal cord (S3–4) and has been shown to cause an increase in urethral pressure in animal models. The drug has been licensed in some countries (2004).

Surgical Treatment

For USI this should be directed at one or other of the two basic causes of incontinence after proper assessment by vaginal examination and urodynamic testing.

Urethral hypermobility. This is best treated by repositioning procedures. There are three main classes of operation:

- *Retropubic techniques* including the Burch colposuspension, vagino-obturator shelf procedure and Marshall Marchetti Krantz operation have the best long-term results.
- *Needle suspension procedures* include the Pereyra, Stamey, Raz and Gittes operations. These have good initial results but on longer-term follow-up have shown an increasing failure rate from one to five years.

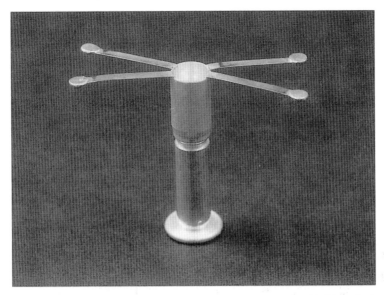

Fig. 6.3 Stainless steel intraurethral device inserted *per urethram*: the "wings" hold the device on the bladder base. The patient voids by straining and activating a sophisticated valve system. 📖

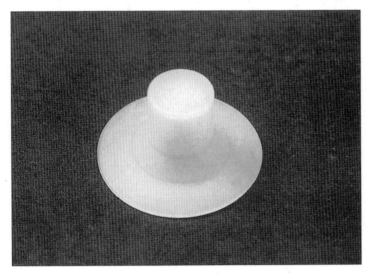

Fig. 6.4 Small "sucker" device applied directly over the external urinary meatus to be removed for voiding. 📖

- *Vaginal procedures* such as the Kelly procedure are the least effective class of operation for the relief of USI. Vaginal or anterior repair is the operation of choice for simple anterior vaginal wall descent.
- *Minimally invasive slings* have been developed since the late 1990s. These use the low tension principle and either mimic the Aldridge sling or are placed using a trans obturator foramen technique.

There must be adequate vaginal mobility for repositioning procedures to be used.

Intrinsic urethral sphincter weakness. This is usually not associated with anterior vaginal wall descent, being due to either neurogenic causes or trauma, for example after repeated procedures for USI Treatment may be by:

- *Periurethral injection.* Teflon (polytetrafluoroethylene) and Silastic (silicone rubber) are not now widely used because of fears over particle migration. Collagen has been the most popular injected substance, but additional compounds have been introduced and more are currently being investigated.
- *Sling procedures.* The original procedure (Aldridge sling) used the patient's own rectus fascia. This has an excellent reputation for cure of incontinence. but may produce voiding dysfunction. Formerly these procedures had adverse publicity due to urethral erosion when artificial sling material was used. But by using fascial material, either from the patient or from porcine sources, and by using low-tension techniques these problems have been largely overcome.
- *Artificial urinary sphincter (AUS).* Most of the treatments for USI can only be used in women, although the sling procedure and injections have been used in men. The AUS can be used in men, women and children, and produces excellent results. Because the AUS (Fig. 6.5) is made from artificial material, infection can be a problem, in that an infected sphincter has to be removed.

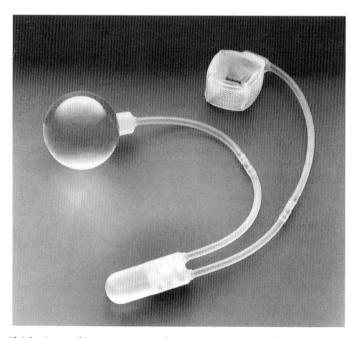

Fig. 6.5 Artificial urinary sphincter consisting of a pressure-regulating balloon, a periurethral cuff and an intrascrotal (or intralabial) control pump. 📖

Management of Intractable Incontinence

If age, physical status, mental state or disease prevents the use of the techniques described above then other methods of treatment may be needed. These methods can be divided into conservative and surgical.

Conservative Techniques

Included among these are:

- *Pads.* These vary in type from dribble pouches for the man with small-volume incontinence to a full-sized nappy for the incontinent adult. All patients should be properly assessed as to their pad needs, with the appropriate size of pad being given together with suitable incontinence pants to support the pad. All-in-one washable pants with fitted pads are preferred by many patients. Patients may require different protection at night from that used in the daytime. Better bed protection in the form of disposable or washable, reusable protective sheets should be provided.
- *Indwelling catheter.* There is a longstanding prejudice against permanent catheterisation, but it may be the only practical way of managing some patients. The situation has been improved by the use of long-term catheters and by proper systematic catheter care. Suprapubic catheterisation is preferable to the urethral route, although catheter blockage and leakage around the catheter are relatively common problems.

Surgical Techniques

If conservative methods fail then surgical techniques may be needed:

- *Urethral closure.* If despite an effective suprapubic catheter there is troublesome urethral leakage then the urethra may need to be closed surgically.
- *Urinary diversion.* Intractable incontinence in a patient with a normal life expectancy is a huge burden to both the patient and any carers. Formation of an ileal conduit can transform the life of a patient who has suffered urinary incontinence for years. It is easier for most carers to change or drain the urine drainage bag of a conduit than to change both the clothes and the bedclothes of an incontinent patient. The main indications for ileal diversion are in wheelchair-bound meningomyelocele patients with significant skeletal deformity and in multiple sclerosis patients.

The proper management of incontinence depends on a nurse continence service which is properly integrated into not only the urodynamic but also the urological, gynaecological, neurological, paediatric and geriatric services.

Other Storage Phase Problems: Nocturia

Nocturia is a common and troublesome problem. Its causes are several (see Chapter 4). Treatment should be directed at the cause or causes. Where bladder outlet obstruction with associated residual urine has reduced functional capacity, then effective surgery will reduce nocturia. Similarly, effective treatment of detrusor overactively will reduce nocturia if it is responsible for that symptom. Congestive cardiac failure (CCF) is a potent cause of nocturia and is often subclinical. If CCF is the cause of nocturia there will be nocturnal polyuria (more than one-third of urine produced during the eight night hours). If nocturnal polyuria is due to cardiac dysfunction then synthetic antidiuretic hormone (DDAVP) should not be used; treatment should aim to induce a relative diuresis in the second half of the day so that the patient goes to bed without oedema fluid. It should be remembered that at least a litre of oedema fluid must be present in the legs before it is clinically obvious. We use frusemide in a dose of at least 40 mg given at teatime (approximately 4 PM to 6 PM). DDAVP is useful in nocturia if there is no other obvious cause and may help in patients with detrusor over-activity: care should be taken in the elderly because of its potential for causing fluid reten-tion, resulting in a low serum sodium.

Management of Voiding Problems

Voiding problems may be due to bladder outlet obstruction (BOO) or to detrusor underac-tivity (DUA). Most patients with BOO are male, although neurological conditions cause outlet obstruction in both males and females.

Bladder Outlet Obstruction

BOO either can be due to anatomical causes or may result from a functional obstruction to the bladder outlet. Treatment may be demanded by a variety of anatomical causes, for example in a child with a congenital abnormality such as urethral valves, a young man with a stricture or an elderly man who has developed acute retention of urine. However most causes of BOO present with symptoms which can be managed conservatively, medically or by surgery.

Conservative Management

This may consist of:

- General advice such as regulation of the volume, type and timing of fluids.
- Bladder training: If BOO is associated with symptoms of detrusor overactivity, for example, urgency incontinence, then bladder training may be very helpful.
- Catheterisation: if the patient is unfit or unwilling to have definitive treatment then either intermittent self-catheterisation or an indwelling catheter can be used to allow proper bladder drainage when the residual urine is having a deleterious effect on LUTS.

Medical Therapy

If conservative treatment has failed after a reasonable trial period of three months then medical treatment can be considered. There are only two classes of drug that have been shown to be effective:

- *Alpha-adrenergic blocking agents.* These drugs act on alpha-receptors at the bladder neck, in the prostatic capsule and in the prostatic stoma.

- *5-alpha-reductase inhibitors* are used when prostate volume is greater than 40ccs. The prostatic epithelial tissue shrinks when the conversion of testosterone to 5-dihydrotestosterone is blocked.

Drugs produce a moderate decrease in symptoms and some change in BOO with increased flow rates and some reduction in voiding pressure. Alpha-blockers are effective immediately, whereas 5-alpha reductase inhibitors take six months to have full effect. Although 5-alpha reductase inhibitors have little in the way of side-effects, the older alpha-blockers cause some problems by producing postural hypertension with dizziness and loss of energy. However, the newer alpha-blockers are more "prostate-specific" and have fewer side-effects. Neither class of drug has a dramatic effect and tends only to move patients from the obstructed group to the equivocal zone on the ICS pressure-flow nomogram, whereas surgery in the form of transurethral resection of the prostate (TURP) moves most obstructed patients into the unobstructed zone. There is little evidence to support the use of other classes of drugs in BOO. Plant extracts, homoeopathic remedies and aromatase inhibitors have been investigated to a limited extent: none of these drug groups shows convincing evidence of efficacy.

It has been the view that in patients with BOO and detrusor overactivity (DO) the use of antimuscarinic drugs is dangerous. There is little evidence for this view and a careful trial of an antimuscarinic in 200 men with BOO and DO has shown no significant differences between the treated group and those receiving placebo.

Surgical Treatment

For BOO, surgery is the most effective treatment in reducing symptoms and obtaining relief of outlet obstruction. When there is a stricture then optical urethrotomy and urethroplasty in the male and urethral dilatation in the female are the treatments of choice. In the largest group of patients, the older males with BPO, there has been great interest in alternative methods of treating BPO in particular. Whilst (TURP) (see above) remains "*le beau idéal*", a number of other options have been assessed:

- Laser prostatectomy (LAP); techniques include non-contact and contact side-firing, interstitial laser therapy, and holmium laser resection
- High-intensity focused ultrasound (HIFU).
- Transurethral needle ablation (TUNA) using high-frequency radio waves.
- Thermotherapy (TUMT), hypothermia and thermal ablation: these methods deliver microwave energy to the prostate from a urethral source.

Transurethral incision of the prostate (TUIP) is rather better established and is useful in small glands (less than 30 ml). Bladder neck obstruction is quickly and easily dealt with by bladder neck incision (BNI) and it seems unlikely that laser incisions have more to offer.

Prostatic stenting and prostatic dilatation have been used but have few real indications. If patients are unfit then LAP offers a "blood-free" and safe alternative to TURP. The ultimate place of therapies such as laser prostatectomy, HIFU, TUNA and TUMT remain to be defined. It is safe to say that, at present, none of these techniques with the exception of holmium laser prostatectomy, has the ability to reduce symptoms and relieve obstruction as effectively as TURP.

Treatment of Functional Obstruction

Functional causes of BOO are a good deal less common than anatomical causes, and functional BOO is generally associated with neurological disease (see Chapter 5), but there are two small but important groups of patients with no neurological signs who have voiding dysfunction:

- Dysfunctional voiding due to pelvic floor overactivity is normally seen in children (see Chapter 5). Its treatment is by biofeedback using either the flow traces or perineal surface electromyography. The patient by understanding the mechanism of their interrupted stream learns to relax the pelvic floor during voiding.
- Idiopathic urinary retention (Fowler's Syndrome): this syndrome is usually seen in women 20 to 40 years of age and often results in the inability to void. At present there are no effective curative treatments and management is usually by intermittent self-catheterisation, although sacral neuromodulation is proving successful in the majority of women with this condition.

As discussed in Chapter 5, two relatively common conditions produce functional BOO in neurological patients:

- Detrusor-sphincter dyssynergia, classically seen in spinal cord injury patients and in multiple sclerosis.
- Non-relaxing urethral sphincter obstruction: this is found in meningomyelocele patients and in patients after radical pelvic surgery associated with denervation (for example, after Wertheim's hysterectomy or abdominoperineal resection of the rectum).
Treatments of functional BOO can be classed as conservative, medical or surgical.

Conservative Therapies

These include biofeedback as described above, and catheterisation. ISC is used when possible, but in some patients an indwelling catheter will be necessary. ISC has revolutionised the management of functional BOO. It can be used by both sexes and all ages. If the patient is too young or too disabled then intermittent catheterisation can be performed by the parent, relative or carer. The technique is remarkably free of complications, although urinary infections can be a problem in the first few weeks, and this has led clinicians to prescribe low-dose antibiotics for the first four to eight weeks of ISC.

Medical Therapy

This is rarely successful, although alpha-adrenergic blockers have been used in spinal cord injury patients. Occasionally women with idiopathic urinary retention benefit from alpha-blocker therapy and a trial of treatment is worth while, particularly if it means avoiding the need for ISC.

Surgical Therapy

This was formerly the routine for functional obstructions: meningomyelocele girls were diverted and boys were subjected to urethral sphincterotomy. These procedures were usually performed for intractable incontinence or because of recurrent infections and or upper tract deterioration. With the advent of intermittent self-catheterisation (ISC) most surgical interventions can be avoided. Nevertheless, there is still a small place for surgery when patients are unable to perform ISC and have problems with indwelling catheters (either urethral or suprapubic). The ileal conduit is still appropriate in some patients, although an alternative is offered by the Mitrofanoff procedure, in which the bladder or augmented bladder is joined to the anterior abdominal wall by a conduit fashioned from appendix, small bowel, fallopian tube or ureter. Instead of performing ISC through the urethra the patient can catheterise using the Mitrofanoff stoma.

Some reputable centres perform VY plasty of the bladder neck if video studies show that the bladder neck fails to open and if the patient is unhappy to do ISC.

Treatment of Detrusor Underactivity

Detrusor underactivity (DUA) occurs in patients both with and without neurological disease. In men the symptom complex in patients with DUA is indistinguishable from that suffered by patients with BOO. In the neurological patients it is common for DUA, to occur in combination with neurogenic detrusor overactivity during filling, and BOO due to sphincter overactivity during voiding. DUA can be managed as follows:

- Conservative therapy is possible if there are no complications and the patient's symptoms are not troublesome. However if symptoms or complications occur and there is significant post-void residual urine (PVR) then ISC and the other measures discussed under the section on management of BOO may be required.

- Medical therapy aimed at increasing detrusor activity, for example by cholinergic drugs, is not effective. Some believe that DUA may be secondary to sphincter overactivity and would use alpha-adrenergic blockers to try to improve sphincter relaxation and thereby enhance bladder emptying.

- Surgical therapy can be considered if there is evidence of significant PVR and conservative therapy has failed. However there is little evidence that surgery will improve voiding function in men with DUA, although it is possible that bladder neck incision, prostatic incision or TURP may improve voiding by allowing more effective straining.

Management of Post-Micturition Symptoms

Post-micturition dribble (PMD) is a common symptom in elderly men but is not due to BOO. PMD is due to urine left in the bulbous and penile urethra, at the end of micturition. This urine dribbles out and wets the underpants and occasionally the trousers after the man has dressed and left the toilet. Treatment is by explaining the cause and by suggesting that the man takes a little more care and time in voiding. If this fails to work, pelvic floor exercises help, as they lead to contraction of the periurethral musculature. Finally the patient should be taught how to manually express the subsphincteric urethra by exerting upward perineal pressure and slowly moving the pressure point down the urethra towards the tip of the penis.

This chapter has attempted to provide a frame work of management of LUTD, but readers are advised to consult other texts aiming more directly at treatment rather than investigation such as the ICI books.

References

Abrams P (1994). Managing lower urinary tract symptoms in older men. Br Med J 310:1113–1118.

Anthuber C, Pigny A, Schussler B, Lacock J, Norton P, Stanton S. editors (1994). Pelvic floor re-education. Principles and practice, first edn 4.4.3. Clinical results neuromuscular electrical stimulation. London: Springer-Verlag pp 163–167.

Bakke A, Brun OH, Høisæter PA (1992). Clinical background of patients treated with clean intermittent catheterisation in Norway. Scand J Urol Nephrol 26:211–217.

Fall M, Lindstrøm S (1991). Electrical stimulation. A physiologic approach to the treatment of urinary incontinence. Urol Clin N Am 18:393–407.

Fantl JA, Wyman JF, McClish DK et al. (1991). Efficacy of bladder training in older women with urinary incontinence. JAMA 256:609.

Frewin WK (1979). Role of bladder training in the treatment of the unstable bladder in the female. Urol Clin N Am 6:273.

Kegel AH (1951). Physiologic therapy for urinary incontinence. JAMA 146:915–917.

Peattie AB, Plevnick S, Stanton SL (1988). Vaginal cones: a conservative method of treating genuine stress incontinence. Br J Obstet Gynaecol 95:1049.

Swami SK, Abrams P (1996). Urge incontinence. Urol Clin N Am II 23:417–426.

The Third Edition of Incontinence (2005). Eds. Abrams P, Cardozo L, Khoury S, Wein A. Health Publications Ltd. Editions 21-76, rue de la Pompe, 75116 Paris (+33 1 45 03 31 96; FAX: +33 1 45 72 89; e-mail: progress.urologie@wanadoo-fr. Also available through www. amazon.com.

Wilson PD, Samarrai TA, Deakin M, Kolbe E, Brown ADG (1987). An objective assessment of physiotherapy for female genuine stress incontinence. Br J Obstet Gynaecol 94:575–582.

Chapter 7
Organisation of the Urodynamic Unit

The urodynamic unit must respond to the need for patient investigation from a variety of sources and must ensure that the studies are carried out to a consistently high standard. There is a need for three levels of urodynamic investigation:

- Basic urodynamics, including urine flow studies, filling cystometry, pressure-flow studies and pad testing.
- Advanced urodynamics, including urethral pressure profilometry and video-urodynamics.
- Complex urodynamics, including ambulatory urodynamics and neurophysiological testing.

The requirements for each level is different, although all have common needs:

- Secretarial staff
- Technical/nursing support
- Medical physics backing
- Medical involvement
- Urodynamic records system

The basic organisation of our department can be illustrated by tracing a patient through the department.

Patient Referral

After reviewing the referral letter from the patient's general practitioner (family physician) or specialist, the patient is assigned to either the urgent category or the routine list. The patient details are entered into the patient administration system of the hospital if the patient has not yet received a hospital number. The recorded details are shown on the front sheet of the patient's urodynamic data proforma (Appendix 3, Part 1).

Making the Patient's Appointment

The individual patient's requirements are assessed so that an appointment of appropriate length and timing can be given. Appointment lengths are:

- *60 minutes:* for routine appointments for either basic or advanced UDS in the neurologically normal patient.
- *90 minutes:* for advanced UDS in neurological or disabled patients and children.
- *120 minutes:* for complex UDS and for ambulatory UDS. The patient is warned they need to set aside 2 to 4 hours for the appointment.

For male patients who have not had screening uroflow in the referring centre, a morning appointment is made for the flow clinic and a 60-minute appointment for urodynamics in the afternoon. Female patients in whom there is a possibility that ambulatory studies (AUDS) may be needed are often investigated by video UDS in the morning with a provisional appointment for AUDS in the afternoon. If patients have to travel some distance to reach us then a late morning appointment is given.

All patients are sent a seven-day frequency-volume chart (Appendix 2, Part 1) for completion before attending their appointment. We offer appointments four weeks in advance and if the patient does not confirm the appointment, then it is offered by telephone to another patient. In the British system we have a problem with "no-shows" or "DNAs" (did-not-attends) as we call them: by insisting on confirmation of appointment we have significantly increased our efficiency.

For the urine flow clinic the patient is also sent a frequency-volume chart with their clinic appointment. Both urodynamic patients and flow clinic patients are sent information leaflets (Appendix 3, Part 1) which describe the investigations. All patients are sent the relevant information sheet (Appendix 2, Part 2).

The Patient's Hospital Attendance

On arrival the patient presents at the clinic reception and the urodynamic technician or flow clinic nurse is informed.

Urodynamic Studies

The patient is shown to the urodynamic room where the technician describes the test procedure to the patient, emphasising the points raised in the information leaflet. The following sequence is then followed:

- *Urodynamic history.* We use a standard proforma which can be entered into our computer database either online or offline. We have computer terminals in each urodynamic room (Fig. 7.1, *overleaf*). The screens on the terminal follow the urodynamics answer sheet (Appendix 3, Part 2). If the clinician is unfamiliar with the computer system then he or she can complete an answer sheet and the technician will enter the data into the database later that day. A master questionnaire (Appendix 3, Part 1) is available in each room to aid the clinician if necessary.
- After the history has been taken, the patient undresses.

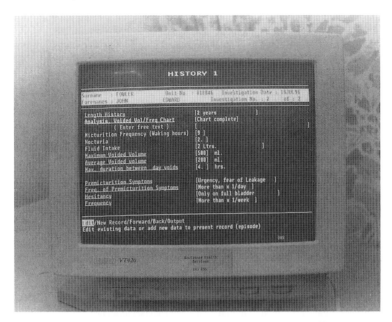

Fig. 7.1 Computer terminal within the urodynamic room. 📖

- *Urodynamic examination.* The examination as detailed in Chapter 3 is carried out and the findings entered into the computer or on the answer sheet.
- *Urodynamic investigations.* After the investigations the technician analyses the urodynamic traces and enters the urodynamic data into the computer.
- *Urodynamic report generation.* The doctor is given the skeleton urodynamic report (Fig. 7.2) by the technician so that the clinical information from the history and physical examination can be entered into the upper part of the report form while the urodynamic findings, management recommendations and arrangements for follow-up are detailed in the lower part of the report. The report is sent to the referring clinicians as well as other relevant doctors including the family physician (GP) and other appropriate persons such as the continence advisor.
- After completing the test the patient dresses and then the physician explains the finding of the tests to the patient, outlining the suggested management plan which will be communicated to the patient's doctor.

Urine Flow Clinic

We set up the flow clinic because of an awareness that we were often unable to get patients to do a flow study in the regular outpatients: usually the patient did not expect to be in the outpatients for more than half an hour and as we also wanted urine for microscopy and culture they were not prepared to stay for an additional test. As with UDS we follow a set protocol:

- Patients are sent their appointment 3 to 4 weeks in advance together with a frequency-volume chart.

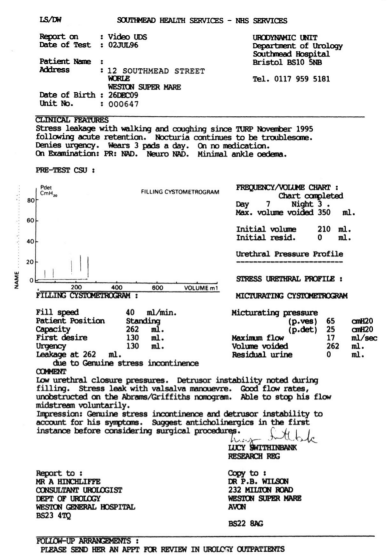

LS/DW   SOUTHMEAD HEALTH SERVICES - NHS SERVICES

Report on   : Video UDS   URODYNAMIC UNIT
Date of Test   : 02JUL96   Department of Urology
                                                  Southmead Hospital
Patient Name   :   Bristol BS10 5NB
Address   : 12 SOUTHMEAD STREET
                 WORLE   Tel. 0117 959 5181
                 WESTON SUPER MARE
Date of Birth : 26DEC09
Unit No.   : 000647

CLINICAL FEATURES
Stress leakage with walking and coughing since TURP November 1995
following acute retention. Nocturia continues to be troublesome.
Denies urgency. Wears 3 pads a day. On no medication.
On Examination: PR: NAD. Neuro NAD. Minimal ankle oedema.

PRE-TEST CSU :

FILLING CYSTOMETROGRAM

FREQUENCY/VOLUME CHART :
                    Chart completed
Day   7   Night 3 .
Max. volume voided 350   ml.

Initial volume   210   ml.
Initial resid.   0   ml.

Urethral Pressure Profile

STRESS URETHRAL PROFILE :

FILLING CYSTOMETROGRAM :   MICTURATING CYSTOMETROGRAM

Fill speed   40   ml/min.   Micturating pressure
Patient Position   Standing   (p.ves)   65   cmH20
Capacity   262 ml.   (p.det)   25   cmH20
First desire   130 ml.   Maximum flow   17   ml/sec
Urgency   130 ml.   Volume voided   262 ml.
Leakage at 262 ml.   Residual urine   0   ml.
     due to Genuine stress incontinence
COMMENT
Low urethral closure pressures. Detrusor instability noted during
filling. Stress leak with valsalva manouevre. Good flow rates,
unobstructed on the Abrams/Griffiths nomogram. Able to stop his flow
midstream voluntarily.
Impression: Genuine stress incontinence and detrusor instability to
account for his symptoms. Suggest anticholinergics in the first
instance before considering surgical procedures.
                                       LUCY SWITHINBANK
                                       RESEARCH REG

Report to :   Copy to :
MR A HINCHLIFFE   DR P.B. WILSON
CONSULTANT UROLOGIST   232 MILTON ROAD
DEPT OF UROLOGY   WESTON SUPER MARE
WESTON GENERAL HOSPITAL   AVON
BS23 4TQ
                                       BS22 8AG

FOLLOW-UP ARRANGEMENTS :
PLEASE SEND HER AN APPT FOR REVIEW IN UROLOGY OUTPATIENTS

Fig. 7.2 Completed urodynamic report form. ▢

- The patient is asked to drink normally at home on the day of the appointment.
- On arrival at the hospital the patient is shown the flow room and the tests are explained.
- The first flow is taken when the patient has a comfortably full bladder – or in other words is getting slightly uncomfortable!
- Soft drinks or water are provided at the clinic and the patient is encouraged to drink.
- Three flow studies are recorded, with post-void residual urines measured by ultrasound.
- Report preparation: the flow results and PVR volumes are presented on one of three flow nomograms, for men under the age of 50 years, men over 50, or women (Fig. 7.3) (see "Uroflowmetry" in Chapter 3).

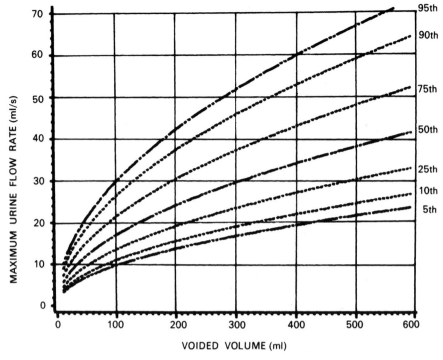

Fig. 7.3 Liverpool nomogram for women. 📖

If the patient has not been seen in the urology outpatients then the flow clinic appointment is arranged to coincide with the relevant urological clinic allowing the patient a single hospital visit. Flow clinic appointments for morning urology clinics are made for 9 AM and those for afternoon urology clinics at 11 AM.

Planning a New Urodynamic Service

Since the first edition of this book, urodynamics has become widely accepted and established in most centres in western countries. In some centres the organisation is suboptimal and below are suggestions for the basic structures that will determine the shape of a new unit.

What size of population will you serve? There is little point in establishing a unit if there are units in surrounding areas offering an efficient and comprehensive service. If your hospital serves a population of 250 000, then it is likely that you will need to perform basic urodynamics on six patients per week and flow studies on 12 to 15 patients per week.

What investigations do you plan to offer? Again the breadth of services will depend on existing services in surrounding areas and on the population you serve. It is probably unnecessary to offer advanced urodynamics (video-urodynamics etc.) unless the referrals for urodynamics amount to the equivalent of 15 patients per week. If there are 30 urodynamic referrals per week then complex urodynamics should be offered.

Where will you do the urodynamic studies? This will depend on the quantity and type of studies you offer. Our urodynamic unit is a separate part of a specialised urology outpatients. All patients – children, women and men – attend our unit with referrals from all specialities. If you do not have your own outpatient building then it may be more convenient to have the urodynamic unit close to the urology or gynaecology ward. Other suitable sites are in continence care areas or clinical investigation units which might also offer investigations, such as gastrointestinal studies and cardiac tests. Videourodynamics must be done either in the X-ray department or in a suitably screened room, in outpatients or on the ward, if an image intensifier is used. If imaging is by ultrasound then these limitations do not apply.

Above all, a friendly sympathetic atmosphere with proper privacy for the patient must be offered.

The unit must have:

- Changing facilities: these may be a curtained area in the investigation room (Fig. 7.4, *below*).
- Sluicing facilities for disposal of urine and occasional faeces (Fig. 7.5, *overleaf*).
- Adequate storage space for catheters, catheter packs and other essential items.

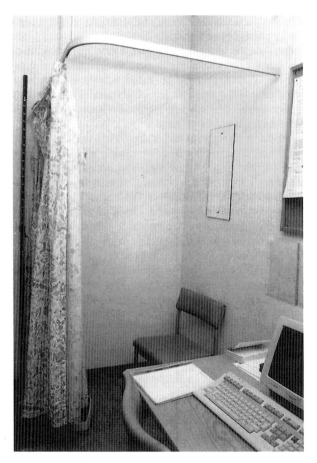

Fig. 7.4 Changing facilities: a curtained-off area of the investigation room. 📖

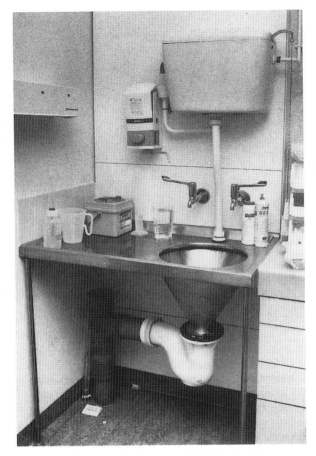

Fig. 7.5 Sluice for disposing of body fluids. 📖

- Adequate space for the urodynamic table, commode and equipment. The minimum size for basic urodynamics is 20 square metres and for video-urodynamics 30 square metres; Fig. 7.6 shows why a relatively large room is needed.
- Waiting area for patients.

It is highly desirable to have the urodynamic area solely for urodynamic use. This enables the equipment to be left ready for use with tests being done at times convenient for the patients and staff: this also allows a more relaxed approach to UDS. If the studies have to be done in shared space then there is pressure to complete the tests at a set time, resulting in an incomplete test if more time is needed than was appreciated. Similarly, if UDS are done in the X-ray department then it is necessary to fit into the timetable of the X-ray department where the expensive equipment and limited number of rooms demand highly efficient usage. UDS are an investigation that demands sensitivity and privacy and everything should be done to ensure that these quality issues are addressed.

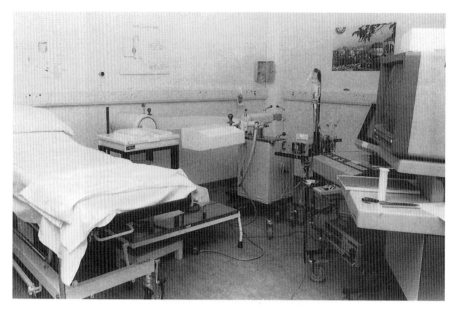

Fig. 7.6 Videourodynamics room. 📖

Who will perform the urodynamic studies? We believe that a doctor must be involved in the urodynamic investigations and that technical assistance is also required. The doctor has to be suitably qualified and suitably trained. The best units have a variety of medical input:

- There should be a consultant (specialist) who leads, providing the link between investigation and therapy.
- In large units permanent medical staff should provide a continuity that ensures good quality control for the studies and enables doctors coming to the department to receive proper training in urodynamic theory and technique.
- Training-grade doctors may perform many of the tests in departments that are large or in small departments if the consultant is too busy to perform all UDS him or herself. Herein lies a danger, because relatively inexperienced doctors require supervision for several months before they are able to report reliably on the urodynamic findings.

In many departments the key personnel will be the technicians or nurses who assist with the tests and, like the consultant or other permanent staff, provide a continuity that allows the maintenance of an efficient and effective unit.

Who should assist at urodynamics? It is probably not important whether it is a nurse or a technician. The nurse brings the advantages of training, whilst the technician brings technical background into an investigation area where this is vital. Our unit started with technicians only but now has a mixture of nurses and technicians. As medicine has become more complex most recently trained nurses are very comfortable with urodynamic apparatus. The principle responsibilities of the nurse/technician are to:

- Maintain and calibrate the urodynamic equipment.
- Ensure proper standards of cleanliness and sterility.
- Be responsible for the general care of patients.

- Work the urodynamic equipment during UDS.
- Analyse the urodynamic tracing and prepare the report.
- Be responsible for restocking the urodynamic room with disposables, catheters, infusion fluids and sterile gloves, and so on.
- Liaise with the medical physics department.

In our department all the technicians and nurses have been women. This has arisen from the need to have a female to chaperone female patients when the investigating clinician is male.

What record system should be used? We have always kept our own records and now have 25 000 urodynamic patient files in our secretarial area. These files are separate from the general hospital patient record files. Hence we can obtain urodynamic records without delay. The urodynamic record files contain:

- The referral letter.
- The completed frequency-volume chart.
- The urodynamic tracing.
- The urodynamic report.

In addition the records may contain the urodynamic data sheet if the details of patient history, examination and urodynamic findings were put into the computer database offline.

Several of the new computer-based systems have a database and report generation capacity. It is useful if the system can link into the hospital patient administration system so that double data entry can be avoided. This should become possible with the increasing flexibility of computer systems and software and with the refocusing of these systems on the user rather than the organisation.

What equipment should you buy? The decision as to which system to buy depends on a number of factors:

- First decide what range of urodynamic tests will be offered.
- It is wise to involve the medical physics department of your hospital whose help can prove invaluable at times of crisis.
- It is sensible to talk to and visit colleagues who are using the equipment you wish to buy.
- Attend meetings which have trade exhibitions, because you will be able to have a demonstration and to handle the equipment on the commercial stand.
- Establish what service facility the company can offer. In a busy department losing a machine for a week, due to a breakdown, is a disaster!
- Ask for a demonstration in your own hospital so that you can invite colleagues including medical physics staff to see the equipment.
- Lastly make a cost-benefit assessment, going for reliability and service rather than equipment with a myriad of computer functions you are unlikely to use. The computerisation of urodynamics has brought problems as well as benefits. Computers allow the manipulation of data, but this facility can be a weakness as well as a strength. The raw data must be accurate and relevant to that patient: if it is not then any manipulation of data for the purpose of diagnosis, as in pressure-flow studies, will lead to the wrong diagnosis and possibly to inappropriate management. The key data points must be verified before computer programmes are used for diagnosis.

What relationships should exist with other departments? The urodynamic unit is a service department for other departments. However as discussed above, the lead specialist and permanent doctors will have or will develop the skills to advise on management. The important relationships will be with:

- Urology, which provides more than 50% of our referrals. In particular the flow clinic is largely used by male patients.
- Gynaecology, the next largest referral source. The former director of our unit is a gynaecologist and she established excellent relationships with the neighbouring departments of gynaecology.
- Paediatrics, since an increasing source of referrals come from paediatric urologists, paediatric surgeons (for example problems associated with anorectal anomalies), paediatricians, and paediatric nephrologists (with referrals of children who may have a lower urinary tract cause for renal impairment).
- Neurology/neurosurgery, which refers a significant number of patients with proven or suspected neurological abnormalities associated with vesicourethral dysfunction.
- Geriatrics, a declining primary source of referral, and we have found it useful to screen the elderly in outpatients before requesting UDS.
- Gastro-enterology, and in particular surgeons with an interest in lower bowel dysfunction, who are moving into closer relationships with urodynamic units. They are forming collaborative links with gynaecologists and urologists interested in pelvic floor function. In our department ano-rectal measurements are carried out by our technicians with the colo-rectal surgeon.
- Nephrology, particularly where patients have renal failure which cannot clearly be attributed to intrinsic renal disease, and who often need to be assessed urodynamically prior to being transplanted.
- Radiology, an important link because it is often necessary to organise additional tests such as urethrography, micturating cystourethrography, pyelography and isotope scanning (DMSA and MAG 3 renography)
- Medical physics, who are useful friends and allies both for emergencies and for basic maintenance and problem-solving. They can also be useful in discussion with the equipment manufacturers.

The Investigating and Therapeutic Team

In terms of therapy the team approach should be continued and should consist of:
- Nurse Continence care staff under the direction of the nurse continence adviser.
- A specialist physiotherapist.
- A urologist.
- A paediatric urologist.
- A gynaecologist.
- A colo-rectal surgeon.

The facilities should exist for joint outpatient sessions and joint operating lists where necessary.

Summary of Equipment Needs

Basic Urodynamics

Uroflow

- Uroflowmeter, commode, examination couch, ultrasound machine.
    - Private room with lockable door (Fig. 3.3).
    - Nurse/technician.

Pressure-Flow Studies

- Uroflowmeter, examination couch, commode, transducer stand, basic urodynamic equipment with transducers and infusion pump.
    - Room with 20 square metres of floor area (Fig. 7.7).
    - Doctor plus nurse/technician.

Advanced Urodynamics (Additional Requirements)

- Imaging apparatus (image intensifier, fixed X-ray unit or ultrasound machine). Motorised withdrawal pump for urethral pressure profilometry. Advanced urodynamic equipment.
    - Room with 30 square metres of floor area (Fig. 7.6).
    - Radiographer if studies performed in the X-ray department.

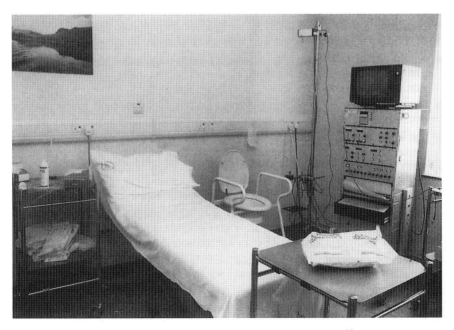

Fig. 7.7 Urodynamics room for basic pressure-flow tests.

Complex Urodynamics (Additional Requirements)

- Electrophysiological equipment. Ambulatory urodynamic equipment.
  – Input from neurophysiologist/neurologist.

Appendix 1, Part 1
List of ICS Standardisation Committee Reports 1973 to 2002

1. Report on Urodynamic Equipment, Technical Aspects.
   Rowan D, James ED, Kramer AEJL, Sterling AM, Suhel PF.
   J Med Eng Technol 11(2):57-64 (1987)

2. The Standardisation of Terminology of lower urinary tract function.
   Abrams P, Blaivas JG, Stanton S, Andersen JT.
   Neurourol Urodyn 7:403-26 (1988)

3. Lower Urinary Tract Rehabilitation Techniques: Seventh Report on the Standardisation of Terminology of Lower Urinary Tract Function.
   Andersen JT, Blaivas JG, Cardozo L, Thüroff J.
   Neurourol Urodyn 11:593-603 (1992)

4. The Standardisation of Terminology of Female Pelvic Organ Prolapse and Pelvic Floor Dysfunction.
   Bump RC, Mattiasson A, Bo K, Brubaker LP, DeLancey JOL, Klarskov P, Shull BL, Smith ARB.
   Am J Obstet Gynecol 175:10-1 (1996)

5. The Standardisation of Terminology and Assessment of Functional Characteristics of Intestinal Reservoirs.
   Joachim W, Thòroff J, Mattiasson A, Thorup Andersen J, Hedlund H, Hinman F, Hohenfellner M, Mµnsson W, Mundy AB, Rowland RG, Steven K.
   Neurourol Urodyn 15:499-511 (1996)

6. The Standardisation of Terminology in Lower Urinary Tract Function: Pressure-Flow Studies of Voiding, Urethral Resistance and Urethral Obstruction.
   Griffiths D, HØfner K, van Mastrigt R, Rollema HJ, Spangberg A, Gleason D.
   Neurourol Urodyn 16:521-532 (1997)

7. Standardisation of Outcome Studies in Patients with Lower Urinary Tract Dysfunction: a report on general principles.
   Mattiasson A, Djurhuus JC, Fonda D, Lose G, Nordling J, StØhrer M.
   Neurourol Urodyn 17:249-253 (1998)

8. Outcome Measures for Research in Adult Women with Symptoms of Lower Urinary Tract Dysfunction.
   Lose G, Fantl JA, Victor A, Walter S, Wells TL, Wyman J, Mattiasson A.
   Neurourol Urodyn 17:255-262 (1998)

9. Outcome Measures for research of Lower Urinary Tract Dysfunction in Frail and Older People.
   Fonda D, Resnick NM, Colling J, Burgio K, Ouslander JG, Norton C, Ekelund P, Versi E, Mattiasson A.
   Neurourol Urodyn 17:273-281

10. Outcome Measures for Research in Treatment of Adult Males with Symptoms of Lower Urinary Tract Dysfunction.
    Nordling J, Abrams P, Ameda K, Andersen JT, Donovan J, Griffiths D, Kobayashi S, Koyanagi T, Schafer W, Yalla S, Mattiasson A.
    Neurourol Urodyn 17:263-271 (1998)

11. The Standardisation of Terminology in Neurogenic Lower Urinary Tract Dysfunction.
    StØhrer M, Goepel M, Kondo A, Kramer G, Madersbacher H, Millard R, Rossier A, Wyndaele JJ.
    Neurourol Urodyn 18:139-158 (1999)

12. The Standardisation of Ambulatory Urodynamic Monitoring.
    van Waalwijk van Doorn E, Anders K, Khullar V, Kulseng Hansen S, Pesce F, Robertson A, Rosario D, Schafer W.
    Neurourol Urodyn 19:113-125 (2000)

13. The Standardisation of Terminology in Lower Urinary Tract Function.
    Abrams P, Cardozo L, Fall M, Griffiths D, Rosier P, Ulmsten U, van Kerrebroeck P, Victor A, Wein A.
    Neurourol Urodyn 21:167-178 (2002)

14. The Standardisation of Terminology in Nocturia.
    van Kerrebroeck P, Abrams P, Chaikin D, Donovan J, Fonda D, Jackson S, Jennum P, Johnson T, Lose G, Mattiasson A, Robertson G, Weiss J.
    Neurourol Urodyn 21:179-183 (2002)

15. The Standardisation of Urethral Pressure Measurement.
    Lose G, Griffiths D, Hosker G, Kulseng-Hanssen S, Perucchini D, Schafer W, Thind P, Versi E.
    Neurourol Urodyn 2002;21(3):258-60

16. Report on Good Urodynamic Practice
    Schafer W, Abrams P, Liao L, Mattiasson A, Pesce F, Spangberg A, Sterling AM, Zinner NR, van Kerrebroeck P.
    Neurourol Urodyn 2002;21(3):261-74

Appendix 1, Part 2
The Standardisation of Terminology of Female Pelvic Organ Prolapse and Pelvic Floor Dysfunction

Am J Obstet Gynec (1996) 175:10–17
Richard C. Bump, Anders Mattiasson, Kari Bø, Linda P. Brubaker, John O. L. DeLancey, Peter Klarskov, Bob L. Shull and Anthony R. B. Smith
Produced by the International Continence Society Committee on Standardisation of Terminology (Anders Mattiasson, chairman), Subcommittee on Pelvic Organ Prolapse and Pelvic Floor Dysfunction (Richard Bump, chairman) in collaboration with the American Urogynecologic Society and the Society of Gynecologic Surgeons.

Condensation

A system of standard terminology for the description and evaluation of pelvic organ prolapse and pelvic floor dysfunction, adopted by several professional societies, is presented.

1. Introduction

The International Continence Society (ICS) has been at the forefront in the standardisation of terminology of lower urinary tract function since the establishment of the Committee on Standardisation of Terminology in 1973. This committee's efforts over the past two decades have resulted in the world-wide acceptance of terminology standards that allow clinicians and researchers interested in the lower urinary tract to communicate efficiently and precisely. While female pelvic organ prolapse and pelvic floor dysfunction are intimately related to lower urinary tract function, such accurate communication using standard terminology has not been possible for these conditions since there has been no universally accepted system for describing the anatomic position of the pelvic organs. Many reports use terms for the description of pelvic organ prolapse which are undefined; none of the many aspiring grading systems has been adequately validated with respect either to reproducibility or to the clinical significance of different grades. The absence of standard, validated definitions prevents comparisons of published series from different institutions and longitudinal evaluation of an individual patient.

In 1993, an international, multidisciplinary committee composed of members of the ICS, the American Urogynecologic Society (AUGS), and Society of Gynecologic Surgeons (SGS) drafted this standardisation document following the committee's initial meeting at the ICS meeting in Rome. In late 1994 and early 1995, the final draft was circulated to members of all three societies for a one-year review and trial. During that year several minor revisions were made and reproducibility studies in six centres in the United States and Europe were completed, documenting the inter- and intrarater reliability and clinical utility of the system in 240 women.[1-5] The standardisation document was formally adopted by the ICS in October 1995, by the AUGS in January 1996, and by the SGS in March 1996. The goal of this report is to introduce the system to clinicians and researchers.

Acknowledgement of these standards in written publications and scientific presentations should be indicated in the Methods Section with the following statement: "Methods, definitions and descriptions conform to the standards recommended by the International Continence Society except where specifically noted."

2. Description of Pelvic Organ Prolapse

The clinical description of pelvic floor anatomy is determined during the physical examination of the external genitalia and vaginal canal. The details of the examination technique are not dictated by this document but authors should precisely describe their technique. Segments of the lower reproductive tract will replace such terms as "cystocele, rectocele, enterocele, or urethrovesical junction" because these terms may imply an unrealistic certainty as to the structures on the other side of the vaginal bulge particularly in women who have had previous prolapse surgery.

2.1. Conditions of the Examination

It is critical that the examiner sees and describes the maximum protrusion noted by the individual during her daily activities. Criteria for the end point of the examination and the full development of the prolapse should be specified in any report. Suggested criteria for demonstration of maximum prolapse should include one or all of the following: (a) Any protrusion of the vaginal wall has become tight during straining by the patient. (b) Traction on the prolapse causes no further descent. (c) The subject confirms that the size of the prolapse and extent of the protrusion seen by the examiner is as extensive as the most severe protrusion which she has experienced. The means of this confirmation should be specified. For example, the subject may use a small hand-held mirror to visualise the protrusion. (d) A standing, straining examination confirms that the full extent of the prolapse was observed in other positions used.

Other variables of technique that should be specified during the quantitative description and ordinal staging of pelvic organ prolapse include the following: (a) the position of the subject; (b) the type of examination table or chair used; (c) the type of vaginal specula, retractors, or tractors used; (d) diagrams of any customised devices used; (e) the type (e.g., Valsalva manoeuvre, cough) and, if measured, intensity (e.g. vesical or rectal pressure) of straining used to develop the prolapse maximally; (f) fullness of bladder and, if the bladder was empty, whether this was by spontaneous voiding or by catheterisation; (g) content of rectum; (f) the method by which any quantitative measurements were made.

2.2. Quantitative Description of Pelvic Organ Position

This descriptive system is a tandem profile in that it contains a series of component measurements grouped together in combination, but listed separately in tandem, without being fused into a distinctive new expression or "grade". It allows for the precise description of an individual woman's pelvic support without assigning a "severity value". Second, it allows accurate site-specific observations of the stability or progression of prolapse over time by the same or different observers. Finally, it allows similar judgements as to the outcome of surgical repair of prolapse. For example, noting that a surgical procedure moved the leading edge of a prolapse from 0.5 cm beyond the hymeneal ring to 0.5 cm above the hymeneal ring denotes more meagre improvement than stating that the prolapse was reduced from Grade 3 to Grade 1 as would be the case using some current grading systems.

2.2.1. Definition of Anatomic Landmarks

Prolapse should be evaluated by a standard system relative to clearly defined anatomic points of reference. These are of two types, a fixed reference point and defined points which are located with respect to this reference.

(a) *Fixed Point of Reference.* Prolapse should be evaluated relative to a fixed anatomic landmark which can be consistently and precisely identified. The hymen will be the fixed point of reference used throughout this system of quantitative prolapse description. Visually, the hymen provides a precisely identifiable landmark for reference. Although it is recognised that the plane of the hymen is somewhat variable depending upon the degree of levator ani dysfunction, it remains the best landmark available. "Hymen" is preferable to the ill-defined and imprecise term "introitus". The anatomic position of the six defined points for measurement should be centimetres above or proximal to the hymen (negative number) or centimetres below or distal to the hymen (positive number) with the plane of the hymen being defined as zero (0). For example, a cervix that protruded 3 cm distal to the hymen would be +3 cm.

(b) *Defined Points*. This site-specific system has been adapted from several classifications developed and modified by Baden and Walker.[6] Six points (two on the anterior vaginal wall, two in the superior vagina, and two on the posterior vaginal wall) are located with reference to the plane of the hymen.

Anterior Vaginal Wall. Because the only structure directly visible to the examiner is the surface of the vagina, anterior prolapse should be discussed in terms of a segment of the vaginal wall rather than the organs which lie behind it. Thus, the term "anterior vaginal wall prolapse" is preferable to "cystocele" or "anterior enterocele" unless the organs involved are identified by ancillary test two anterior sites are as follows:

Point Aa. A point located in the midline of the anterior vaginal wall three (3) cm proximal to the external urethral meatus. This corresponds to the approximate location of the "urethro-vesical crease", a visible landmark of variable prominence that is obliterated in many patients. By definition, the range of position of Point Aa relative to the hymen is –3 to + 3 cm.

Point Ba. A point that represents the most distal (i.e., most dependent) position of any part of the upper anterior vaginal wall from the vaginal cuff or anterior vaginal fornix to Point Aa. By definition, Point Ba is at -8 cm in the absence of prolapse and would have a positive value equal to the position of the cuff in women with total post-hysterectomy vaginal eversion.

Superior Vagina. These points represent the most proximal locations of the normally positioned lower reproductive tract. The two superior sites are as follows:

Point C. A point that represents either the most distal (i.e., most dependent) edge of the cervix or the leading edge of the vaginal cuff (hysterectomy scar) after total hysterectomy.

Point D. A point that represents the location of the posterior fornix (or pouch of Douglas) in a woman who still has a cervix. It represents the level of uterosacral ligament attachment to the proximal posterior cervix. It is included as a point of measurement to differentiate suspensory failure of the uterosacral-cardinal ligament complex from cervical elongation. When the location of Point C is significantly more positive than the location of Point D, this is indicative of cervical elongation which may be symmetrical or eccentric. Point D is omitted in the absence of the cervix.

Posterior Vaginal Wall. Analogous to anterior prolapse, posterior prolapse should be discussed in terms of segments of the vaginal wall rather than the organs which lie behind it. Thus, the term "posterior vaginal wall prolapse" is preferable to "rectocele" or "enterocele" unless the organs involved are identified by ancillary tests. If small bowel appears to be present in the rectovaginal space, the examiner should comment on this fact and should clearly describe the basis for this clinical impression (e.g., by observation of peristaltic activity in the distended posterior vagina, by palpation of loops of small bowel between an examining finger in the rectum and one in the vagina, etc.). In such cases, a "pulsion" addendum to the point Bp position may be noted (e.g., Bp = +5 [pulsion]; see Sections 3.1(a) and 3.1(b) for further discussion). The two posterior sites are as follows:

Point Bp. A point that represents the most distal (i.e., most dependent) position of any part of the upper posterior vaginal wall from the vaginal cuff or posterior vaginal fornix to Point Ap. By definition, Point Bp is at -3 cm in the absence of prolapse and would have a

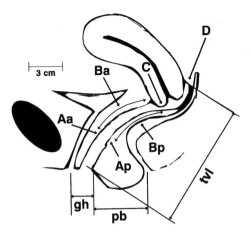

Fig. A.1.2.1 The six sites (Aa, Ba, C, D, Bp and Bp), the genital hiatus (gh), perineal body (pb) and total vaginal length (tvl) used of pelvic organ support quantitation.

positive value equal to the position of the cuff in a women with total post-hysterectomy vaginal eversion.

Point Ap. A point located in the midline of the posterior vaginal wall three (3) cm proximal to the hymen. By definition, the range of position of Point Ap relative to the hymen is -3 to +3 cm.

(c) *Other Landmarks and Measurements*. The genital hiatus (GH) is measured from the middle of the external urethral meatus to the posterior midline hymen. If the location of the hymen is distorted by a loose band of skin without underlying muscle or connective tissue, the firm palpable tissue of the perineal body should be substituted as the posterior margin for this measurement. The perineal body (PB) is measured from the posterior margin of the genital hiatus to the midanal opening. Measurements of the genital hiatus and perineal body are expressed in centimetres. The total vaginal length (TVL) is the greatest depth of the vagina in cm when Point C or D is reduced to its full normal position. *Note:* Eccentric elongation of a prolapsed anterior or posterior vaginal wall should not be included in the measurement of total vaginal length. The points and measurements are represented in Fig. A.1.2.1.

2.2.2. Making and Recording Measurements

The position of Points Aa, Ba, Ap, Bp, C, and (if applicable) D with reference to the hymen should be measured and recorded. Positions are expressed as centimetres above or proximal to the hymen (negative number) or centimetres below or distal to the hymen (positive number) with the plane of the hymen being defined as zero (0). While an examiner may be able to make measurements to the nearest half (0.5) cm, it is doubtful that further precision is possible. All reports should clearly specify how measurements were derived. Measurements may be recorded as a simple line of numbers (e.g., –3, –3, –7, –9, –3, –3, 9, 2, 2 for Points Aa, Ba, C, D, Bp, Ap, total vaginal length, genital hiatus, and perineal body respectively). Note that the last three numbers have no + or – sign attached to them because they denote lengths and not positions relative to the hymen. Alternatively, a three by three

anterior wall	anterior wall	cervix or cuff
Aa	**Ba**	**C**
genital hiatus	perineal body	total vaginal length
gh	**pb**	**tvl**
posterior wall	posterior wall	posterior fornix
Ap	**Bp**	**D**

Fig. A.1.2.2 A three-by-three grid for recording the quantitative description of pelvic organ support.

"tic-tac-toe" grid can be used to organise concisely the measurements as noted in Fig. A.1.2.2 and/or a line diagram of the configuration can be drawn as noted in Figs A.1.2.3 and A.1.2.4. Figure A.1.2.3 is a grid and line diagram contrasting measurements indicating normal support to those of post hysterectomy vaginal eversion. Figure A.1.2.4 is a grid and line diagram representing predominant anterior and posterior vaginal wall prolapse with partial vault descent.

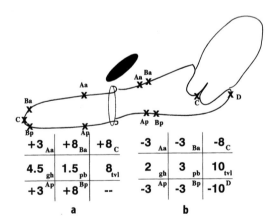

+3 (Aa)	+8 (Ba)	+8 (C)
4.5 (gh)	1.5 (pb)	8 (tvl)
+3 (Ap)	+8 (Bp)	--

a

-3 (Aa)	-3 (Ba)	-8 (C)
2 (gh)	3 (pb)	10 (tvl)
-3 (Ap)	-3 (Bp)	-10 (D)

b

Fig. A.1.2.3 a Example of a grid and line diagram of complete eversion of the vagina. The most distal point of the anterior wall (Point Ba), the vaginal cuff scar (Point C) and the most distal point of the posterior wall (Bp) are all at the same position (+8) and Points Aa and Ap are maximally distal (both at +3). The fact that the total vagina length equals the maximum protrusion makes this a Stage IV prolapse. b Example of normal support. Points Aa and Ba and Points Ap and Bp are all –3 since there is no anterior or posterior wall descent. The lowest point of the cervix is 8 cm above the hymen (–8) and the posterior fornix is 2 cm above this (–10). The vaginal length is 10 cm and the genital hiatus and perineal body measure 2 and 3 cm respectively. This represents Stage 0 support.

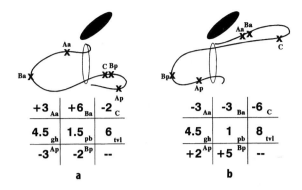

Fig. A.1.2.4 a Example of a grid and line diagram of a predominant anterior support defect. The leading point of the prolapse is the upper anterior vaginal wall, Point Ba (+6). Note that there is significant elongation of the bulging anterior wall. Point Aa is maximally distal (+3) and the vaginal cuff scar is 2 cm above the hymen (C = –2). The cuff scar has undergone 4 cm of descent since it would be at –6 (the total vaginal length) if it were perfectly supported. In this example, the total vaginal length is not the maximum depth of the vagina with the elongated anterior vaginal wall maximally reduced, but rather the depth of the vagina at the cuff with Point C reduced to its normal full extent as specified in Section 2.2.1(c). This represents Stage III-Ba prolapse. b Example of a predominant posterior support defect. The leading point of the prolapse is the upper posterior vaginal wall, Point Bp (+5). Point Ap is 2 cm distal to the hymen (+2) and the vaginal cuff scar is 6 cm above the hymen (–6). The cuff has undergone only 2 cm of descent since it would be at –8 (the total vaginal length) if it were perfectly supported. This represents Stage III-Bp prolapse.

2.3. Ordinal Stages of Pelvic Organ Prolapse

The tandem profile for quantifying prolapse provides a precise description of anatomy for individual patients. However, because of the many possible combinations, such profiles cannot be directly ranked; the many variations are too numerous to permit useful analysis and comparisons when populations are studied. Consequently they are analogous to other tandem profiles such as the TNM Index for various cancers. For the TNM description of individual patient's cancers to be useful in population studies evaluating prognosis or response to therapy, they are clustered into an ordinal set of stages. Ordinal stages represent adjacent categories that can be ranked in an ascending sequence of magnitude, but the categories are assigned arbitrarily and the intervals between them cannot be actually measured. While the committee is aware of the arbitrary nature of an ordinal staging system and the possible biases that it introduces, we conclude such a system is necessary if populations are to be described and compared, if symptoms putatively related to prolapse are to be evaluated, and if the results of various treatment options are to be assessed and compared.

Stages are assigned according to the most severe portion of the prolapse when the full extent of the protrusion has been demonstrated. In order for a stage to be assigned to an individual subject, it is essential that her quantitative description be completed first. The 2 cm buffer related to the total vaginal length in Stages 0 and IV is an effort to compensate for vaginal distensibility and the inherent imprecision of the measurement of total vaginal length. The 2 cm buffer around the hymen in Stage II is an effort to avoid confining a stage to a single plane and to acknowledge practical limits of precision in this assessment. Stages can be subgrouped according to which portion of the lower reproductive tract is the *most distal* part of the prolapse using the following letter qualifiers: a = anterior vaginal wall, p = posterior vaginal wall, C = vaginal cuff, Cx = cervix, and Aa, Ap, Ba, Bp, and D for the points of measurement already defined. The five stages of pelvic organ support (0 through IV) are as follows:

Stage 0. No prolapse is demonstrated. Points Aa, Ap, Ba, and Bp are all at -3 cm and either Point C or D is between – TVL cm and – (TVL -2) cm) (i.e., the quantitation value for point C or D is = – (TVL -2) cm). Figure 3a represents Stage 0.

Stage I. The criteria for Stage 0 are not met but the most distal portion of the prolapse is more than 1 cm above the level of the hymen (i.e., its quantitation value is < -1 cm).

Stage II. The most distal portion of the prolapse is 1 cm or less proximal to or distal to the plane of the hymen (i.e., its quantitation value is = -1 cm but = + 1 cm).

Stage III. The most distal portion of the prolapse is more than 1 cm below the plane of the hymen, but protrudes no further than two centimetres less than the total vaginal length in cm (i.e., its quantitation value is > + 1 cm but < + (TVL -2) cm). Figure A.1.4.4a represents Stage III-Ba and Figure A.1.4.4b represents Stage III-Bp prolapse.

Stage IV. Essentially complete eversion of the total length of the lower genital tract is demonstrated. The distal portion of the prolapse protrudes to at least (TVL -2) cm (i.e., its quantitation value is = + (TVL -2) cm). In most instances, the leading edge of stage IV prolapse will be the cervix or vaginal cuff scar. Figure 3B represents Stage IV-C prolapse.

3. Ancillary Techniques for Describing Pelvic Organ Prolapse

This series of procedures may help further characterise pelvic organ prolapse in an individual patient. They are considered ancillary either because they are not yet standardised or validated or because they are not universally available to all patients. Authors utilising these procedures should include the following information in their manuscripts: (a) Describe the objective information they intended to generate and how it enhanced their ability to evaluate or treat prolapse. (b) Describe precisely how the test was performed, any instruments that were used, and the specific testing conditions so that other authors can reproduce the study. (c) Document the reliability of the measurement obtained with the technique.

3.1. Supplementary Physical Examination Techniques

Many of these techniques are essential to the adequate pre-operative evaluation of a patient with pelvic organ prolapse. While they do not directly affect either the tandem profile or the ordinal stage, they are important for the selection and performance of an effective surgical repair. These techniques include, but are not necessarily limited to, the following: (a) performance of a digital rectal-vaginal examination while the patient is straining and the prolapse is maximally developed to differentiate between a high rectocele and an enterocele; (b) digital assessment of the contents of the rectal-vaginal septum during the examination noted in 3.1(a) to differentiate between a "traction" enterocele (the posterior cul-de-sac is pulled down with the prolapsing cervix or vaginal cuff but is not distended by intestines) and a "pulsion" enterocele (the intestinal contents of the enterocele distend the rectal-vaginal septum and produce a protruding mass); (c) Q-tip testing for the measurement of urethral axial mobility; (d) measurements of perineal descent; (e) measurements of the transverse diameter of the genital hiatus or of the protruding prolapse; (f) measurements of vaginal volume; (g) description and measurement of rectal prolapse; (h) examination techniques for differentiating between various types of defects (e.g., central versus paravaginal defects of the anterior vaginal wall).

3.2. Endoscopy

Cystoscopic visualisation of bowel peristalsis under the bladder base or trigone may identify an anterior enterocele in some patients. The endoscopic visualisation of the bladder base and rectum and observation of the voluntary constriction and dilation of the urethra, vagina and rectum has, to date, played a minor role in the evaluation of pelvic floor anatomy and function. When such techniques are described, authors should include the type, size and lens angle of the endoscope used, the doses of any analgesic, sedative or anaesthetic agents used, and a statement of the level of consciousness of the subjects in addition to a description of the other conditions of the examination.

3.3. Photography

Still photography of Stage II and greater prolapse may be utilised both to document serial changes in individual patients and to illustrate findings for manuscripts and presentations. Photographs should contain an internal frame of reference such as a centimetre ruler or tape.

3.4. Imaging Procedures

Different imaging techniques have been used to visualise pelvic floor anatomy, support defects and relationships among adjacent organs. These techniques may be more accurate than physical examination in determining which organs are involved in pelvic organ prolapse. However, they share the limitations of the other techniques in this section, i.e., a lack of standardisation, validation and/or availability. For this reason, no specific technique can be recommended but guidelines for reporting various techniques will be considered.

3.4.1. General Guidelines for Imaging Procedures

Landmarks should be defined to allow comparisons with other imaging studies and the physical examination. The lower edge of the symphysis pubis should be given high priority. Other examples of bony landmarks include the superior edge of the public symphysis, the ischial spine and tuberosity, the obturator foramen, the tip of the coccyx and the promontory of the sacrum. All reports on imaging techniques should specify the following: (a) position of the patient including the position of her legs; (Images in manuscripts should be oriented to reflect the patient's position when the study was performed and should not be oriented to suggest an erect position unless the patient was erect.) (b) specific verbal instructions given to the patient; (c) bladder volume and content and bowel content, including any pre-study preparations; and (d) the performance and display of simultaneous monitoring such as pressure measurements.

3.4.2. Ultrasonography

Continuous visualisation of dynamic events is possible. All reports using ultrasound should include the following information: (a) transducer type and manufacturer (e.g., sector, linear, MHz); (b) transducer size; (c) transducer orientation; and (d) route of scanning (e.g., abdominal, perineal, vaginal, rectal, urethral).

3.4.3. Contrast Radiography

Contrast radiography may be static or dynamic and may include voiding colpo-cysto-urethrography, defecography, peritoneography and pelvic fluoroscopy among others. All reports of contrast radiography should include the following information: (a) projection (e.g., lateral, frontal, horizontal, oblique); (b) type and amount of contrast media used and sequence of opacification of the bladder, vagina, rectum and colon, small bowel and peritoneal cavity; (c) any urethral or vaginal appliance used (e.g., tampon, catheter, bead-chain); (d) type of exposures (e.g., single exposure, video); and (e) magnification – an internal reference scale should be included.

3.4.4. Computed Tomography and Magnetic Resonance Imaging

These techniques do not currently allow for continuous imaging under dynamic conditions and most equipment dictates supine scanning. Specifics of the technique should be specified including: (a) the specific equipment used, including the manufacturer; (b) the plane of imaging (e.g., axial, sagittal, coronal, oblique); (c) the field of view (d) the thickness of sections and the number of slices; (e) the scan time; (f) the use and type of contrast; and (g) the type of image analysis.

3.5. Surgical Assessment

Intra-operative evaluation of pelvic support defects is intuitively attractive but as yet of unproven value. The effects of anaesthesia, diminished muscle tone and loss of consciousness are of unknown magnitude and direction. Limitations due to the position of the patient must also be evaluated.

4. Pelvic Floor Muscle Testing

Pelvic floor muscles are voluntarily controlled, but selective contraction and relaxation necessitates muscle awareness. Optimal squeezing technique involves contraction of the pelvic floor muscles without contraction of the abdominal wall muscles and without a Valsalva manoeuvre. Squeezing synergists are the intraurethral and anal sphincteric muscles. In normal voiding, defecation and optimal abdominal-strain voiding, the pelvic floor is relaxed, while the abdominal wall and the diaphragm may contract. With coughs and sneezes and often when other stresses are applied, the pelvic floor and abdominal wall are contracted simultaneously.

Evaluation and measurement of pelvic floor muscle function includes (1) an assessment of the patient's ability to contract and relax the pelvic muscles selectively (i.e., squeezing without abdominal straining and vice versa) and (2) measurement of the force (strength) of contraction. There are pitfalls in the measurement of pelvic floor muscle function because the muscles are invisible to the investigator and because patients often simultaneously and erroneously activate other muscles. Contraction of the abdominal, gluteal and hip adductor muscles, Valsalva manoeuvre, straining, breath holding and forced inspirations are typically seen. These factors affect the reliability of available testing modalities and have to be taken into consideration in the interpretation of these tests.

The individual types of tests cited in this report are based both on the scientific literature and on current clinical practice. It is the intent of the committee neither to endorse specific tests or techniques nor to restrict evaluations to the examples given. The standards recommended are intended to facilitate comparison of results obtained by different investigators and to allow investigators to replicate studies precisely. For all types of measuring techniques the following should be specified: (a) patient position, including the position of the legs; (b) specific instructions given to the patient; (c) the status of bladder and bowel fullness; (d) techniques of quantification or qualification (estimated, calculated, directly measured); and (e) the reliability of the technique.

4.1. Inspection

A visual assessment of muscle integrity, including a description of scarring and symmetry, should be performed. Pelvic floor contraction causes inward movement of the perineum and straining causes the opposite movement. Perineal movements can be observed directly or assessed indirectly by movement of an externally visible device placed into the vagina or urethra. The abdominal wall and other specified regions might be watched simultaneously. The type, size and placement of any device used should be specified as should the state of undress of the patient.

4.2. Palpation

Palpation may include digital examination of the pelvic floor muscles through the vagina or rectum as well as assessment of the perineum, abdominal wall and/or other specified regions. The number of fingers and their position should be specified. Scales for the description of the strength of voluntary and reflex (e.g., with coughing) contractions and of the degree of voluntary relaxation should be clearly described and intra- and inter-observer reliability documented. Standardised palpation techniques could also be developed for the semi-quantitative estimation of the bulk or thickness of pelvic floor musculature around the circumference of the genital hiatus. These techniques could allow for the localisation of any atrophic or asymmetric segments.

4.3. Electromyography

Electromyography from the pelvic floor muscles can be recorded alone or in combination with other measurements. Needle electrodes permit visualisation of individual motor unit action potentials, while surface or wire electrodes detect action potentials from groups of adjacent motor units underlying or surrounding the electrodes. Interpretation of signals from these letter electrodes must take into consideration that signals from erroneously contracted adjacent muscles may interfere with signals from the muscles of interest. Reports of electromyographic recordings should specify the following: (a) type of electrode; (b) placement of electrodes; (c) placement of reference electrode; (d) specifications of signal processing equipment; (e) type and specifications of display equipment; (f) muscle in which needle electrode is placed; and (g) description of decision algorithms used by the analytic software.

4.4. Pressure Recording

Measurements of urethral, vaginal and anal pressures may be used to assess pelvic floor muscle control and strength. However, interpretations based on these pressure measurements must be made with a knowledge of their potential for artefact and their unproven or limited reproducibility. Anal sphincter contractions, rectal peristalsis, detrusor contractions and abdominal straining can affect pressure measurements. Pressures recorded from the proximal vagina accurately mimic fluctuations in abdominal pressure. Therefore it may be important to compare vaginal pressures to simultaneously measured vesical or rectal pressures. Reports using pressure measurements should specify the following: (a) the type and size of the measuring device at the recording site (e.g., ballon, open catheter, etc.); (b) the exact placement of the measuring device; (c) the type of pressure transducer; (d) the type of display system; and (e) the display of simultaneous control pressures.

As noted in Section 4.1, observation of the perineum is an easy and reliable way to assess for abnormal straining during an attempt at a pelvic muscle contraction. Significant straining or a Valsalva manoeuvre causes downward/caudal movement of the perineum; a correctly performed pelvic muscle contraction causes inward/cephalad movement of the perineum. Observation for perineal movement should be considered as an additional validation procedure whenever pressure measurements are recorded.

5. Description of Functional Symptoms

Functional deficits caused by pelvic organ prolapse and pelvic floor dysfunction are not well characterised or absolutely established. There is an ongoing need to develop, standardise, and validate various clinimetric scales such as condition-specific quality of life questionnaires for each of the four functional symptom groups thought to be related to pelvic organ prolapse.

Researchers in this area should try to use standardised and validated symptom scales whenever possible. They must always ask precisely the same questions regarding functional symptoms before and after therapeutic intervention. The description of functional symptoms should be directed toward four primary areas: (1) lower urinary tract, (2) bowel, (3) sexual, and (4) other local symptoms.

5.1. Urinary Symptoms

This report does not supplant any currently approved ICS terminology related to lower urinary tract function.[7] However, some important prolapse related symptoms are not included in the current standards (e.g., the need to manually reduce the prolapse or assume an unusual position to initiate or complete micturition). Urinary symptoms that should be considered for dichotomous, ordinal, or visual analogue scaling include, but are not limited to, the following: (a) stress incontinence, (b) frequency (diurnal and nocturnal), (c) urgency, (d) urge incontinence, (e) hesitancy, (f) weak or prolonged urinary stream, (g) feeling of incomplete emptying, (h) manual reduction of the prolapse to start or complete bladder emptying, and (f) positional changes to start or complete voiding.

5.2. Bowel Symptoms

Bowel symptoms that should be considered for dichotomous, ordinal or visual analog scaling include, but are not limited to, the following: (a) difficulty with defecation, (b) incontinence of flatus, (c) incontinence of liquid stool, (d) incontinence of solid stool, (e) faecal staining of underwear, (f) urgency of defecation, (g) discomfort with defecation, (h) digital manipulation of vagina, perineum or anus to complete defecation, (i) feeling of incomplete evacuation and (j) rectal protrusion during or after defecation.

5.3. Sexual Symptoms

Research is needed to attempt to differentiate the complex and multifactorial aspects of "satisfactory sexual function" as it relates to pelvic organ prolapse and pelvic floor dysfunction. It may be difficult to distinguish between the ability to have vaginal intercourse and normal sexual function. The development of satisfactory tools will require multidisciplinary collaboration. Sexual function symptoms that should be considered for dichotomous, ordinal, or visual analog scaling include, but are not limited to, the following: (a) Is the patient sexually active? (b) If she is not sexually active, why? (c) Does sexual activity include vaginal coitus? (c) What is the frequency of vaginal intercourse? (d) Does the patient experience pain with coitus? (e) Is the patient satisfied with her sexual activity? (f) Has there been any change in orgasmic response? (g) Is any incontinence experienced during sexual activity?

5.4. Other Local Symptoms

We currently lack knowledge regarding the precise nature of symptoms that may be caused by the presence of a protrusion or bulge. Possible anatomically based symptoms that should be considered for dichotomous, ordinal or visual analog scaling include, but are not limited to, the following: (a) vaginal pressure or heaviness; (b) vaginal or perineal pain; (c) sensation or awareness of tissue protrusion from the vagina; (d) low back pain; (e) abdominal pressure or pain; (f) observation or palpation of a mass.

Acknowledgements

The subcommittee would like to acknowledge the contributions of the following consultants who contributed to the development and revision of this document: W. Glenn Hurt, Bernhard Schüssler, L. Lewis Wall.

References

1. Athanasiou S, Hill S, Gleeson C, Anders K, Cardozo L (1995). Validation of the ICS proposed pelvic organ prolapse descriptive system. Neurourol Urodyn 14:414–415 (abstract of ICS 1995 meeting).
2. Schüssler B, Peschers U (1995). Standardisation of terminology of female genital prolapse according to the new ICS criteria: inter-examiner reproducibility. Neurourol Urodynamics 14:437–438 (abstract of ICS 1995 meeting).
3. Montella JM, Cater JR (1995). Comparison of measurements obtained in supine and sitting position in the evaluation of pelvic organ prolapse (abstract of AUGS 1995 meeting).
4. Kobak WH, Rosenberg K, Walters MD (1995). Interobserver variation in the assessment of pelvic organ prolapse using the draft International Continence Society and Baden grading systems.- (abstract of AUGS 1995 meeting).
5. Hall AF, Theofrastous JP, Cundiff GC, Harris RL, Hamilton LF, Swift SE, Bump RC (1996). Inter- and intra-observer reliability of the proposed International Continence Society, Society of Gynecologic Surgeons, and American Urogynecologic Society pelvic organ prolapse classification system. Am J Obstet Gynecol (submitted through the program of the Society of Gynecologic Surgeons 1996 meeting).
6. Baden W, Walker T (1992). Surgical repair of vaginal defects. Philadelphia: Lippincott, pp 1–7, 51–62.
7. See this volume, Appendix 1, Part 2.

Appendix 1, Part 3
The Standardisation of Terminology of Lower Urinary Tract Function: Pressure-Flow Studies of Voiding, Urethral Resistance and Urethral Obstruction

Neurourol Urodyn (1997) in press

Derek Griffiths (subcommittee chairman), Klaus Höfner, Ron van Mastrigt, Harm Jan Rollema, Anders Spångberg, Donald Gleason and Anders Mattiasson (overall chairman)

International Continence Society Subcommittee on Standardisation of Terminology of Pressure-Flow Studies

1. Introduction

This report has been produced at the request of the International Continence Society. It was approved at the twenty-fifth annual meeting of the society in Sydney, Australia.

The 1988 version of the collated reports on standardisation of terminology, which appeared in *Neurourology and Urodynamics*, vol. 7, pp. 403–427, contains material relevant to pressure-flow studies in many different sections. This report is a revision and expansion of Sections 4.2 and 4.3 and parts of Sections 6.2 and 7 of the 1988 report. It contains a recommendation for a provisional standard method for defining obstruction on the basis of pressure-flow data.

2. Evaluation of Micturition

2.1. Pressure-Flow Studies

At present, the best method of analysing voiding function quantitatively is the pressure-flow study of micturition, with simultaneous recording of abdominal, intravesical and detrusor pressures and flow rate (Fig. A.1.3.1).

Direct inspection of the raw pressure and flow data before, during and at the end of micturition is essential, because it allows artefacts and untrustworthy data to be recognised and eliminated. More detailed analyses of pressure-flow relationships, described below, are advisable to aid diagnosis and to quantify data for research studies.

The flow pattern in a pressure-flow study should be representative of free flow studies in the same patient. It is important to eliminate artefacts and unrepresentative studies before applying more detailed analyses.

Pressure-flow studies contain information about the behaviour of the urethra and the behaviour of the detrusor. Section 2.2 deals with the urethra. Detrusor function is considered in Section 2.3.

2.1.1. Pressure and Flow Rate Parameters

Definitions See Fig. A.1.3.1 and Table A.1.3.I; see also Table A.1.3.II.

Maximum flow rate is the maximum measured value of the flow rate. Symbol Q_{max}.

Maximum pressure is the maximum value of the pressure measured during a pressure-flow study. Note that this may be attained at a moment when the flow rate is zero. Symbols: $p_{abd,max}, p_{ves,max}, p_{det,max}$.

Pressure at maximum flow is the pressure recorded at maximum measured flow rate. If the same maximum value is attained more than once or if it is sustained for a period of time, then the point of maximum flow is taken to be where the detrusor pressure has its lowest value for this flow rate; abdominal, intravesical and detrusor pressures at maximum flow are all read at this same point. Flow delay (see Section 2.1.2) may have a significant influence and should be considered. Symbols: $p_{abd,Qmax}, p_{ves,Qmax}, p_{det,Qmax}$,

Opening pressure is the pressure recorded at the onset of measured flow. Flow delay should be considered. Symbols: $p_{abd,open}, p_{ves,open}, p_{det,open}$.

Closing pressure is the pressure recorded at the end of measured flow. Flow delay should be considered. Symbols: $p_{abd,clos}, p_{ves,clos}, p_{det,clos}$.

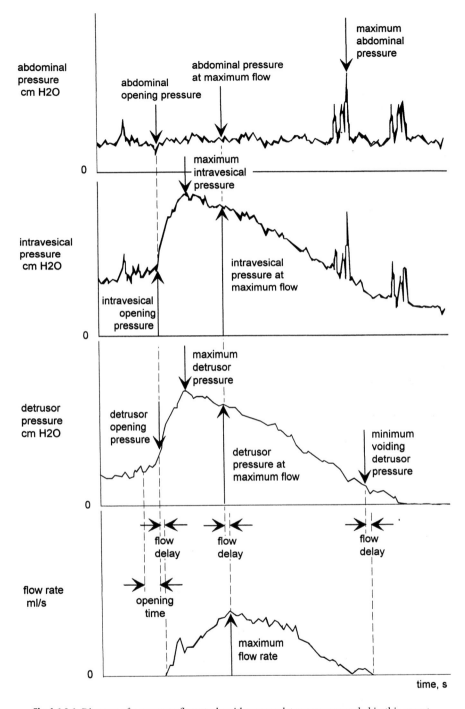

Fig. A.1.3.1 Diagram of a pressure-flow study with nomenclature recommended in this report.

Minimum voiding pressure is the minimum pressure during measurable flow (see Fig. A.1.6.1). It may be, but is not necessarily, equal to the opening pressure or the closing pressure. Example: minimum voiding detrusor pressure, symbol: $p_{det, min, void}$*

2.1.2. Flow Delay

When a pressure-flow study is performed, the flow rate is measured at a location downstream of the bladder pressure measurement and so the flow rate measurement is delayed. The delay is partly physiological, but it also depends on the equipment. It may depend on the flow rate.

When considering pressure-flow relationships, it may be important to take this delay into account, especially if there are rapid changes in pressure and flow rate. In current practice an average value is estimated by each investigator, from observations of the delay between corresponding pressure and flow rate changes in a number of actual studies. Values from 0.5 s to 1.0 s are typical.

Definition. *Flow delay* is the time delay between a change in bladder pressure and the corresponding change in measured flow rate.

2.1.3. Presentation of Results

Pressure-flow plots and the nomograms used for analysis should be presented with the flow rate plotted along the *x*-axis and the detrusor pressure along the *y*-axis (see Fig. A.1.6.2).

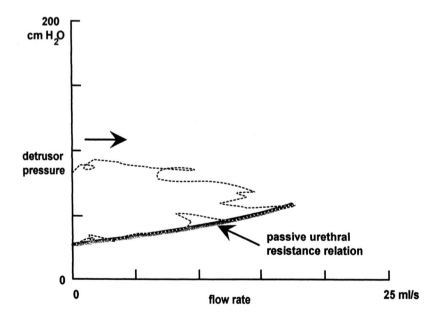

Fig. A.1.3.2 Plot of detrusor pressure against flow rate during voiding (broken curve), providing an indication of the urethral resistance relation (URR). The continuous smooth curve is an estimate of the passive urethral resistance relation.

Specify

The value of the flow delay that is used.

2.2. Urethral Resistance and Bladder Outlet Obstruction

2.2.1. Urethral Function During Voiding

During voiding urethral function may be

(a) normal or

(b) obstructive as a result of

    (i) overactivity or

    (ii) abnormal structure.

Obstruction due to urethral overactivity occurs when the urethral closure mechanism contracts involuntarily or fails to relax during attempted micturition in spite of an ongoing detrusor contraction. Obstruction due to abnormal structure has an anatomical basis, e.g., urethral stricture or prostatic enlargement.

2.2.2. Urethral Resistance

Urethral resistance is represented by a relation between pressure and flow rate, describing the pressure required to propel any given flow rate through the urethra. The relation is called the *urethral resistance relation* (URR).

An indication of the urethral resistance relation is obtained by plotting detrusor pressure against flow rate. The most accurate procedure, which requires a computer or an *x/y* recorder, is a quasi-continuous plot showing many pairs of corresponding pressure and flow rate values (Fig. A.1.3.2). A simpler procedure, which can be performed by hand, is to plot only two or three pressure-flow points connected by straight lines; for example, the points of minimum voiding pressure and of maximum flow may be selected. In whatever way the plot is made, flow delay should be considered.

A further simplification is to plot just one point showing the maximum flow rate and the detrusor pressure at maximum flow. Flow delay should be considered.

Methods of analysing pressure-flow plots are further discussed below.

2.2.3. Urethral Activity

Ideally, the urethra is fully relaxed during voiding. The urethral resistance is then at its lowest and the detrusor pressure has its lowest value for any given flow rate. Under these circumstances the urethral resistance relation is defined by the inherent mechanical and morphological properties of the urethra and is called the *passive urethral resistance relation* (Fig. A.1.3.2).

Urethral activity can only increase the detrusor pressure above the value defined by the passive urethral resistance relation. Therefore, any deviations of the pressure-flow plot from the passive urethral resistance relation toward higher pressures are regarded as due to activity of the urethral or periurethral muscles, striated or smooth.

2.2.4. Bladder Outlet Obstruction

Obstruction is a physical concept which is assessed from measurements of pressure and flow rate, made during voiding. Whether due to urethral over-activity or to abnormal structure, obstruction implies that the urethral resistance to flow is abnormally elevated. Because of natural variation from subject to subject, there cannot be a sharp boundary between normal and abnormal. Therefore the definition of abnormality requires further elaboration.

2.2.5. Methods of Analysing Pressure-Flow Plots

The results of pressure-flow studies may be used for various purposes, for example for objective diagnosis of urethral obstruction or for statistical testing of differences in urethral resistance between groups of patients. For these purposes methods have been developed to quantify pressure-flow plots in terms of one or more numerical parameters. The parameters are based on aspects such as the position, slope or curvature of the plot. Some of these methods are primarily intended for use in adult males with possible prostatic hypertrophy.

Some methods of analysis are shown in Table A.1.3.I.

Quantification of Urethral Resistance.   In all current methods, urethral resistance is derived from the relationship between pressure and flow rate. A commonly used method of demonstrating this relationship is the pressure-flow plot. The lower pressure part of this plot is taken to represent the passive urethral resistance relation (see Fig. A.1.6.2). In general, the higher is the pressure for a given flow rate, and/or the steeper or more sharply curved upward is this part of the plot, the higher is the urethral resistance. The various methods differ in how the position, slope, and/or curvature of the plot are quantified and how and whether they are combined. Some methods grade urethral resistance on a continuous scale; others grade it in a small number of classes (Table A.1.3.I). If there are few classes, small changes in resistance may not be detected. Conversely, a small change on a continuous scale may not be clinically relevant.

Table A.1.3.I. Methods of analysing pressure-flow plots

Method	Aim	Number of p/Q points	Assumed shape of URR	Number of parameters	Number of classes or continuous
Abrams-Griffiths nomogram[1]	diagnosis	1	n/a	n/a	3
Spångberg nomogram[2]	diagnosis	1	n/a	n/a	3
URA[3,4]	resistance	1	curved	1	continuous
linPURR[5]	resistance	1[a]	linear	1	7
Schäfer PURR[6]	resistance	many	curved	2	continuous
CHESS[7]	resistance	many	curved	2	16
OBI[8]	resistance	many	linear	1	continuous
Spångberg *et al.*	resistance	many	linear or curved	3	continuous + 3 categories
DAMPF[9]	resistance	2	linear	1	continuous
A/G number[10]	resistance	1	linear	1	continuous

[a] Schäfer uses 2 points to draw a linear relation but the point at maximum flow determines the resistance grade.

Some methods result in a single parameter; others result in two or more parameters (Table A.1.3.I). A single parameter makes it easy to compare different measurements. A larger number of parameters makes comparison more difficult but potentially gives higher accuracy and validity. If there are too many parameters, however, accuracy may be compromised by poor reproducibility.

Choice of Method.   Some methods in Table A.1.3.I are intended primarily to quantify urethral resistance. Others are intended only for the diagnosis of obstruction. Methods that quantify urethral resistance on a scale can also be used to aid diagnosis of obstruction by comparison with cutoff values. In every case an equivocal zone may be included.

Because of their underlying similarity, all the above methods classify clearly obstructed and clearly unobstructed pressure-flow studies consistently, but there is some lack of agreement in a minority of cases with intermediate urethral resistance.

Any of the methods of analysing pressure-flow studies may be useful for a particular purpose. In selecting a method, investigators should consider carefully what their aims are and which method is best suited to attain them.

Identification of Optimum Methods.   For a subsequent report the International Continence Society will compare the above methods with each other and may also develop new methods, with the aim of reaching a consensus on their use. The Society will continue to seek better ways of clinically validating these methods. The following procedure has been agreed on.

Making use of good-quality data stored in digital format, the following databases will be examined:

1. Pressure-flow studies in untreated men with lower urinary tract symptoms and signs suggestive of benign prostatic obstruction.
2. Pressure-flow studies repeated after a time interval with no intervention.
3. Pressure-flow studies before and after TURP.
4. Pressure-flow studies before and after alternative therapeutical intervention that causes a small change in urethral resistance.

Database I will be used to determine which existing or new methods adequately describe the actual pressure-flow plots of male patients with lower urinary tract symptoms. Database 2 will be used to determine the reproducibility of the various methods. Database 3 will be used to determine in which groups of patients TURP significantly reduces urethral resistance, and hence which patients are indeed obstructed. Database 4 will be used to test the sensitivity of the various methods to small changes of urethral resistance.

On the basis of these analyses, the International Continence Society will attempt to identify:

(i)   A simple and reproducible method with high validity of diagnosing obstruction.
(ii) A sensitive and reproducible method with high validity of measuring urethral resistance and changes in resistance.

Provisional Recommendation.   Pending the results of these procedures, it is recommended that investigators reporting pressure-flow studies in adult males, particularly those with benign prostatic hyperplasia, use one simple standard method of analysis in addition to any other method that they have selected, so that results from different centres can be compared.

For this provisional method it is recommended that urethral resistance is specified by the maximum flow rate and the detrusor pressure at maximum flow, i.e., by the pair of values $(Q_{max}, p_{det}, Q_{max})$. A provisional diagnostic classification may be derived from these values as follows:

- If $(p_{det}, Q_{max} - 2Q_{max})$ *bg 40 the pressure-flow study is obstructed.
- If $(p_{det}, Q_{max} - 2Q_{max})$ *bl 20 the pressure-flow study is unobstructed.
- Otherwise the study is equivocal.

In these formulae pressure and flow rate are expressed in cmH_2O and ml/s respectively. This method is illustrated graphically in Fig. A.1.3.3. It may be referred to as the *provisional ICS method for definition of obstruction*.

The equivocal zone of the provisional method (Fig. A.1.3.3) is similar but not identical to those of the Abrams-Griffiths and Spa[o]ngberg nomograms and to the region defining linPURR grade II. For micturitions with low to moderate flow rates it is consistent with cutoff values used to define obstruction in the URA and CHESS methods.

2.3. The Detrusor During Micturition

During micturition the detrusor may be

(a) Acontractile
(b) Underactive

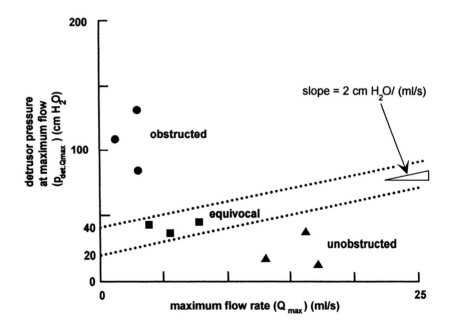

Fig. A.1.3.3 Provisional ICS method for definition of obstruction. The points represent schematically the values of maximum flow rate and detrusor pressure at maximum flow for 9 different voids, 3 in each class.

(c) Normal

(a) The acontractile detrusor is one that cannot be demonstrated to contract during urodynamic studies.

(b) Detrusor underactivity is defined as a detrusor contraction of inadequate magnitude and/or duration to effect complete bladder emptying in the20absence of urethral obstruction. (Concerning the elderly see (c). Both magnitude and duration should be considered in the evaluation of detrusor contractility.

(c) Normal detrusor contractility. In the absence of obstruction, a normal detrusor contraction will effect complete bladder emptying. Detrusor contractility in the elderly may need special consideration.

For a given detrusor contraction, the magnitude of the recorded pressure rise will depend on the outlet resistance. In general, the higher the detrusor pressure and/or the higher the flow rate, the stronger is the detrusor contraction. The magnitude of the detrusor contraction may be approximately quantified by means of a nomogram applied to the pressure-flow plot or by calculation.

3. Additional Symbols

Qualifiers that can be used to form symbols for variables relevant to voiding are shown in Table A.1.3.II. These are additions to those in Table A.1.5.II of the 1988 standardisation report.

Table A.1.3.II. Qualifiers that can be used to indicate pressure and flow variables relevant to voiding

Qualifiers	
At maximum flow	Q_{max}
During voiding	void
Opening	open
Closing	clos
Examples	
$p_{det,\ Q_{max}}$	Detrusor pressure at maximum flow
$p_{det\ min,\ void}$	Minimum voiding detrusor pressure
$p_{ves,\ open}$	Intravesical opening pressure
$p_{ves,\ clos}$	Intravesical closing pressure

When possible, qualifiers should be printed as subscripts (see above). Note that the preferred symbol for pressure is lower-case p, while the symbol for flow rate is capital (upper-case) Q.

References

1. Abrams PH, Griffiths DJ (1979). The assessment of prostatic obstruction from urodynamic measurements and from residual urine. Br J Urol 51:129–134.
2. Spa[o]ngberg A, Teriö H, Ask P, Engberg A (1991). Pressure/flow studies preoperatively and post-operatively in patients with benign prostatic hypertrophy: estimation of the urethral pressure/flow relation and urethral elasticity. Neurourol Urodyn 10:139–167.

3. Griffiths D, Van Mastrigt R, Bosch R (1989). Quantification of urethral resistance and bladder function during voiding, with special reference to the effects of prostate size reduction on urethral obstruction due to benign prostatic hypertrophy. Neurourol Urodyn 8:17–27.
4. Rollema HJ, van Mastrigt R (1992). Improved indication and follow-up in transurethral resection of the prostate (TUR) using the computer program CLIM. J Urol 148:111–116.
5. Schäfer W (1990). Basic principles and clinical application of advance analysis of bladder voiding function. Urol Clin N Am 17:553–566.
6. Schäfer W (1983). The contribution of the bladder outlet to the relation between pressure and flow rate during micturition. In: Hinman F Jr (ed) Benign prostatic hypertrophy. New York: Springer-Verlag, pp. 470–496.
7. Höfner K, Kramer AEJL, Tan HK, Krah H, Jonas U (1995). CHESS classification of bladder outflow obstruction. A consequence in the discussion of current concepts. World J Urol 13:59–64.
8. Kranse M, Van Mastrigt R (1991). The derivation of an obstruction index from a three parameter model fitted to the lowest part of the pressure flow plot. J Urol 145:261A.
9. Schäfer W (1995). Analysis of bladder-outlet function with the linearized passive urethral resistance relation, linPURR, and a disease-specific approach for grading obstruction: from complex to simple. World J Urol 13:47–58.
10. Lim CS, Abrams P (1995). The Abrams-Griffiths nomogram. World J Urol 13:34–39.

Appendix: ICS Standard for Digital Exchange of Pressure-Flow Study Data

A1. Introduction

To facilitate exchange of digital urodynamic data a standard file format is required. In this document an ICS standard is summarised. Its primary purpose is to enable data from pressure-flow studies to be exchanged. Enough detail is given to allow exchange of other urodynamic data. Extensions may be made as described in Section A5.

A2. General Description of Signal Storage

For each pressure-flow study, urodynamic signals sampled equidistantly with an A/D converter, and other associated information, are stored in one binary MS-DOS compatible file on a 5.25 or 3.5 inch floppy disk. The stored signals start 10 seconds before a detectable change in the flow rate signal and continue until 10 seconds after the flow rate has finally returned to baseline. Whenever possible, all signals should be stored at the same sample rate. In this case all signals have the same length, i.e., contain the same number of bytes.

The file name and extension are A B C D E F G H. ICS, where A B C D E F G H stands for a unique measurement identification string. In the case of a multicentre study requiring exchange of data, "unique" implies that this string is defined by the coordinating centre. In the ICS-BPH study for instance this would be a number consisting of (first) 3 digits for centre number, (next) 3 digits for patient number and (finally) 2 digits for identification of successive measurements made on this one patient in one or more sessions.

The file consists of a number of records of various types. In the ICSMFF proposal on which this document is partly based (see Section A8: Acknowledgements) 14 different types of record are defined, numbered -1 and 1 to 13. Existing record types may not be modified but extensions may be implemented by defining new types of record. For ICS purposes 6 additional types of record, types 14 to 19, are required and are defined in Section A5. In addition, the structures of records of types 8 and 9 are further elaborated in Section A5.

A3. Variable Values and Types

In this report actual values for bytes or words may be given in hexadecimal notation as follows: Hex:DD for 8-bit bytes, Hex:DDDD for 16-bit words, and so on, where D stands for a hexadecimal digit.

The following variable types are used in the definitions in the following sections:

Byte	unsigned 8-bit value
word	unsigned 16-bit value
integer	signed 16-bit value
dword	unsigned 32-bit value
string [N]	N bytes including a terminating Hex:00
word [N]	N words

A4. General Structure of File and Records

Each file A B C D E F G H. ICS consists of a number of records. The number of records is not predefined. Records may be of different types, containing different kinds of data. For example a record may contain a description of a urodynamic signal or information about the patient.

Each record starts with a descriptor containing the record type, the size of the data block in bytes and a checksum. The descriptor is followed by the block containing the actual data (see Fig. A.1.3.A1).

The record type and the block size are integers. The checksum is an integer such that the 16-bit sum of the record type, the data block size and the checksum is zero.

A5. Definitions of Record Types

The record type defines what kind of data is contained by the data block in the record. The only constraint is that the record type is unique.

Backward compatibility is preserved by the requirement that previously defined record types may not be modified. Extensions are implemented by defining new types of record. New types of signal may be implemented by defining new signal IDs, together with signal names and units. Forward compatibility will be insured if the user does not try to handle unknown types of record or unknown signal IDs.

A register of the types of record in use, and a register of signal IDs, signal names and units, will be administered centrally by the ICS. This standard contains initial versions of the registers. Proposed extensions should be communicated to the ICS for registration.

Default Values

Empty fields are not permitted. Occasionally, the value for a certain field may not be available. In this case a default value should be stored (see below).

Signal ID

See Section A9: Addendum.

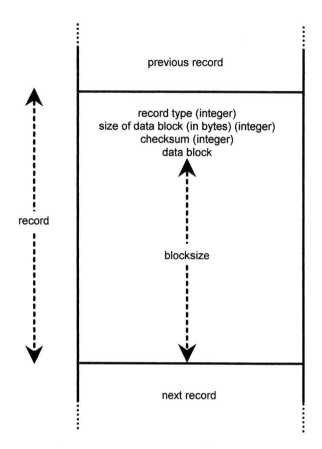

Fig. A.1.3.A1 Schematic structure of file and records.

The following sections describe the types of record needed to implement this ICS standard. Other types are described in the document *ICS Measure File Format (ICSMFF)* version 1.00, dated 14.10.93 (see Section A8: Acknowledgements).

Record Type 8: The Measurement Marker Record

This type of record defines a marker within the measurement and an associated comment.

Record type	8	integer
Blocksize	$1 + N + 1 + 4 + M$	integer
Checksum	$-(8+\text{blocksize})$	integer
Data block	marker type	byte
name	string $[N]$	
signal ID	byte	
Position	dword	
Comment	string $[M]$	

The following information should be stored in these fields:
    In the field:

marker type	0 = default value
	(other types are defined in the ICSMFF document)
name	empty string as default value
	(empty string contains only the terminating Hex:00, so that $N = 1$)
signal ID	as in Section A9: Addendum
position	the number of the sample (16-bit word) with which the marker and comment are associated.
comment	the comment string, terminated with Hex:00

Record Type 9: The Measurement Comment Record

This record stores a comment. For the ICS standard it should be used to identify the patient and the type of the measurement.

Record type	9	integer
Blocksize	N	integer
Checksum	$-(9 + \text{blocksize})$	integer
Data block	measurement comment	string $[N]$

The following information should be stored:
    In the field:

measurement comment	a free format string, terminated with Hex:00, that uniquely identifies patient and measurement for the originating centre. This string would not only include a patient ID, e.g. from the local hospital information system, but also the relation of this measurement to a particular research study, e.g. "post-TURP investigation". For use in a specific multi-centre study, this string may be specified more strictly.

Record Type 14: The ICS Signal Property Record

This record type describes the properties of one stored signal, including its name, the unit of measurement, the zero and full scale values, and the sample rate (which if possible should be identical for all signals).

Record type	14	integer
Blocksize	$1 + N + M + 2 + 4$	integer
Checksum	$-(14 + \text{blocksize})$	integer
Data block	signal id	byte
	signal name	string $[N]$
	unit	string $[M]$
	Binzero	integer
	Binsize	integer
	fullscale	integer
	Sample rate	dword

The following information should be stored in these fields:
In the field:

signal ID	as specified in Section A9: Addendum
signal name	as specified in Section A9: Addendum
unit	as specified in Section A9: Addendum
binzero	the signal value represented in the data samples field of record type 18 by the word 0
binsize	the full scale binary sample value
fullscale	the signal value represented in the data samples field of record type 18 by the full scale binary value
sample rate	sample rate specification in samples/s (Hz). The sample rate is in 16.16 format: i.e., it is a long integer, where bits 16 through 31 specify the integer part of a fixed point number and bits 0 through 15 specify the decimal part.

The following values are recommended:

- Sample rate at least 10 samples/s.
- Pressure signals bipolar up to + 200 cmH_2O with a minimum resolution of 0.5 cmH_2O/bit.
- Flow rate signal unipolar up to 50 ml/s with a minimum resolution of 0.05 ml/s/bit.

Example showing how sample rate is to be specified:

Suppose the rate of sampling is 512.5 Hz. Then the value to be stored in the field sample rate is the 16.16 value Hex:02008000.

Example showing how binzero, binsize and fullscale are to be used:

Suppose the abdominal pressure is sampled bipolarly with a ten bit A/D converter. Then the binary value will range from 0 to 1023. Suppose the A/D converter is configured so that this range represents the pressure range from -50 to 200 cmH_2O, then the three values to be stored are:

binzero	−50
binsize	1023
fullscale	200

Record Type 15: The ICS Patient Data Record

This record type contains the basic demographic data of the patient. It contains the actual text and numerical fields plus an index table to facilitate location of a particular field. The index gives the relative position within the data block.

Record type	15	integer
Blocksize	$17* 2 + N + M + O + P + Q + R + S + T + U + V + W + X + Y + 3 + 2$	integer
Checksum	−(15 + blocksize)	integer
Data block	surname index	word
	first name index	word
	maiden name index	word
	ID index	word
	street index	word
	housenumber index	word
	city index	word
	country index	word
	postcode index	word
	phone index	word

height index	word
weight index	word
sex index	word
comments index	word
birth day index	word
birth month index	word
birth year index	word
surname	string [N]
first name	string [M]
maiden name	string [O]
ID	string [P]
street	string [Q]
housenumber	string [R]
city	string [S]
country	string [T]
postcode	string [U]
phone	string [V]
height	string [W]
weight	string [X]
comments	string [Y]
sex	byte*
birth day	byte
birth month	byte
birth year	word†

* 0 = male, 1 = female.
† Birth year is expressed in full, e.g., 1895, 1995, 2005.

The first name field may contain a middle or other initial in addition to the first name.

As a default, an empty string (containing only Hex:00) may be stored in any of the string fields for which information is not available or may not be disclosed because of ethical considerations. In this case the length (N, M, etc.) of the string is 1.

The index fields contain the position (in bytes) of the corresponding text or numerical field, relative to the start of the data block. Thus the value to be stored in surname index is $17 * 2$; the value to be stored in first name index is $17 * 2 + N$; and so on. All the index fields must be completed.

Record Type 16: The ICS Source Record

This record type specifies the origin of the measurement. It consists of an index table together with the actual text fields.

Record type	16	integer
Blocksize	$10 * 2 + N + M + O + P + Q + R + S + T + U + V$	integer
Checksum	$-(16 + blocksize)$	integer
Data block	clinic name index	word
	investigator name index	word
	street index	word
	streetnumber index	word
	city index	word
	country index	word
	postcode index	word
	phone index	word
	fax index	word
	comments index	word
	clinic name	string [N]

investigator name		string [M]
Street		string [O]
Streetnumber		string [P]
City		string [Q]
Country		string [R]
Postcode		string [S]
Phone		string [T]
Fax		string [U]
Comments		string [V]

The phone and fax fields should include the area code as well as the local number.

An empty string may be stored in any of the string fields for which information is not available. In this case the length (N, M, etc.) of the string is 1.

The index fields contain the position (in bytes) of the corresponding text field, relative to the start of the data block. All the index fields must be completed.

Record Type 17: ICS Volume Record

This record contains the filling volume and the residual volume.

Record type	17	integer
Blocksize	4	integer
Checksum	$-(17 + \text{blocksize})$	integer
Data block	filling volume	integer
	residual volume	integer

The following information should be stored:
  In the field:

filling volume	the calculated volume in the bladder at the beginning of the pressure-flow study (in ml)
residual volume	the volume in the bladder at the end of the study, either calculated or measured directly (in ml); if the calculated volume is negative the value zero should be stored

Record Type 18: The ICS Signal Value Record

The ICS signal value record contains the actual data samples for one of the urodynamic signals. It includes a record number, allowing a signal that is too long to fit into one record to be divided so as to span several records. If the signal spans more than one record the number of the first record should be 1 and the following records should be numbered 2, 3,. ... If there is only one record its record number should be 0.

Record type	18	integer
Blocksize	$2 + N* 2$	integer
Checksum	$-(18 + \text{blocksize})$	integer
Data block	signal ID	byte
	record number	byte
	data samples	word [N]

The following information should be stored in these fields:
   In the field:

signal ID	As specified in Section A9: Addendum.
record number	As described above.
data samples	The binary samples themselves, 1 word = 2 bytes = 1 sample, stored in the order low byte, high byte.

Record Type 19: The ICS Measurement Description Record

This record indicates that the file is an ICS standard file and describes the measurement's start date and time, the number of signals stored and the number of records in the file.

Record type	19	integer	
Blocksize	$1 + N + 5 + 1 + 2$	integer	
Checksum	$-(19 + \text{blocksize})$	integer	
Data block	Measurement type	byte	
	Name	string $[N]$	
	Start	minute	byte
		hour	byte
		day	byte
		month	byte
		year	byte*
	Number of signals	byte	
	Number of records	word	

* Year is expressed modulo 100; e.g. 1995 = 95, 2005 = 05.

The following information should be stored in these fields:
   In the field:

measurement type	the version number of this document, multiplied by 10 (e.g., for this version 70). (Note that the version number may not contain hundredths or smaller decimal fractions.)
name	the string "ICS standard pressure-flow study"
start	the starting time and date of the measurement (if any of these are unavailable, the default value Hex:00 should be stored in the corresponding position: minute, hour, day, month and/or year)
number of signals	the number of signals stored in this file (e.g., 3 if just intravesical pressure, abdominal pressure and flow rate are stored).
number of records	the total number of records stored in this file (including this measurement description record)

A6. Signals and Information to be Stored: Minimal Specification and Optional Extensions

Minimally the following 3 signals should be stored in 3 records of type 18:

intravesical pressure
abdominal pressure
flow rate

   For each signal certain associated information should be stored in a record of type 14.

Optionally the following signals can also be stored in records of type 18, with associated information in records of type 14:

EMG envelope
voided volume

The voided volume signal may be useful if this is the signal measured by the urodynamic system, and the flow rate signal is derived from it.

In addition to the signals, further information about the patient and the measurements should be stored in records of types 16, 17 and 19. Full demographic data for the patient can be stored in a record of type 15. Optionally a free format comment can be stored in a record of type 9, and if detailed comments relating to events during the measurement are available they can be stored in records of type 8.

A7. Typical File Structure

Of the various record types, some are mandatory and some are optional. The structure of the file describing a particular measurement varies according to what records are stored.

The order of the records within the file is arbitrary in principle. However, it may be convenient to place records containing easily recognisable strings near the beginning, so that the file can quickly be identified if it is accidentally renamed or misplaced. In particular, record type 19 should preferably be the first one.

Thus a typical file structure might be:

Record type 19: ICS measurement description record (identifies file as an ICS standard file)
Record type 16: ICS source record (identifies originating clinic and investigator)
Record type 9: Measurement comment record (identifies patient and type of measurement)

Optionally, record type 15: ICS patient data record (contains full demographic data for patient)

Record type 14: ICS signal property record (describes properties of intravesical pressure signal)
Record type 14: ICS signal property record (describes properties of abdominal pressure signal)
Record type 14: ICS signal property record (describes properties of flow rate signal)

Optionally, further records of type 14 for voided volume and EMG envelope Record type 18: ICS signal value record (contains actual intravesical pressure data)

Record type 18: ICS signal value record (contains actual abdominal pressure data)
Record type 18: ICS signal value record (contains actual flow rate data)

Optionally, further records of type 18 for voided volume and EMG envelope
Optionally, record type 8: measurement marker record (identifies position and type of marker in data, the signal with which it is associated and a comment)
Optionally, further records of type 8 with additional markers

Record type 17: ICS volume record (contains filling volume prior to pressure-flow study and residual urine volume after voiding)

A8. Acknowledgements

This draft proposal is based partly on the ICS Measure File Format (ICSMFF) version 1.00 of 14.10.93, which was written by Michael Gondy Jensen, formerly of the Wiest company and now of Andromeda Medical Systems, and also on an earlier proposal for a simple digital pressure-flow standard circulated by Ron van Mastrigt. The Dantec, Laborie, Life-Tech and Wiest companies have agreed in principle to support a standard similar to the ICSMFF. The Life-Tech company has agreed to support the approved ICS standard.

A9. Addendum: Signal IDs

In records of types 8, 14 and 18, a signal ID of the type byte is specified. Corresponding signal names and units of the type string are required in record type 14. The following signal ID values, signal names and units have been defined:

	Signal ID	Signal name	Unit
For intravesical pressure	1	pves	cmH_2O
abdominal pressure	2	p_{abd}	cmH_2O
flow rate	3	Q	ml/s
EMG envelope	4	EMG_{env}	μV
voided volume	5	V_{void}	ml

The following are reserved for possible future use:

	Signal ID	Signal name	Unit
For P_{det} acquired independently	6	p_{det}	cmH_2O
infused volume	7	V_{inf}	ml
direct EMG signal	8	EMG	μV
urethral pressure	9	p_{ura}	cmH_2O
urethral closure pressure	10	p_{clos}	cmH_2O

Additional signal IDs, signal names and units may be introduced; proposed additions should be communicated to the ICS for registration.

Appendix 1, Part 4
Standardisation of Ambulatory Urodynamic Monitoring

Report of the Standardisation Sub-committee of the ICS for ambulatory urodynamic studies. *

Committee

Ernst van Waalwijk van Doorn (Chairman)
Kate Anders
Vik Khullar
Sigurd Kulseng-Hanssen
Francesco Pesce
Andrew Robertson
Derek Rosario
Werner Schafer

Neurourol Urodyn (2000) 19:113-125/

1. Introduction

Ambulatory urodynamic monitoring (AUM) has become an established method of investigating lower urinary tract function. This report recommends standards for terminology, methodology, analysis and reporting of AUM in a uniform fashion to facilitate communication between investigators and to improve the quality of clinical practice and research. The document can be integrated with earlier reports of the International Continence Society committee on Standardisation with special reference to the collated ICS report from 1988 (1) and the ICS recommendations on good urodynamic practice (2).

AUM in contrast to conventional urodynamic studies frees the patient to be more independent of fixed urodynamic apparatus. This allows the patient to perform those activities that, he or she knows from experience, will provoke troublesome urinary symptoms.

2. Indications for AUM

- Lower urinary tract symptoms which conventional urodynamic investigation fails to reproduce or explain
- Situations in which conventional urodynamics may be unsuitable
- Neurogenic lower urinary tract dysfunction.
- Evaluation of therapies for lower urinary tract dysfunction. *bl/BL*bg

3. Terminology

The terminology applied to observations during AUM should wherever possible be consistent with terminology used during conventional urodynamic investigation.

3.1. Definitions

An Ambulatory Urodynamic investigation is defined as any functional test of the lower urinary tract predominantly utilising natural filling of the urinary tract and reproducing subject's normal activity.

The terms introduced by this definition are further explained below.

Ambulatory
This refers to the nature of monitoring rather than the mobility of the subject. Monitoring will usually take place outside a urodynamic laboratory.

Natural
This refers to the natural production of urine rather than an artificial medium. Stimulation by forced drinking or pharmacological manipulation must be stated in the methodology.

Remark: The bladder may be pre-filled with an artificial medium but this is not comparable with natural bladder filling. This method of investigation needs further evaluation.

Normal activity
Refers to the activities of the subject during which symptoms are likely to occur. These may include manoeuvres designed specifically to identify the presence of involuntary detrusor or urethral behaviour or to provoke incontinence.

4. Methodology

4.1. Signals

The following signals have been recorded by AUM
Pressure: intravesical
                abdominal
                urethral
                intrapelvic (renal)
Flowrate
Micturition volume
Urinary leakage
Leakage volume
Urethral electrical conductance
Perineal integrated surface electromyography

As examples of AUM investigations, which have been established home uroflowmetry and ambulatory cystography can be men-tioned: the first recording the flow(time) signal the latter at least recording the intravesical and abdominal pressure(time) signals

Additional information that should be recorded during any AUM investigation as event markers representing the following phenomena:

- initiation of voluntary voids
- cessation of voluntary voids
- episodes of urgency
- episodes of discomfort or pain
- provocative manoeuvres
- time and volume of fluid intake
- time and volume of urinary leakage
- time of pad change

4.2. Signal Quality

AUM is more versatile than equivalent conventional urodynamic investigation, but for the same reasons AUM is associated with a greater risk of losing signal quality. Therefore although all signals should be recorded as recommended in the ICS recommendations on 'Good Urodynamic Practice', there are a number of cautions which apply specifically to AUM. These are described below.

4.3. Intravesical and Abdominal Pressure Measurement

Although it is possible to measure intravesical and abdominal pressures using fluid-filled lines (water or air), the use of catheter mounted microtip transducers allows greater mobility during AUM. In the absence of continuous supervision, stringent checks on signal quality should be incorporated in the measurement protocol. At the start of monitoring, these should include testing of recorded pressure on-line by coughing and abdominal straining in the supine, sitting and erect positions. The investigator must be convinced that signal quality is adequate before proceeding with the ambulatory phase of the investigation. Prior to termination of the investigation and at regular intervals during monitoring similar checks of signal quality such as cough tests should be carried out. Such tests will serve as a useful retrospective quality check during the interpretation of traces. The following considerations must be taken into account when using microtip transducers:

- Transducers should be calibrated prior to every investigation.
- The "zero point" is atmospheric pressure (there is no fixed reference point). All transducers must be "zeroed" at atmospheric pressure prior to insertion of the catheters.
- Water filled pressure catheters have a fixed reference point at the upper edge of symphysis pubis whereas catheter mounted microtip pressure transducers have no fixed reference point.
- Microtip transducers will record direct contact with solid material (the wall of a viscus or faecal material) as a change in pressure. The use of multiple transducers may eliminate this source of artefact
- Under some circumstances, the pressure measured at the transducer surface will result in a discrepancy equal to the difference in vertical height between the two transducers. This can result in the estimated detrusor pressure being less than zero (i.e. negative) with, for instance, the patient in the supine position (see Figs. A.1.4.1 and A.1.4.2).

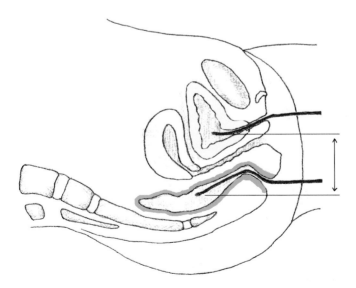

Fig. A.1.4.1 The difference in reference level between the vesical and rectal pressure sensor in supine position is shown schematically.

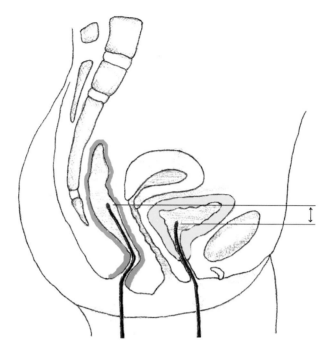

Fig. A.1.4.2 The difference in reference level between the vesical and rectal pressure sensor in upright position is shown schematically.

4.4. Urethral Pressure and Conductance

The recording of urethral pressure is a qualitative measurement with emphasis on changes in pressure rather than absolute values. The use of urethral electrical conductance to identify leakage in association with pressure monitoring facilities interpretation of urethral pressure traces. Precise positioning and secure fixation are essential to maintain signal quality. The orientation of the transducer should be documented.

Remark: The use of multiple pressure transducers facilitates identification of movement artefact but increases catheter stiffness and thereby deformation of the urethra during recording.

4.5. Catheter Fixation

As specified earlier, secure catheter fixation is essential to maintain signal quality. Methods that have been used include adhesive tape, suture fixation and purpose designed silicone-fixation devices

4.6. Recording of Urinary Leakage

The method of urine leakage determination should be recorded. It should be stated whether the urinary leakage is recorded as a signal with the pressure measurements, is dependent on the subject pressing an event marker button or completing a urinary diary.

4.7. Instructions to the Patient

Detailed instructions as to recording of symptoms, identification of catheter displacement and hardware failure should be given to the patient. It is the recommendation of this group that such verbal instructions should be reinforced by written instructions and in addition to the hardware built into the system, the patient is provided with a simple diary to record events. This allows the common primary aim of all urodynamics i.e. to correlate the test outcome with symptoms.

5. Analysis

5.1. Quality Assessment

The first step in the analysis of an AUM traces is the assessment of the quality of data recorded. The specific points that should be addressed with regard to pressure measurement are:

- Is the trace "active" i.e. fine second to second variation in pressure rather than a fine line?
- Is the baseline static or highly variable?
- Are the cough tests or other activities causing abdominal pressure changes that can be used for signal plausibility check, regularly present?
- Is the subtraction adequate, e.g. minimal change in subtracted detrusor pressure with coughing?

If the technical quality of the traces is less than perfect, then, although the investigation may yield valuable clinical information, in the context of accurate measurement, the pressure recordings must be viewed as qualitative and further quantitative analysis can be flawed (see Figures A.1.4.4 to A.1.4.13).

5.2. Phase Identification

Depending on the purpose of the investigation, markers must be placed to identify voluntary voids and allow differentiation of such events from involuntary events, which may be associated with changes in recorded pressure. The protocol of the investigation should specifically state the point at which the markers identifying commencement and cessation of a voluntary void are placed. Analysis of the voiding phase follows the same principles and terminology used during conventional pressure-flow investigation.

5.3. Events

The use of a patient diary considerably improves the detailed analysis of events occurring during AUM and is strongly recommended. The events usually recorded during AUM have been identified in section 4.1. Typical events occurring during the filling phase are detrusor contractions, urethral relaxations and episodes of urgency and incontinence.

Remark: At least for research purposes it is strongly advised to define and validate variables for quantitative interpretation. Validation means to establish data on healthy volunteers and specific patient groups, test retest reproducibility, interrater validity and sensitivity to treatment modalities.

6. Clinical Report

The report should be tailored to the urodynamic indication(s) and can include the following:
   Indication(s) and/or urodynamic question(s) (*obligatory*)

- Duration of recording
- Fill rate, timing, method and volume of any retrograde filling prior to commencing AUM
- Dose and timing of diuretics if administered
- Volume of fluid drunk during the test
- Number of voids
- Total and range of voided volumes and post micturition urinary residual
- Episodes of urgency, urinary incontinence and pain
- Detrusor activity during the filling phase (frequency, time, duration, amplitude, area, form)
- Pressure/flow analysis
- Results of provocative manoeuvres employed during the test
- Reasons for termination of recording if prematurely terminated

7. Scientific Presentation

To facilitate clear communication and evaluation regarding AUM the following guidelines should be applied:
   Description of AUM protocol which should include:

- Planned duration of recording
- Actual duration of recording
- Specification of recording device i.e. manufacturer, type, sampling rates, events button(s)
- Catheter – type, transducer, location, route and fixation technique
- Leakage detection method or device
- Urinary flow transducer
- Protocol for diuresis

- volume and timing of fluid drunk during test
- dose and timing of diuretics administered
- Fill rate, timing, method and volume of any retrograde filling before or during AUM
- Events recorded by diary or electronic markers
- Detrusor activity during the filling phase with any associated urgency, incontinence and pain
- Pressure/flow analysis (according to ICS standards)
- Any provocative manoeuvres employed during the test
- Reasons for premature termination of recording
- Presentation of urodynamic curves should include:
  - channel identification
  - Units of measurement
  - minimum scale for pressures should be two millimetres per five centimetres of water
  - minimum scale for time should be four centimetres per minute

8. Explanatory Examples

This chapter aims to support this report and stimulate the further growth of use of AUM by giving examples of AUM traces with specific events. The examples with the explanatory text will also help to increase ones ability to interpret AUM traces (see Fig. A.1.4.3).

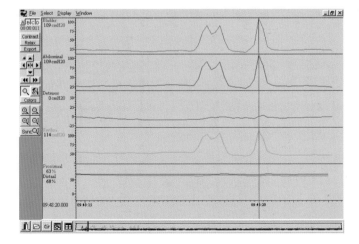

Fig. A.1.4.3 Typical traces of a double and single cough in supine position at 16 samples per second (x-axis 7 seconds).

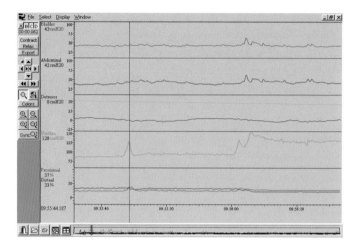

Fig. A.1.4.4 On the left, typical traces of a contraction of the urethral sphincter mechanism, followed on the right by squeezing again combined with a change in position causing displacement of urethral sensor

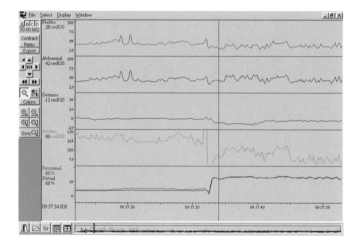

Fig. A.1.4.5 In the middle, typical movement artifact on the urethra pressure trace, causing sensor displacement; after the movement artifact the urethra pressure level has decreased. The conductance signals show an increased level indicating a displacement of the catheter towards the bladderneck.

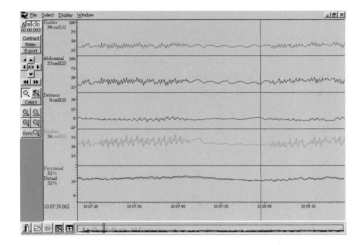

Fig. A.1.4.6 Typical traces showing walking (first half), respiration (third quarter), walking (last quarter). Of course, the pressure waves caused by breathing can also be detected during walking. Generally it can be stated that the pressure waves due to respiration are affected by the type of respiration, the physical activity and patient's stature.

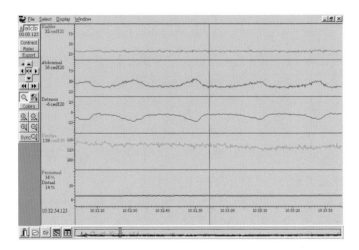

Fig. A.1.4.7 Typical abdominal and detrusor traces during rectal activity. Here, the patient is at rest and hardly any effect of respiration can be detected in the traces.

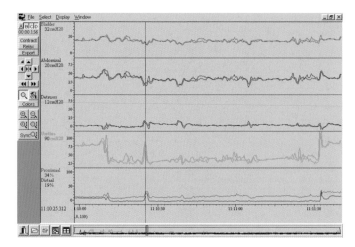

Fig. A.1.4.8 This example shows the traces during about 90 seconds. Because the sample rate for the pressure signals is 16 Hz it is not possible to plot every single sample value in the trace. The double lines represent the envelop of the pressure signals. This means, at every dot on the x-axis, the minimum and maximum pressure values of the time interval, represented by that dot, are plotted. In this plot we see a sequence of events: the patient is sitting (left), stands up (movement artifact urethra signal and abdominal activity in the vesical and abdominal traces), walks a few steps (difference between double lines increases). At the cursor position a 'reaching' phenomenon is seen, where the urethra sensor moves shortly towards the highest pressure region in the urethra and at the same time the abdomen is enlarged causing a pressure dip in the vesical and abdominal pressure signals. At 11:10:40, 11:11:10 and 11:11:25 a same kind of movement phenomenon can be seen. In between the patient walks some steps. At 11:11:30 the patient sits again.

The next two figures show the same events in detail.

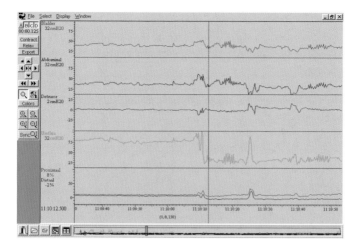

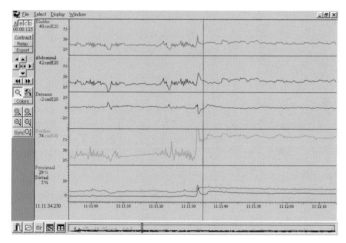

Figs. A.1.4.9 and A.1.4.10 These traces show the sequence of events described at fig . 6 in detail. Depending on the patients activity and the signal quality on should choose an adequate time resolution for analysis.

General information on traces:

- The analysis of AUM traces asks for the ability to look at different time and signal scales. To study these examples, it is necessary to look every time at the x an y-axis scales and the pressure ranges.
- Every example shows from top to bottom: the intravesical, abdominal (rectal), detrusor (subtracted) and urethral pressure signals followed by two urethral conductance signals (proximal and distal)
- For recording Gaeltec micro transducer catheters (5 French) and a Gaeltec MPR3 recorder is applied with the maximum sample frequency for storage set at 16 Hz.
- At the bottom of each figure, one can see which window, where in the complete investigation, is shown.
- Filling and voiding phase are separated by event markers ('E') at the x-axis.
- Detrusor contractions are indicated by a bar under the contraction curve.

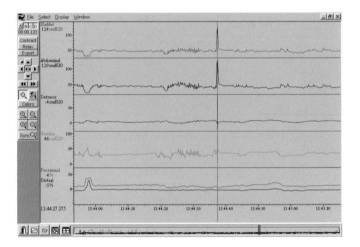

Fig. A.1.4.11 On the left, walking a few steps followed by a reaching movement artifact can be detected, causing a pressure dip in the vesical and rectal traces and a positive wave in the urethral pressure and conductance; at the cough pressure peak there is decreased transmission towards the urethral sensor, due to distal position of the urethral sensor. That the urethral sensor is displaced distally can be concluded, because there is no change in urethral conductance signals during the cough.

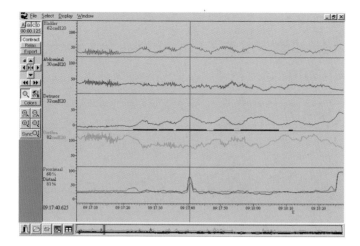

Fig. A.1.4.12 This example shows the most common sequence of events in a patient suffering from bladder overactivity and imperative voiding. On the left the traces start showing with walking, followed by a urethral relaxation and detrusor contractions. Then walking towards the toilet with increasing detrusor activity with a moment of urine loss (see conductance signals). Finally the patient enters the toilet at the E-vent mark (bottom).

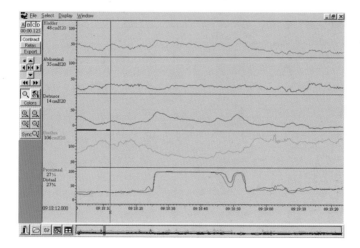

Fig. A.1.4.13 This traces show the continuation of the previous figure; the patient enters the toilet with detrusor activity continuing, sits down and a nice urethra relaxation and voiding contraction can be seen, while the conductance curves show the flow phase. At the end of the voiding the urethra closure pressure recovers to the pre-voiding level.

References

1. Abrams P., Blaivas J.G., Stanton S.L., Anderson J.T. The standardisation of terminology of lower urinary tract function. Scand J Urol Nephrol Supp 114: 5-19, 1989.
2. Good urodynamic practice (in preparation).

Appendix 1, Part 5
The Standardisation of Terminology in Lower Urinary Tract Function

Report from the Standardisation Sub-committee of the International Continence Society*

Committee

Paul Abrams, Linda Cardozo, Magnus Fall, Derek Griffiths, Peter Rosier, Ulf Ulmsten, Philip van Kerrebroeck, Arne Victor, Alan Wein.

This report presents definitions of the symptoms, signs, urodynamic observations and conditions associated with lower urinary tract dysfunction (LUTD) and urodynamic studies (UDS), for use in all patients groups from children to the elderly.

The definitions restate or update those presented in previous International Continence Society Standardisation of Terminology reports (see references) and those shortly to be published on Urethral Function (Lose et al., in press) and Nocturia (van Kerrebroeck et al., 2002). The published ICS report on the technical aspects of urodynamic equipment (Rowen et al., 1987) will be complemented by the new ICS report on urodynamic practice to be published shortly (Schäfer et al., 2002). In addition there are four published ICS outcome reports (Fonda et al., 1998; Lose et al., 1998; Mattiasson et al., 1998; Nordling et al., 1998).*

New or changed definitions are all indicated; however, recommendations concerning technique are not included in the main text of this report.

The definitions have been written to be compatible with the WHO publication ICIDH-2 (International Classification of Functioning, Disability and Health) published in 2001 and ICD10, the International Classification of Diseases. As far as possible, the definitions are descriptive of observations, without implying underlying assumptions that may later prove to be incorrect or incomplete. By following this principle, the International Continence Society (ICS) aims to facilitate comparison of results and enable effective communication by investigators who use urodynamic methods. This report restates the ICS principle that symptoms, signs and conditions are separate categories and adds a category of urodynam-

Neurourol Urodyn (2002) 21:167-178

ic observations. In addition, terminology related to therapies is included (Andersen et al., 1992).

When a reference is made to the whole anatomical organ the vesica urinaria, the correct term is the bladder. When the smooth muscle structure known as the m.detrusor urinae is being discussed, then the correct term is detrusor.

It is suggested that acknowledgement of these standards in written publications be indicated by a footnote to the section "Methods and Materials" or its equivalent, to read as follows:

"Methods, definitions and units conform to the standards recommended by the International Continence Society, except where specifically noted".

The report covers the following areas:

1. *Lower Urinary Tract Symptoms (LUTS)*
   Symptoms are the subjective indicator of a disease or change in condition as perceived by the patient, carer or partner and may lead him/her to seek help from health care professionals. **(NEW)**

   Symptoms may either be volunteered or described during the patient interview. They are usually qualitative. In general, Lower Urinary Tract Symptoms cannot be used to make a definitive diagnosis. Lower Urinary Tract Symptoms can also indicate pathologies other than lower urinary tract dysfunction, such as urinary infection.

2. *Signs suggestive of Lower Urinary Tract Dysfunction (LUTD)*
   Signs are observed by the physician including simple means, to verify symptoms and quantify them. **(NEW)**

   For example, a classical sign is the observation of leakage on coughing. Observations from frequency volume charts, pad tests and validated symptom and quality of life questionnaires are examples of other instruments that can be used to verify and quantify symptoms.

3. *Urodynamic Observations*
   Urodynamic observations are observations made during urodynamic studies. **(NEW)**

   For example, an involuntary detrusor contraction (detrusor overactivity) is a urodynamic observation. In general, a urodynamic observation may have a number of possible underlying causes and does not represent a definitive diagnosis of a disease or condition and may occur with a variety of symptoms and signs, or in the absence of any symptoms or signs.

4. *Conditions*
   Conditions are defined by the presence of urodynamic observations associated with characteristic symptoms or signs and/or non-urodynamic evidence of relevant pathological processes. **(NEW)**

5. *Treatment*
   Treatment for lower urinary tract dysfunction: these definitions are from the 7th ICS report on Lower Urinary Tract Rehabilitation Techniques (3).

1. Lower Urinary Tract Symptoms (LUTS)

Lower urinary tract symptoms are defined from the individual's perspective who is usually, but not necessarily, a patient within the healthcare system. Symptoms are either volunteered by, or elicited from, the individual or may be described by the individual's caregiver.

Lower urinary tract symptoms are divided into three groups: storage, voiding, and post micturition symptoms.

1.1. Storage Symptoms are experienced during the storage phase of the bladder and include daytime frequency and nocturia. (NEW)

- *Increased daytime frequency* is the complaint by the patient who considers that he/she voids too often by day. (NEW)
  This term is equivalent to pollakisuria used in many countries.
- *Nocturia* is the complaint that the individual has to wake at night one or more times to void. (NEW)[1]
- *Urgency* is the complaint of a sudden compelling desire to pass urine which is difficult to defer. (CHANGED)
- *Urinary incontinence* is the complaint of any involuntary leakage of urine. (NEW)[2]

In each specific circumstance, urinary incontinence should be further described by specifying relevant factors such as type, frequency, severity, precipitating factors, social impact, effect on hygiene and quality of life, the measures used to contain the leakage and whether or not the individual seeks or desires help because of urinary incontinence.[3]

Urinary leakage may need to be distinguished from sweating or vaginal discharge.

- *Stress urinary incontinence* is the complaint of involuntary leakage on effort or exertion, or on sneezing or coughing. (CHANGED)[4]
- *Urge urinary incontinence* is the complaint of involuntary leakage accompanied by or immediately preceded by urgency. (CHANGED)[5]
- *Mixed urinary incontinence* is the complaint of involuntary leakage associated with urgency and also with exertion, effort, sneezing or coughing. (NEW)

---

[1] The term night time frequency differs from that for nocturia, as it includes voids that occur after the individual has gone to bed, but before he/she has gone to sleep, and voids which occur in the early morning which prevent the individual from getting back to sleep as he/she wishes. These voids before and after sleep may need to be considered in research studies, for example, in nocturnal polyuria. If this definition were used then an adapted definition of daytime frequency would need to be used with it.

[2] In infants and small children the definition of Urinary Incontinence is not applicable. In scientific communications the definition of incontinence in children would need further explanation.

[3] The original ICS definition of incontinence " Urinary incontinence is the involuntary loss of urine that is a social or hygienic problem", relates the complaint to quality of life (QoL) issues. Some QoL instruments have been and are being developed in order to assess the impact of both incontinence and other LUTS on QoL.

[4] The committee considers the term "stress incontinence" to be unsatisfactory in the English language because of its mental connotations. The Swedish, French and Italian expression "effort incontinence" is preferable. However, words such as "effort" or "exertion" still do not capture some of the common precipitating factors for stress incontinence such as coughing or sneezing. For this reason the term is left unchanged.

[5] Urge incontinence can present in different symptomatic forms; for example, as frequent small losses between micturitions or as a catastrophic leak with complete bladder emptying.

- *Enuresis* means any involuntary loss of urine. If it is used to denote incontinence during sleep, it should always be qualified with the adjective 'nocturnal'. **(ORIGINAL)**

If it is used to denote incontinence during sleep, it should always be qualified with the adjective "nocturnal".

- *Nocturnal enuresis* is the complaint of loss of urine occurring during sleep. **(NEW)**
- *Continuous urinary incontinence* is the complaint of continuous leakage. **(NEW)**
- *Other types of urinary incontinence* may be situational, for example the report of incontinence during sexual intercourse, or giggle incontinence.
- *Bladder sensation* can be defined, during history taking, by five categories.

    Normal: the individual is aware of bladder filling and increasing sensation up to a strong desire to void. **(NEW)**

    Increased: the individual feels an early and persistent desire to void. **(NEW)**

    Reduced: the individual is aware of bladder filling but does not feel a definite desire to void. **(NEW)**

    Absent: the individual reports no sensation of bladder filling or desire to void. **(NEW)**

    Non-specific: the individual reports no specific bladder sensation but may perceive bladder filling as abdominal fullness, vegetative symptoms, or spasticity. **(NEW)**[6]

1.2. Voiding Symptoms are experienced during the voiding phase. (NEW)

- *Slow stream* is reported by the individual as his or her perception of reduced urine flow, usually compared to previous performance or in comparison to others. **(NEW)**
- *Splitting or spraying* of the urine stream may be reported. **(NEW)**
- *Intermittent stream (Intermittency)* is the term used when the individual describes urine flow which stops and starts, on one or more occasions, during micturition. **(NEW)**
- *Hesitancy* is the term used when an individual describes difficulty in initiating micturition resulting in a delay in the onset of voiding after the individual is ready to pass urine. **(NEW)**
- *Straining* to void describes the muscular effort used to either initiate, maintain or improve the urinary stream. **(NEW)**[7]
- *Terminal dribble* is the term used when an individual describes a prolonged final part of micturition, when the flow has slowed to a trickle/dribble. **(NEW)**

1.3. Post Micturition Symptoms are experienced immediately after micturition. (NEW)

- *Feeling of incomplete emptying* is a self-explanatory term for a feeling experienced by the individual after passing urine. **(NEW)**

---

[6] These non-specific symptoms are most frequently seen in neurological patients, particularly those with spinal cord trauma and in children and adults with malformations of the spinal cord.

[7] Suprapubic pressure may be used to initiate or maintain urine flow. The Credé manoeuvre is used by some spinal cord injury patients, and girls with detrusor underactivity sometimes press suprapubically to help empty the bladder.

- *Post micturition dribble* is the term used when an individual describes the involuntary loss of urine immediately after he or she has finished passing urine, usually after leaving the toilet in men, or after rising from the toilet in women. (NEW)

1.4. Symptoms Associated with Sexual Intercourse

Dyspareunia, vaginal dryness and incontinence are amongst the symptoms women may describe during or after intercourse. These symptoms should be described as fully as possible. It is helpful to define urine leakage as: during penetration, during intercourse, or at orgasm.

1.5. Symptoms Associated with Pelvic Organ Prolapse

The feeling of a lump ("something coming down"), low backache, heaviness, dragging sensation, or the need to digitally replace the prolapse in order to defaecate or micturate, are amongst the symptoms women may describe who have a prolapse.

1.6. Genital and Lower Urinary Tract Pain[8]

Pain, discomfort and pressure are part of a spectrum of abnormal sensations felt by the individual. Pain produces the greatest impact on the patient and may be related to bladder filling or voiding, may be felt after micturition, or be continuous. Pain should also be characterised by type, frequency, duration, precipitating and relieving factors and by location as defined below:

- *Bladder pain* is felt suprapubically or retropubically, and usually increases with bladder filling, it may persist after voiding. (NEW)
- *Urethral pain* is felt in the urethra and the individual indicates the urethra as the site. (NEW)
- *Vulval pain* is felt in and around the external genitalia. (NEW)
- *Vaginal pain* is felt internally, above the introitus. (NEW)
- *Scrotal pain* may or may not be localised, for example to the testis, epididymis, cord structures or scrotal skin. (NEW)
- *Perineal pain* is felt: in the female, between the posterior fourchette (posterior lip of the introitus) and the anus, and in the male, between the scrotum and the anus. (NEW)
- *Pelvic pain* is less well defined than, for example, bladder, urethral or perineal pain and is less clearly related to the micturition cycle or to bowel function and is not localised to any single pelvic organ. (NEW)

---

[8] The terms "strangury", "bladder spasm", and "dysuria" are difficult to define and of uncertain meaning and should not be used in relation to lower urinary tract dysfunction, unless a precise meaning is stated. Dysuria literally means 'abnormal urination' and is used correctly in some European countries. However, it is often used to describe the stinging/burning sensation characteristic of urinary infection. It is suggested that these descriptive words should be used in future.

1.7. Genito-Urinary Pain Syndromes and Symptom Syndromes Suggestive of LUTD

Syndromes describe constellations, or varying combinations of symptoms, but cannot be used for precise diagnosis. The use of the word 'syndrome' can only be justified if there is at least one other symptom in addition to the symptom used to describe the syndrome. In scientific communications the incidence of individual symptoms within the syndrome should be stated, in addition to the number of individuals with the syndrome.

The syndromes described are functional abnormalities for which a precise cause has not been defined. It is presumed that routine assessment (history taking, physical examination, and other appropriate investigations) has excluded obvious local pathologies such as those that are infective, neoplastic, metabolic or hormonal in nature.

1.7.1. Genito-Urinary Pain Syndromes are all chronic in their nature. Pain is the major complaint but concomitnat complaints are of lower urinary tract, bowel, sexual or gynaecological nature.

- *Painful bladder syndrome* is the complaint of suprapubic pain related to bladder filling, accompanied by other symptoms such as increased daytime and night-time frequency, in the absence of proven urinary infection or other obvious pathology. (NEW)[9]

- *Urethral pain syndrome* is the occurrence of recurrent episodic urethral pain usually on voiding, with daytime frequency and nocturia, in the absence of proven infection or other obvious pathology. (NEW)

- *Vulval pain syndrome* is the occurrence of persistent or recurrent episodic vulval pain, which is either related to the micturition cycle or associated with symptoms suggestive of urinary tract or sexual dysfunction. There is no proven infection or other obvious pathology. (NEW)[10]

- *Vaginal pain syndrome* is the occurrence of persistent or recurrent episodic vaginal pain which is associated with symptoms suggestive of urinary tract or sexual dysfunction. There is no proven vaginal infection or other obvious pathology.

- *Scrotal pain syndrome* is the occurrence of persistent or recurrent episodic scrotal pain which is associated with symptoms suggestive of urinary tract or sexual dysfunction. There is no proven epididimo-orchitis or other obvious pathology.

- *Perineal pain syndrome* is the occurrence of persistent or recurrent episodic perineal pain which is either related to the micturition cycle or associated with symptoms suggestive of urinary tract or sexual dysfunction. There is no proven infection or other obvious pathology. (NEW)[11]

---

[9] The ICS believes this to be a preferable term to "interstitial cystitis". Interstitial cystitis is a specific diagnosis and requires confirmation by typical cystoscopic and histological features. In the investigation of bladder pain it may be necessary to exclude conditions such as carcinoma in situ and endometriosis.

[10] The ICS suggests that the term vulvodynia (vulva – pain) should not be used, as it leads to confusion between a single symptom and a syndrome.

[11] The ICS suggests that in men, the term prostatodynia (prostate-pain) should not be used as it leads to confusion between a single symptom and a syndrome.

- *Pelvic pain syndrome* is the occurrence of persistent or recurrent episodic pelvic pain associated with symptoms suggestive of lower urinary tract, sexual, bowel or gynaeco-logical dysfunction. There is no proven infection or other obvious pathology. (**NEW**)

1.7.2. Symptom Syndromes Suggestive of Lower Urinary Tract Dysfunction

In clinical practice, empirical diagnoses are often used as the basis for initial management after assessing the individual's lower urinary tract symptoms, physical findings and the results of urinalysis and other indicated investigations.

- *Urgency,* with or without urge incontinence, usually with frequency and nocturia, can be described as the <u>overactive bladder syndrome</u>, <u>urge syndrome</u> or <u>urgency-frequency syndrome</u>. (**NEW**)
  These symptom combinations are suggestive of urodynamically demonstrable detru-sor overactivity but can be due to other forms of urethro-vesical dysfunction. These terms can be used if there is no proven infection or other obvious pathology.
- *Lower urinary tract symptoms suggestive of bladder outlet obstruction* is a term used when a man complains predominately of voiding symptoms in the absence of infection or obvious pathology other than possible causes of outlet obstruction. (**NEW**)[12]

2. Signs Suggestive of Lower Urinary Tract Dysfunction (LUTD)

2.1. Measuring the Frequency, Severity and Impact of Lower Urinary Tract Symptoms

Asking the patient to record micturitions and symptoms[13] for a period of days provides invaluable information. The recording of micturition events can be in three main forms:

- *Micturition time chart:* this records only the times of micturitions, day and night, for at least 24 hours. (**NEW**)
- *Frequency volume chart (FVC):* this records the volumes voided as well as the time of each micturition, day and night, for at least 24 hours. (**CHANGED**)
- *Bladder diary:* this records the times of micturitions and voided volumes, incontinence episodes, pad usage and other information such as fluid intake, the degree of urgency and the degree of incontinence. (**NEW**)[14]

---

[12] in women voiding symptoms are usually thought to suggest detrusor underactivity rather than bladder outlet obstruction.

[13] Validated questionnaires are useful for recording symptoms, their frequency, severity and bother, and the impact of LUTS on QoL. The instrument used should be specified.

[14] It is useful to ask the individual to make an estimate of liquid intake. This may be done precisely by measuring the volume of each drink or crudely by asking how many drinks are taken in a 24 hour period. If the individual eats significant quantities of water containing foods (vegetables, fruit, salads) then an appreciable effect on urine production will result. The time that diuretic therapy is taken should be marked on a chart or diary.

The following measurements can be abstracted from frequency volume charts and bladder diaries:

- *Daytime frequency* is the number of voids recorded during waking hours and includes the last void before sleep and the first void after waking and rising in the morning. **(NEW)**
- *Nocturia* is the number of voids recorded during a night's sleep: each void is preceded and followed by sleep. **(NEW)**
- *24-hour frequency* is the total number of daytime voids and episodes of nocturia during a specified 24 hours period. **(NEW)**
- *24-hour production* is measured by collecting all urine for 24 hours. **(NEW)**
  This is usually commenced <u>after</u> the first void produced after rising in the morning and is completed by including the first void on rising the following morning.
- *Polyuria* is defined as the measured production of more than 2.8 litres of urine in 24 hours in adults. It may be useful to look at output over shorter time frames (van Kerrebroeck et al., 2002). **(NEW)**[15]
- *Nocturnal urine volume* is defined as the total volume of urine passed between the time the individual goes to bed with the intention of sleeping and the time of waking with the intention of rising. **(NEW)** Therefore, it excludes the last void before going to bed but includes the first void after rising in the morning.
- *Nocturnal polyuria* is present when an increased proportion of the 24-hour output occurs at night (normally during the 8 hours whilst the patient is in bed). **(NEW)** The night time urine output excludes the last void before sleep but includes the first void of the morning.[16]
- *Maximum voided volume* is the largest volume of urine voided during a single micturition and is determined either from the frequency/volume chart or bladder diary. **(NEW)**
  The maximum, mean and minimum voided volumes over the period of recording may be stated.[17]

2.2. Physical Examination is essential in the assessment of all patients with lower urinary tract dysfunction. It should include abdominal, pelvic, perineal and a focussed neurological examination. For patients with possible neurogenic lower urinary tract dysfunction, a more extensive neurological examination is needed.

---

[15] The causes of polyuria are various and reviewed elsewhere but include habitual excess fluid intake. The figure of 2.8 is based on a 70kg person voiding > 40ml/kg.

[16] The normal range of nocturnal urine production differs with age and the normal ranges remain to be defined. Therefore, nocturnal polyuria is present when greater than 20% (young adults) to 33% (over 65 years) is produced at night. Hence the precise definition is dependent on age.

[17] The term "functional bladder capacity" is no longer recommended, as "voided volume" is a clearer and less confusing term, particularly if qualified e.g. 'maximum voided volume'. If the term "bladder capacity" is used, in any situation, it implies that this has been measured in some way, if only by abdominal ultrasound. In adults, voided volumes vary considerably. In children, the "expected volume" may be calculated from the formula (30+ (age in years x 30) in ml). Assuming no residual urine, this will be equal to the "expected bladder capacity".

2.2.1. Abdominal: the bladder may be felt by abdominal palpation or by suprapubic percussion. Pressure suprapubically or during bimanual vaginal examination may induce a desire to pass urine.

2.2.2. Perineal / Genital Inspection allows the description of the skin, for example the presence of atrophy or excoriation, any abnormal anatomical features and the observation of incontinence.

- *Urinary incontinence (the sign)* is defined as urine leakage seen during examination: this may be urethral or extraurethral.

- *Stress urinary incontinence* is the observation of involuntary leakage from the urethra, synchronous with exertion/effort, or sneezing or coughing. **(CHANGED)**[18]
  Stress Leakage is presumed to be due to raised abdominal pressure.

- *Extra-urethral incontinence* is defined as the observation of urine leakage through channels other than the urethra. **(ORIGINAL)**

- *Uncategorised incontinence* is the observation of involuntary leakage that cannot be classified into one of the above categories on the basis of signs and symptoms. **(NEW)**

2.2.3. Vaginal Examination allows the description of observed and palpable anatomical abnormalities and the assessment of pelvic floor muscle function, as described in the ICS report on Pelvic Organ Prolapse. The definitions given are simplified versions of the definitions in that report. (Bump et al., 1996)

- *Pelvic organ prolapse* is defined as the descent of one or more of: the anterior vaginal wall, the posterior vaginal wall, and the apex of the vagina (cervix/uterus) or vault (cuff) after hysterectomy. Absence of prolapse is defined as stage 0 support; prolapse can be staged from stage I to stage IV. **(NEW)**
  Pelvic organ prolapse can occur in association with urinary incontinence and other lower urinary tract dysfunction and may on occasion mask incontinence.

- *Anterior vaginal wall prolapse* is defined as descent of the anterior vagina so that the urethrovesical junction (a point 3cm proximal to the external urinary meatus) or any anterior point proximal to this is less than 3cm above the plane of the hymen. **(CHANGED)**

- *Prolapse of the apical segment of the vagina* is defined as any descent of the vaginal cuff scar (after hysterectomy) or cervix, below a pointwhich is 2cm less than the total vaginal length above the plane of the hymen. **(CHANGED)**

- *Posterior vaginal wall prolapse* is defined as any descent of the posterior vaginal wall so that a midline point on the posterior vaginal wall 3cm above the level of the hymen or any posterior point proximal to this, less than 3cm above the plane of the hymen. **(CHANGED)**

---

[18] Coughing may induce a detrusor contraction, hence the sign of stress incontinence is only a reliable indication of urodynamic stress incontinence when leakage occurs synchronously with the first proper cough and stops at the end of that cough.

2.2.4. Pelvic Floor Muscle Function can be qualitatively defined by the tone at rest and the strength of a voluntary or reflex contraction as strong, weak or absent or by a validated grading system (e.g. Oxford 1-5). A pelvic muscle contraction may be assessed by visual inspection, by palpation, electromyography or perineometry. Factors to be assessed include strength, duration, displacement and repeatability. (**NEW**)

2.2.5. Rectal Examination allows the description of observed and palpable anatomical abnormalities and is the easiest method of assessing pelvic floor muscle function in children and men. In addition, rectal examination is essential in children with urinary incontinence to rule out faecal inpaction.

- *Pelvic floor muscle function* can be qualitatively defined, during rectal examination, by the tone at rest and the strength of a voluntary contraction, as strong, weak or absent. (**NEW**)

2.3. Pad Testing may be used to quantify the amount of urine lost during incontinence episodes and methods range from a short provocative test to a 24-hour pad test.

3. Urodynamic Observations and Conditions

3.1. Urodynamic Techniques There are two principal methods of urodynamic investigation:

- *Conventional urodynamic studies* normally take place in the urodynamic laboratory and usually involve artificial bladder filling. (**NEW**)
  - *Artificial bladder filling* is defined as filling the bladder, via a catheter, with a specified liquid at a specified rate. (**NEW**)
- *Ambulatory urodynamic studies* are defined as a functional test of the lower urinary tract, utilising natural filling, and reproducing the subject's every day activities.[19]
  - *Natural filling* means that the bladder is filled by the production of urine rather than by an artificial medium.

Both filling cystometry and pressure flow studies of voiding require the following measurements:

- *Intravesical pressure* is the pressure within the bladder. (**ORIGINAL**)
- *Abdominal pressure* is taken to be the pressure surrounding the bladder. In current practice it is estimated from rectal, vaginal or, less commonly, from extraperitoneal pressure or a bowel stoma. The simultaneous measurement of abdominal pressure is essential for the interpretation of the intravesical pressure trace. (**ORIGINAL**)
- *Detrusor pressure* is that component of intravesical pressure that is created by forces in the bladder wall (passive and active). It is estimated by subtracting abdominal pressure from intravesical pressure. (**ORIGINAL**)

---

[19] The term Ambulatory Urodynamics is used to indicate that monitoring usually takes place outside the urodynamic laboratory, rather than the subject's mobility using natural filling.

3.2. Filling Cystometry

The word "cystometry" is commonly used to describe the urodynamic investigation of the filling phase of the micturition cycle. To eliminate confusion, the following definitions are proposed:

- *Filling cystometry* is the method by which the pressure/volume relationship of the bladder is measured during bladder filling. **(ORIGINAL)**
  The filling phase starts when filling commences and ends when the patient and urodynamicist decide that "permission to void" has been given.[20]

Bladder and urethral function, during filling, need to be defined separately.
  The rate at which the bladder is filled is divided into:

- *Physiological filling rate* is defined as a filling rate less than the predicted maximum–predicted maximum body weight in kg divided by 4 expressed as ml/min (Klevmark, 1999) **(CHANGED)**
- *Non-physiological filling rate* is defined as a filling rate greater than the predicted maximum filling rate–predicted maximum body weight in kg divided by 4 expressed as ml/min (Klevmark, 1999) **(CHANGED)**

Bladder storage function should be described according to bladder sensation, detrusor activity, bladder compliance and bladder capacity.[21]

3.2.1. Bladder Sensation During Filling Cystometry

- *Normal bladder sensation* can be judged by three defined points noted during filling cystometry and evaluated in relation to the bladder volume at that moment and in relation to the patient's symptomatic complaints.
- *First sensation of bladder filling* is the feeling the patient has, during filling cystometry, when he/she first becomes aware of the bladder filling. **(NEW)**
- *First desire to void* is defined as the feeling, during filling cystometry, that would lead the patient to pass urine at the next convenient moment, but voiding can be delayed if necessary. **(CHANGED)**
- *Strong desire to void* this is defined, during filling cystometry, as a persistent desire to void without the fear of leakage. **(ORIGINAL)**
- *Increased bladder sensation* is defined, during filling cystometry, as an early first sensation of bladder filling (or an early desire to void) and/or an early strong desire to void, which occurs at low bladder volume and which persists. **(NEW)**[22]

---

[20] The ICS no longer wishes to divide filling rates into slow, medium and fast. In practice almost all investigations are performed using medium filling rates which have a wide range. It may be more important during investigations to consider whether or not the filling rate used during conventional urodynamic studies can be considered physiological.

[21] Whilst bladder sensation is assessed during filling cystometry the assumption that it is sensation from the bladder alone, without urethral or pelvic components may be false.

[22] The assessment of the subject's bladder sensation is subjective and it is not, for example, possible to quantify "low bladder volume" in the definition of "increased bladder sensation".

- *Reduced bladder sensation* is defined, during filling cystometry, as diminished sensation throughout bladder filling. **(NEW)**

- *Absent bladder sensation* means that, during filling cystometry, the individual has no bladder sensation. **(NEW)**

- *Non-specific bladder sensations,* during filling cystometry, may make the individual aware of bladder filling, for example, abdominal fullness or vegetative symptoms. **(NEW)**

- *Bladder pain,* during filling cystometry, is a self explanatory term and is an abnormal finding. **(NEW)**

- *Urgency,* during filling cystometry, is a sudden compelling desire to void. **(NEW)**[23]

- *The vesical/urethral sensory threshold* is defined as the least current which consistently produces a sensation perceived by the subject during stimulation at the site under investigation. (Andersen et al., 1992) **(ORIGINAL)**

3.2.2. Detrusor Function During Filling Cystometry

In everyday life the individual attempts to inhibit detrusor activity until he or she is in a position to void. Therefore, when the aims of the filling study have been achieved, and when the patient has a desire to void, normally the 'permission to void' is given (see Filling Cystometry). That moment is indicated on the urodynamic trace and all detrusor activity before this 'permission' is defined as 'involuntary detrusor activity'.

- *Normal detrusor function:* allows bladder filling with little or no change in pressure. No involuntary phasic contractions occur despite provocation. **(ORIGINAL)**

- *Detrusor overactivity* is a urodynamic observation characterised by involuntary detrusor contractions during the filling phase which may be spontaneous or provoked. **(CHANGED)**[24]

There are certain patterns of detrusor overactivity:

- *Phasic detrusor overactivity* is defined by a characteristic wave form and may or may not lead to urinary incontinence. **(NEW)**[25]

- *Terminal detrusor overactivity* is defined as a single, involuntary detrusor contraction, occurring at cystometric capacity, which cannot be suppressed and results in incontinence usually resulting in bladder emptying (voiding). **(NEW)**[26]

---

[23] The ICS no longer recommends the terms "motor urgency" and "sensory urgency". These terms are often misused and have little intuitive meaning. Furthermore, it may be simplistic to relate urgency just to the presence or absence of detrusor overactivity when there is usually a concomitant fall in urethral pressure.

[24] There is no lower limit for the amplitude of an involuntary detrusor contraction but confident interpretation of low pressure waves (amplitude smaller than 5cm of H_2O) depends on "high quality" urodynamic technique. The phrase "which the patient cannot completely suppress" has been deleted from the old definition.

[25] Phasic detrusor contractions are not always accompanied by any sensation or may be interpreted as a first sensation of bladder filling or as a normal desire to void.

[26] "Terminal detrusor overactivity" is a new ICS term: it is typically associated with reduced bladder sensation, for example, in the elderly stroke patient when urgency may be felt as the voiding contraction occurs. However, in complete spinal cord injury patients there may be no sensation whatsoever.

- *Detrusor overactivity incontinence* is incontinence due to an involuntary detrusor contraction. (**NEW**)

In a patient with normal sensation, urgency is likely to be experienced just before the leakage episode.[27]

Detrusor Overactivity may also be qualified, when possible, according to cause, for example:

● *Neurogenic detrusor overactivity* when there is a relevant neurological condition. This term replaces the term "detrusor hyperreflexia". (**NEW**)

● *Idiopathic detrusor overactivity* when there is no defined cause. (**NEW**)

This term replaces "detrusor instability".[28]

In clinical and research practice, the extent of neurological examination/investigation varies. It is likely that the proportion of neurogenic:idiopathic detrusor overactivity will increase if a more complete neurological assessment is carried out.

Other patterns of detrusor overactivity are seen, for example, the combination of phasic and terminal detrusor overactivity, and the sustained high pressure detrusor contractions seen in spinal cord injury patients when attempted voiding occurs against a dyssynergic sphincter.

● *Provocative manoeuvres* are defined as techniques used during urodynamics in an effort to provoke detrusor overactivity, for example, rapid filling, use of cooled or acid medium, postural changes and hand washing. (**NEW**)

3.2.3. Bladder Compliance During Filling Cystometry

● *Bladder compliance* describes the relationship between change in bladder volume and change in detrusor pressure. (**CHANGED**)[29]

Compliance is calculated by dividing the volume change(?V) by the change in detrusor pressure (?pdet) during that change in bladder volume (C= V. ?pdet). It is expressed in ml/cm H_2O.

A variety of means of calculating bladder compliance has been described. The ICS recommends that two standard points should be used for compliance calculations: the investigator may wish to define additional points. The standards points are:

1. *the detrusor pressure at the start of bladder filling and the corresponding bladder volume (usually zero), and*

2. *the detrusor pressure (and corresponding bladder volume) at cystometric capacity or immediately before the start of any detrusor contraction that causes significant leakage*

---

[27] ICS recommends that the terms "motor urge incontinence" and "reflex incontinence" should no longer be used as they have no intuitive meaning and are often misused.

[28] The terms "detrusor instability" and "detrusor hyperreflexia" were both used as generic terms, in the English speaking world and Scandinavia, prior to the first ICS report in 1976. As a compromise they were allocated to idiopathic and neurogenic overactivity respectively. As there is no real logic or intuitive meaning to the terms, the ICS believes they should be abandoned.

[29] The observation of reduced bladder compliance during conventional filling cystometry is often related to relatively fast bladder filling: the incidence of reduced compliance is markedly lower if the bladder is filled at physiological rates, as in ambulatory urodynamics.

(and therefore causes the bladder volume to decrease, affecting compliance calculation). Both points are measured excluding any detrusor contraction.

3.2.4. Bladder Capacity: During Filling Cystometry

- *Cystometric capacity* is the bladder volume at the end of the filling cystometrogram, when "permission to void" is usually given. The end point should be specified, for example, if filling is stopped when the patient has a normal desire to void. The cystometric capacity is the volume voided together with any residual urine. (CHANGED)[30]
- *Maximum cystometric capacity,* in patients with normal sensation, is the volume at which the patient feels he/she can no longer delay micturition (has a strong desire to void). (ORIGINAL)
- *Maximum anaesthetic bladder capacity* is the volume to which the bladder can be filled under deep general or spinal anaesthetic and should be qualified according to the type of anaesthesia used and the speed, the length of time, and the pressure at which the bladder is filled. (CHANGED)

3.2.5. Urethral Function During Filling Cystometry

The urethral closure mechanism during storage may be competent or incompetent.

- *Normal urethral closure mechanism* maintains a positive urethral closure pressure during bladder filling even in the presence of increased abdominal pressure, although it may be overcome by detrusor overactivity. (CHANGED)
- *Incompetent urethral closure mechanism* is defined as one which allows **leakage of urine in the absence of a detrusor contraction.** (ORIGINAL)
- *Urethral relaxation incontinence* is defined as leakage due to urethral relaxation in the absence of raised abdominal pressure or detrusor overactivity. (NEW)[31]
- *Urodynamic stress incontinence* is noted during filling cystometry and is defined as the involuntary leakage of urine during increased abdominal pressure, in the absence of a detrusor contraction. (CHANGED)

Urodynamic stress incontinence is now the preferred term to "genuine stress incontinence".[32]

---

[30] In certain types of dysfunction, the cystometric capacity cannot be defined in the same terms. In the absence of sensation the cystometric capacity is the volume at which the clinician decides to terminate filling. The reason (s) for terminating filling should be defined, e.g. high detrusor filling pressure, large infused volume or pain. If there is uncontrollable voiding, it is the volume at which this begins. In the presence of sphincter incompetence the cystometric capacity may be significantly increased by occlusion of the urethra e.g. by Foley catheter.

[31] Fluctuations in urethral pressure have been defined as the "unstable urethra". However, the significance of the fluctuations and the term itself lack clarity and the term is not recommended by the ICS. If symptoms are seen in association with a decrease in urethral pressure a full description should be given.

[32] In patients with stress incontinence, there is a spectrum of urethral characteristics ranging from a highly mobile urethra with good intrinsic function to an immobile urethra with poor intrinsic function. Any delineation into categories such as "urethral hypermobility" and "intrinsic sphincter deficiency" may be simplistic and arbitrary, and requires further research.

3.2.6. Assessment of Urethral Function During Filling Cystometry

- **Urethral pressure measurement**
  - *Urethral pressure* is defined as the fluid pressure needed to just open a closed urethra. **(ORIGINAL)**
  - *The Urethral pressure profile* is a graph indicating the intraluminal pressure along the length of the urethra. **(ORIGINAL)**
  - *The Urethral closure pressure profile* is given by the subtraction of intravesical pressure from urethral pressure. **(ORIGINAL)**
  - *Maximum urethral pressure* is the maximum pressure of the measured profile. **(ORIGINAL)**
  - *Maximum urethral closure pressure (MUCP)* is the maximum difference between the urethral pressure and the intravesical pressure. **(ORIGINAL)**
  - *Functional profile length* is the length of the urethra along which the urethral pressure exceeds intravesical pressure in women.
  - *Pressure "transmission" ratio* is the increment in urethral pressure on stress as a percentage of the simultaneously recorded increment in intravesical pressure.
- **Abnormal leak point pressure** is the intravesical pressure at which urine leakage occurs due to increased abdominal pressure in the absence of a detrusor contraction. **(NEW)**[33]
- **Detrusor leak point pressure** is defined as the lowest detrusor pressure at which urine leakage occurs in the absence of either a detrusor contraction or increased abdominal pressure. **(NEW)**[34]

3.3. Pressure Flow Studies

Voiding is described in terms of detrusor and urethral function and assessed by measuring urine flow rate and voiding pressures.

- **Pressure flow studies** of voiding are the method by which the relationship between pressure in the bladder and urine flow rate is measured during bladder emptying. **(ORIGINAL)**

The voiding phase starts when 'permission to void' is given, or when uncontrollable voiding begins, and ends when the patient considers voiding has finished.

---

[33] The Leak Pressure Point should be qualified according to the site of pressure measurement (rectal, vaginal or intravesical) and the method by which pressure is generated (cough or valsalva). Leak point pressures may be calculated in three ways from the three different baseline values which are in common use: zero (the true zero of intravesical pressure), the value of p_{ves} measured at zero bladder volume, or the value of p_{ves} immediately before the cough or valsalva (usually at 200 or 300ml bladder capacity). The baseline used, and the baseline pressure, should be specified.

[34] Detrusor leak point pressure has been used most frequently to predict upper tract problems in neurological patients with reduced bladder compliance. ICS has defined it "in the absence of a detrusor contraction" although others will measure DLPP during involuntary detrusor contractions.

3.3.1. Measurement of Urine Flow

Urine flow is defined either as **continuous**, that is without interruption, or as **intermittent**, when an individual states that the flow stops and starts during a single visit to the bathroom in order to void. The continuous flow curve is defined as a smooth arc-shaped curve or fluctuating when there are multiple peaks during a period of continuous urine flow.[35]

– *Flow rate* is defined as the volume of fluid expelled via the urethra per unit time. It is expressed in ml/s. (**ORIGINAL**)
– *Voided volume* is the total volume expelled via the urethra. (**ORIGINAL**)
– *Maximum flow rate* is the maximum measured value of the flow rate after correction for artefacts. (**CHANGED**)
– *Voiding time* is total duration of micturition, i.e. includes interruptions. When voiding is completed without interruption, voiding time is equal to flow time. (**ORIGINAL**)
– *Flow time* is the time over which measurable flow actually occurs. (**ORIGINAL**)
– *Average flow rate* is voided volume divided by flow time. The average flow should be interpreted with caution if flow is interrupted or there is a terminal dribble. (**CHANGED**)
– *Time to maximum flow* is the elapsed time from onset of flow to maximum flow. (**ORIGINAL**)

3.3.2. Pressure Measurements During Pressure Flow Studies (PFS)

The following measurements are applicable to each of the pressure curves: intravesical, abdominal and detrusor pressure.

– *Premicturition pressure* is the pressure recorded immediately before the initial isovolu-metric contraction. (**ORIGINAL**)
– *Opening pressure* is the pressure recorded at the onset of urine flow (consider time delay). (**ORIGINAL**)
– *Opening time* is the elapsed time from initial rise in detrusor pressure to onset of flow. (**ORIGINAL**)

This is the initial isovolumetric contraction period of micturition. Flow measurement delay should be taken into account when measuring opening time.

– *Maximum pressure* is the maximum value of the measured pressure. (**ORIGINAL**)
– *Pressure at maximum flow* is the lowest pressure recorded at maximum measured flow rate. (**ORIGINAL**)
– *Closing pressure* is the pressure measured at the end of measured flow. (**ORIGINAL**)
– *Minimum voiding pressure* is the minimum pressure during measurable flow but is not necessarily equal to either the opening or closing pressures.
– *Flow delay* is the time delay between a change in bladder pressure and the corresponding change in measured flow rate.

---

[35] The precise shape of the flow curve is decided by detrusor contractility, the presence of any abdominal straining and by the bladder outlet. (11)

3.3.3. Detrusor Function During Voiding

- *Normal detrusor function*
  Normal voiding is achieved by a voluntarily initiated continuous detrusor contraction that leads to complete bladder emptying within a normal time span, and in the absence of obstruction. For a given detrusor contraction, the magnitude of the recorded pressure rise will depend on the degree of outlet resistance. **(ORIGINAL)**
- *Abnormal detrusor activity* can be subdivided:
  - *Detrusor underactivity* is defined as a contraction of reduced strength and/or duration, resulting in prolonged bladder emptying and/or a failure to achieve complete bladder emptying within a normal time span. **(ORIGINAL)**
  - *Acontractile detrusor* is one that cannot be demonstrated to contract during urodynamic studies. **(ORIGINAL)**[36]
- *Post void residual (PVR)* is defined as the volume of urine left in the bladder at the end of micturition. **(ORIGINAL)**[37]

3.3.4. Urethral Function During Voiding

During voiding:

Normal urethra function is defined as urethra that opens and is continuously relaxed to allow the bladder to be emptied at a normal pressure. **(CHANGED)**

Abnormal urethra function may be due to either obstruction to urethral overactivity or the urethra cannot open due to anatomic abnormality, such as an enlarged prostate or a urethral stricture.

- *Bladder outlet obstruction* is the generic term for obstruction during voiding and is characterised by increased detrusor pressure and reduced urine flow rate. It is usually diagnosed by studying the synchronous values of flowrate and detrusor pressure. **(CHANGED)**[38]
- *Dysfunctional voiding* is characterised by an intermittent and/or fluctuating flow rate due to involuntary intermittent contractions of the peri-urethral striated muscle during voiding in neurologically normal individuals. **(CHANGED)**[39]

---

[36] A normal detrusor contraction will be recorded as: high pressure if there is high outlet resistance, normal pressure if there is normal outlet resistance: or low pressure if urethral resistance is low.

[37] If after repeated free flowmetry no residual urine is demonstrated, then the finding of a residual urine during urodynamic studies should be considered an artifact, due to the circumstances of the test.

[38] Bladder Outlet Obstruction has been defined for men but, as yet, not adequately in women and children.

[39] Although dysfunctional voiding is not a very specific term, it is preferred to terms such as "non-neurogenic neurogenic bladder". Other terms such as " idiopathic detrusor sphincter dyssyergia", or " sphincter overactivity voiding dysfunction", may be preferable. However, the term dysfunctional voiding is very well established. The condition occurs most frequently in children. Whilst it is felt that pelvic floor contractions are responsible, it is possible that the intra-urethral striated muscle may be important.

- *Detrusor sphincter dyssynergia* is definec as a detrusor contraction concurrent with an involuntary contraction of the urethral and/or periurethral striated muscle. Occasionally, flow may be prevented altogether. (ORIGINAL)[40]
- *Non-relaxing urethral sphincter obstruction* usually occurs in individuals with a neurological lesion and is characterised by a non relaxing, obstructing urethra resulting in reduced urine flow. (NEW)[41]

4. Conditions

- *Acute retention of urine* is defined as a painful, palpable or percussable bladder, when the patient is unable to pass any urine. (NEW)[42]
- *Chronic retention of urine* is defined as a non-painful bladder, which remains palpable or percussable after the patient has passed urine. Such patients may be incontinent. (NEW)[43]
- *Benign prostatic obstruction* is a form of *bladder outlet obstruction* and may be diagnosed when the cause of outlet obstruction is known to be benign prostatic enlargement, due to histologic benign prostatic hyperplasia. (NEW)
- *Benign prostatic hyperplasia* is a term used (and reserved for) the typical histological pattern which defines the disease. (NEW)
- *Benign prostatic enlargement* is defined as prostatic enlargement due to histologic benign prostatic hyperplasia. The term "prostatic enlargement" should be used in the absence of prostatic histology. (NEW)

5. Treatment

The following definitions were published in the 7th ICS report on Lower Urinary Tract Rehabilitation Techniques [Andersen et al] and remain in their original form.

---

[40] Detrusor sphincter dyssynergia typically occurs in patients with a supra-sacral lesion, for example after high spinal cord injury, and is uncommon in lesions of the lower cord. Although the intraurethral and periurethral striated muscles are usually held responsible, the smooth muscle of the bladder neck or urethra may also be responsible.

[41] Non-relaxing sphincter obstruction is found in sacral and infra-sacral lesions, such as meningomyelocoele, and after radical pelvic surgery. In addition, there is often urodynamic stress incontinence during bladder filling. This term replaces "isolated distal sphincter obstruction".

[42] Although acute retention is usually thought of as painful, in certain circumstances pain may not be a presenting feature, for example when due to prolapsed intervertebral disc, post partum, or after regional anaesthesia such as an epidural anaesthetic. The retention volume should be significantly greater than the expected normal bladder capacity. In patients after surgery, due to bandaging of the lower abdomen or abdominal wall pain, it may be difficult to detect a painful, palpable or percussable bladder.

[43] The ICS no longer recommends the term "overflow incontinence". This term is considered confusing and lacking a convincing definition. If used, a precise definition and any associated pathophysiology, such as reduced urethral function, or detrusor overactivity/low bladder compliance, should be stated. The term chronic retention excludes transient voiding difficulty, for example after surgery for stress incontinence, and implies a significant residual urine; a minimum figure of 300mls has been previously mentioned.

5.1. Lower Urinary Tract Rehabilitation is defned as non-surgical, non-pharmaco-
logical treatment for lower urinary tract function and includes;

- *Pelvic floor training*, defined as repetitive selective voluntary contraction and relaxation of specific pelvic floor muscles.

- *Biofeedback*, the technique by which information about a normally unconscious physiological process is presented to the patient and/or the therapist as a visual, auditory or tactile signal.

- *Behavioural modification*, defined as the analysis and alteration of the relationship between the patient's symptoms and his or her environment for the treatment of maladaptive voiding patterns.

This may be achieved by modification of the behaviour and/or environment of the patient.

5.2. Electrical Stimulation is the application of electrical current to stimulate the
pelvic viscera or their nerve supply.

The aim of electrical stimulation may be to directly induce a therapeutic response or to modulate lower urinary tract, bowel or sexual dysfunction.

5.3. Catheterization is a technique for bladder emptying employing a catheter to drain
the bladder or a urinary reservoir.

5.3.1. Intermittent (in/out) Catheterisation is defined as drainage or aspiration of
the bladder or a urinary reservoir with subsequent removal of the catheter.

The following types of intermittent catheterization are defined:

- **Intermittent self-catheterisation** is performed by the patient himself/herself.

- **Intermittent catheterisation** is performed by an attendant (e.g. doctor, nurse or relative).

- **Clean intermittent catheterisation:** use of a clean technique. This implies ordinary washing techniques and use of disposable or cleansed reusable catheters.

- **Aseptic intermittent catheterisation:** use of a sterile technique. This implies genital disinfection and the use of sterile catheters and instruments/gloves.

5.3.2. Indwelling catheterisation: an indwelling catheter remains in the bladder,
urinary reservoir or urinary conduit for a period of time longer than one emptying.

5.4. Bladder Reflex Triggering comprises various manoeuvres performed by the patient
or the therapist in order to elicit reflex detrusor contraction by exteroceptive stimuli.

The most commonly used manoeuvres are; suprapubic tapping, thigh scratching and anal/rectal manipulation.

5.5. Bladder Expression comprises various manoeuvres aimed at increasing intravesi-
cal pressure in order to facilitate bladder emptying.

The most commonly used manoeuvres are abdominal straining, Valsalva's manoeuvre and Credé manoeuvre.

ACKNOWLEDGEMENTS:
The authors of this report are very grateful to Vicky Rees, Administrator of the ICS, for her typing and editing of numerous drafts of this document.

ADDENDUM:
Formation of the ICS Terminology Committee

The terminology committee was announced at the ICS meeting in Denver 1999 and expressions of interest were invited from those who wished to be active members of the committee. They were asked to comment in detail on the preliminary draft (the discussion paper published in *Neurourology and Urodynamics*). The nine authors replied with a detailed critique by 1st April 2000 and constitute the committee: **Paul Abrams, Linda Cardozo, Magnus Fall, Derek Griffiths, Peter Rosier, Ulf Ulmsten, Philip van Kerrebroeck, Arne Victor and Alan Wein.**

We thank other individuals who later offered their written comments: **Jens Thorup Andersen, Walter Artibani, Jerry Blaivas, Linda Brubaker, Rick Bump, Emmanuel Chartier-Kastler, Grace Dorey, Clare Fowler, Kelm Hjalmas, Gordon Hosker, Vik Khullar, Guus Kramer, Gunnar Lose, Joseph Macaluso, Anders Mattiasson, Richard Millard, Rien Nijman, Arwin Ridder, Werner Schäfer, David Vodusek, Jean Jacques Wyndaele.**

A $^1/_2$ day workshop was held at the ICS Annual Meeting in Tampere (August 2000) and a two-day meeting in London, January 2001. This produced draft 5 of the report which was then placed on the ICS website (www.icsoffice.org). Discussions on draft 6 took place at the ICS meeting in Korea September 2001; draft 7 then remained on the ICS website until final submission to journals in November 2001.

References

1. Abrams P (Chair), Blaivas J G, Stanton S, Andersen J T– ICS Standardisation of Terminology of Lower Urinary Tract Function 1988 – Scand J Urol Nephrol, Supp 114, 1988 pages 5 – 19.
2. Abrams P, Blaivas J G, Stanton S L, Andersen J (Chair)–ICS 6th Report on the Standardisation of Terminology of Lower Urinary Tract Function – Neurourol. Urodyn. 11:593-603 (1992).
3. Andersen J.T (Chair), Blaivas J G, Cardozo L, Thuroff J – ICS 7th Report on the Standardisation of Terminology of Lower Urinary Tract Function -Lower Urinary Tract Rehabilitation Techniques–Neurourol. Urodyn. 11:593-603 (1992)
4. Bump R C, Mattiasson A, Bo K, Brubaker L P, DeLancey J O L, Klarskov P, Shull B L, Smith A R B – The Standardisation of Terminology of Female Pelvic Organ Prolapse and Pelvic Floor Dysfunction–Am J Obstet Gynecol. 1996;175:10-1.
5. Griffiths D, Hofner K, van Mastrigt R, Rollema H J, Spangberg A, Gleason D – ICS Report on the Standardisation of Terminology of Lower Urinary Tract Function: Pressure-Flow Studies of Voiding, Urethral Resistance and Urethral Obstruction – Neurourol. Urodyn. 16:1-18 (1997).
6. Stohrer M, Goepel M, Kondo A, Kramer G, Madersbacher H, Millard R, Rossier A Wyndaele J J – ICS Report on the Standardisation of Terminology in Neurogenic Lower Urinary Tract Dysfunction – Neurourol. Urodyn. 18:139-158 (1999).
7. van Waalwijk van Doorn E, Anders K, Khullar V, Kulseng-Hansen S, Pesce F, Robertson A, Rosario D, Schäfer W. Standardisation of Ambulatory Urodynamic Monitoring: Report of the Standardisation Sub-committee of the International Continence Soceity for Ambulatory Urodynamic Studies – Neurourol. Urodyn. 19:113-125 (2000).
8. Gunnar L, Griffiths D, Hosker G, Kulseng-Hanssen S, Perucchini D, Schäfer W, Thind P and Versi E–Standardisation of Urethral Pressure Measurement: Report from the Standardisation Sub-committee of the International Continence Society – Neurourol. Urodyn. 21 (2002).
9. van Kerrebroeck P, Abrams P, Chaikin D, Donovan J, Fonda D, Jackson S, Jennum P, Johnson T, Lose G, Mattiasson A, Robertson G and Weiss J–ICS Standardisation Report on Nocturia – Neurourol. Urodyn. 21 (2002).

10. Rowan D (Chair), James E D, Kramer A E J L, Sterling A M, Suhel P F–ICS Report on Urodynamic Equipment: Technical Aspects – J Med Eng & Tch. Vol 11, No 2, Pages 57-64 (Mar/Apr 1987).

11. Schäfer W, Sterling A M, Liao L, Spangberg A, Pesce F, Zinner N R, van Kerrebroeck P, Abrams P and Mattiasson A – Good Urodynamic Practice: Report from the Standardisation Sub-committee of the International Continence Society – Neurourol. Urodyn. In press (2002).

12. Mattiasson A, Djurhuus J C, Fonda D, Lose G, Nordling J and Stöhrer M – Standardisation of Outcome Studies in Patients with Lower Urinary Dysfunction: A Report on General Principles from the Standardisation Committee of the International Continence Society – Neurourol. Urodyn. 17:249-253 (1998).

13. Lose G, Fanti J A, Victor A, Walter S, Wells T L, Wyman J and Mattiasson A – Outcome Measures for Research in Adult Women with Symptoms of Lower Urinary Tract Dysfunction – Neurourol. Urodyn. 17:255-262 (1998).

14. Nordling J, Abrams P, Ameda K, Andersen J T, Donovan J, Griffiths D, Kobayashi S, Koyanagi T, Schäfer W, Yalla S and Mattiasson A – Outcome Measures for Research in Treatment of Adult Males with Symptoms of Lower Urinary Tract Dysfunction – Neurourol. Urodyn. 17:263-271 (1998).

15. Fonda D, Resnick N M, Colling J, Burgio K, Ouslander J G, Norton C, Ekelund P, Versi E and Mattiasson A – Outcome Measures for Research of Lower Urinary Tract Dysfunction in Frail and Older People – Neurourol. Urodyn. 17:273-281 (1998).

16. International Classification of Functioning, Disability and Health – ICIDH-2 website http://www.who.int/icidh.

17. Klevmark B – Natural Pressure-Volume Curves and Conventional Cystometry – Scand J Urol Nephrol Suppl 201:1-4 (1999).

Appendix 1, Part 6
Good Urodynamic Practices: Uroflowmetry, Filling Cystometry and Pressure-Flow Studies

Werner Schäfer,* Paul Abrams, Limin Liao, Anders Mattiasson, Francesco Pesce, Anders Spangberg, Arthur M. Sterling, Norman R. Zinner, and Philip van Kerrebroeck
International Continence Society Office, Southme Hospital, Bristol, BSIO SNB, United Kingdom

This is the first report of the International Continence Society (ICS) on the development of comprehensive guidelines for Good Urodynamic Practice for the measurement, quality control, and documentation of urodynamic investigations in both clinical and research environments. This report focuses on the most common urodynamics examinations; uroflowmetry, pressure recording during filling cystometry, and combined pressure–flow studies. The basic aspects of good urodynamic practice are discussed and a strategy for urodynamic measurement, equipment set-up and configuration, signal testing, plausibility controls, pattern recognition, and artifact correction are proposed. The problems of data analysis are mentioned only when they are relevant in the judgment of data quality. In general, recommendations are made for one specific technique. This does not imply that this technique is the only one possible. Rather, it means that this technique is well-established, and gives good results when used with the suggested standards of good urodynamic practice. *Neurourol. Urodynam. 21:261–274, 2002.* @ 2002 Wiley-Liss, Inc.

Key words: urodynamics; standardisation; uroflowmetry; cystometry; pressure-flow studies

Urodynamic techniques were performed according to the 'Good Urodynamic Practice' recommended by the International Continence Society.

This report is from the Standardization Committee of the International Continence Society.

* Correspondence to: Werner Schäfer, International Continence Society Office, Southme Hospital, Bristol, BSIO 5NB, United Kingdom. E-mail: Vicky@icsoffice.org.

DOI 10.1002/nau.10066

Published online in Wiley InterScience (www.interscience.wiley.com).

Introduction

A Good Urodynamic Practice comprises three main elements:

- A clear indication for and appropriate selection of, relevant test measurements and procedures
- Precise measurement with data quality control and complete documentation
- Accurate analysis and critical reporting of results

The aim of clinical urodynamics is to reproduce symptoms whilst making precise measurements in order to identify the underlying causes for the symptoms, and to quantify the related pathophysiological processes. By doing so, it should be possible to establish objectively the presence of a dysfunction and understand its clinical implications. Thus, we may either confirm a diagnosis or give a new, specifically urodynamic, diagnosis. The quantitative measurement may be supplemented by imaging (video-urodynamics).

Urodynamic measurements cannot yet be completely automated, except for the most simple urodynamic procedure, uroflowmetry. This is not an inherent problem of the measurement itself, but is due to the current limitations of urodynamic equipment and the lack of a consensus on the precise method of measurement, signal processing, quantification, documentation, and interpretation. With the publication of this ICS Standardisation document on good urodynamic practice, it is expected that the necessary technological developments in automation will follow.

Urodynamics allows direct assessment of lower urinary tract (LUT) function by the measurement of relevant physiological parameters. The first step is to formulate the 'urodynamic question or questions' from a careful history, physical examination, and standard urological investigations. The patient's recordings of micturitions and symptoms on a frequency volume chart, and repeated free uroflowmetry with determination of post-void residual volume provide important noninvasive, objective information that helps to define the specific 'urodynamic question' or questions, prior to invasive urodynamics such as filling cystometry and pressure-flow studies.

Recommendations for good urodynamic practice are bullet pointed, inset, and printed in bold.

Recording Micturitions and Symptoms

A *Micturition Time Chart* records the time of each micturition. The usefulness of such a record is significantly enhanced when the voided volumes are recorded in a *Frequency Volume Chart*. The *Bladder Diary* adds to this the relevant symptoms and events such as urgency, pain, incontinence episodes, and pad usage. Recording for a minimum of 2 days is recommended. From the recordings, the average voided volume, voiding frequency, and if, the patient's time in bed is recorded, day/night urine production and nocturia can be determined. This information provides objective verification of the patient's symptoms, and furthermore, key values for plausibility control of subsequent urodynamic studies, for example, in order to prevent over-filling of the patient's bladder.

Uroflowmetry

Uroflowmetry is noninvasive and relatively inexpensive. Therefore, it is an indispensable, first-line screening test for most patients with suspected LUT dysfunction. Objective and quantitative information, which helps one to understand both storage and voiding symptoms are provided by this simple urodynamic measurement.

Adequate privacy should be provided and patients should be asked to void when they feel a "normal" desire to void. Patients should be asked if their voiding was representative of their usual voiding and their view should be documented. Automated data analysis must be verified by inspection of the flow curve, artifacts must be excluded, and verification must be documented. The results from uroflowmetry should be compared with the data from the patient's own recording on a frequency/volume chart. Sonographic estimation of post-void residual volume completes the noninvasive assessment of voiding function.

Normal Uroflow

Normal voiding occurs when the bladder outlet relaxes (is passive) and the detrusor contracts (is active). An easily distensible bladder outlet with a normal detrusor contraction results in a smooth arc-shaped flow rate curve with high amplitude. Any other shapes, such as curves that are flat, asymmetric, or have multiple peaks (fluctuating and/or intermittent), indicate abnormal voiding, but are not specific for it's cause.

It is assumed that it is normal for the mechanical properties of a relaxed outlet to be constant, and that the properties can be defined by the dependency of the cross-sectional area of the urethral lumen on the intraurethral pressure at the flow rate controlling zone (FRCZ). Typically, below the minimum urethral opening pressure (pmuo), the urethral lumen is closed. The lumen then opens widely with little additional pressure increase. With normal detrusor contractility and low intraurethral pressure, the normal flow curve is arc-shaped with a high maximum flowrate. (Fig. A.1.6.1, top)

A normal flow curve is a smooth curve without any rapid changes in amplitude, because the shape of the flow curve is determined by the kinetics of the detrusor contraction, which arising from smooth muscle, does not show rapid variations. A decreased detrusor power and/or a constant increased urethral pressure will both result in a lower flowrate and a smooth flat flow curve. A constrictive obstruction (e.g., urethral stricture), with reduced lumen size results in a plateaulike flow curve. (Fig. A.1.6.1, broken line)

A compressive obstruction with increased urethral opening pressure (e.g., benign prostatic obstruction) shows a flattened asymmetric flow curve with a slowly declining end part. (Fig. A.1.6.1, bottom)

The same pattern may also originate from a weak detrusor in aging males and females. Fluctuations in detrusor contractility or abdominal straining, as well as variable outlet conditions, (e.g., intermittent sphincter activity) will lead to complex flow rate patterns.

Rapid changes in flowrate may have physiological or physical causes that owe to either changes in outlet resistance, for example, sphincter/pelvic floor contraction or relaxation, mechanical compression of the urethral lumen, or interference at the meatus, or to changes in driving energy, for example, abdominal straining. These intracorporeal causes lead to true flowrate changes. Rapid changes in flowrate may also be artifacts, when the flowrate

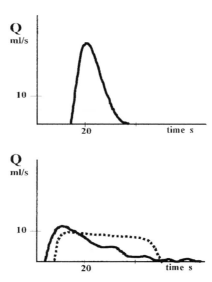

Fig. A.1.6.1. Typical normal flow (**top**), constrictive flow (**bottom**, dotted line), compressive flow curve (**bottom**).

signal is extracorporeally modified through interference between the stream and the collecting funnel, the flowmeter, movement of the stream across the surface of the funnel, or patient movements. (See flow-curves in Figs. A.1.6.3–A.1.6.8)

Accuracy of Uroflowmeters

Uroflowmetry measures the flow rate of the external urinary stream as volume per unit time in milliliters per second, (ml/s). The ICS Technical Report [Rowon et al., 1984] made technical recommendations with respect to uroflowmetry, but did not compare different flowmeters by specific testing. There are, however, differences in the accuracy and precision of the flow rate signals that depend on the type of flowmeter, on internal signal processing, and on the proper use and calibration of the flowmeter. The desired and actual accuracy of uroflowmetry should be assessed in relation to the potential information that could be obtained from the urinary stream compared to the information actually abstracted for clinical and research purposes. Some relevant aspects of the physiological and physical information contained in the urinary stream are outlined here.

The desired clinical accuracy may differ from the technical accuracy of a flow meter. The ICS Technical report recommended the following standards: a range of 0–50 ml/s for Q_{max}, and 0–1,000 ml for voided volume, maximum time constant of 0.75 s; an accuracy of + 5% relative to full scale, although a calibration curve representing the percentage error over the entire range of measurement should be made available. However, technical specifications from the manufacturers are rare and often not in accordance with ICS recommendations: this situation should be rectified.

Furthermore, as most flowmeters are mass flow meters (e.g., a weight transducer or rotating disk), variations in the specific gravity of the fluid will have a direct influence on the measured flow rate. For example, urine of high concentration may increase apparent flow rate by 3%. With X-ray medium, the flow rate may be overestimated by as much as 10%. These effects should be corrected by calibration software.

Thus, since the overall accuracy of flow rate signals will not be better than ± 5%, it would not be meaningful to report a maximum flow rate to a resolution better than a full milliliter per second (ml/s). Under carefully controlled research conditions, a better resolution may be possible by flowmeter calibration and instrument selection. However, such improvements in resolution may not be required for routine clinical applications. The dynamic properties of most flowmeters will be good enough for free uroflowmetry. When pressure flow data are analyzed, however, the limitation in signal dynamics should be taken into account because they will be different for pressure than for flow. Flow signals have a much slower response, and are less accurate than pressure signals.

Problems in Urine Flow Rate Measurement

The problems in measurement, as well as the information that can be abstracted from the flow rate signal are rather different for free uroflowmetry compared to combined pressure/flow recordings.

In free uroflowmetry, the shape of the flow curve may suggest specific types of abnormality, but reliable, specific, and detailed information about the cause for abnormal voiding cannot be derived from a flow curve alone. Only when uroflowmetry is combined with intravesical and abdominal pressure recordings does it become possible, from the pressure—flow relationship, to analyze separately the contributions of detrusor contractility and bladder outlet function to the overall voiding pattern. (Figs. A.1.6.3–A.1.6.8)

Urine flow rate measurement is affected by a number of important factors.

Detrusor Contractility

As the voiding function reflects the interaction between the relaxed outlet and the contracting detrusor, variation of both will affect the flow. For steady outflow conditions, all variations in flowrate are related to changes in detrusor activity alone. The detrusor contraction strength varies neurogenically and myogenically, and can cause significant variability in urine flow rate measurements. (Fig. A.1.6.5)

Bladder Outflow Resistance

If detrusor, contractility is constant, then changes in outflow resistance will lead to changes in flow rate, for example, in patients with detrusor–sphincter dyssynergia (Figs. A.1.6.3, A.1.6.7, A.1.6.8).

Bladder Volume

As the bladder volume increases and the detrusor muscle fibers become more stretched, there is an increase in the potential bladder power and work associated with a contraction. This is most pronounced in the range from empty up to 150–250 ml bladder filling volume. It appears that at volumes higher than 400–500 ml, the detrusor may become overstretched and contractility may decrease again. Therefore, Q_{max} is physiologically dependent on the bladder volume. This dependency will vary between individuals and with the type and degree of pathology, for example, in constrictive obstruction, Q_{max} is almost independent of volume, and in compressive obstruction, the dependency becomes weaker with increasingly obstructed outlet conditions and lower flow rate.

Technical Considerations

The flow rate signal is influenced by the technique of measurement and by signal processing. The external urinary stream should reach the flowmeter unaltered and with minimal delay. However, any funnel or collecting device, as well as the flowmeter, will inevitably introduce modifications to the flow rate recording. Physically, the external urinary stream breaks into drops not far from the meatus. This fine structure of the stream has a high frequency, which can be assessed by drop spectrometry, and contains interesting information. For standard uroflowmetry, however, such high frequencies should be eliminated by signal processing.

For free uroflowmetry, all intracorporeal modulations of the flow rate are physiological artifacts and should be minimized, for example by asking the patient to relax and not to strain. Nevertheless, certain dynamic patterns of intracorporeal modulations can provide information about functional obstruction, for example, typical patterns of the detrusor—sphincter dyssynergia, or abnormal straining. This information may be lost by excessive filtering or during analog to digital A/D conversion with a filter speed of less than 10 Hz. The precise interpretation of dynamic variations in the flow rate signal is only possible when the flow rate is viewed together with the simultaneously recorded pressure signals. Thus, only in combined pressure—flow recordings can the details of the flow signal be fully understood.

For the determination of the 'true' maximum flow rate value, particularly during free flow, such high frequency signal variations are more likely to be misleading, and consequently they should be suppressed electronically.

Recommendations for Uroflowmetry

In order to facilitate the recording of urine flow rate and pattern recognition of flow curves, it is recommended that graphical scaling should be standardized as follows:

● one millimeter should equal 1 s on the x-axis and 1 ml/s and 10 ml voided volume on the y-axis.

With respect to the technical accuracy of uroflowmeters, it is meaningful for routine clinical measurements to read flowrate values only to the nearest full ml/s and volumes to the nearest 10 ml.

In order to make electronically-read Q_{max} values more reliable, comparable, and clinically useful, we recommend internal electronic smoothing of the flow rate curve. It is recommended that:

● a sliding average over 2 s should be used to remove positive and negative spike artifacts.

If curves are smoothed by hand, the same concept should be applied. That is, when reading Q_{max} graphically, the line should be smoothed by eye into a continuous curve so that in each period of 2 s, there are no rapid changes. Such a smoothed, clinically-meaningful maximum free flow Q_{max} will be different (lower) from the peak value in the flow rate recording of electronic instruments currently available. (See Figs. A.1.6.2, A.1.6.5, A.1.6.6, A.1.6.8)

It is recommended that:

- only flow rate values, which have been 'smoothed', either electronically or manually, should be reported.

If a maximum flow value is determined electronically by simple signal peak detection without the recommended electronic smoothing, it should be labeled differently, $Q_{max.raw}$. Such raw data has meaning only if a detailed specification of the type of flowmeter used is given.

The interpretation of any dynamic variation (signal patterns) in free flow will rely on personal experience, can be only descriptive, and in general will remain speculative.

For the documentation of the results of uroflowmetry, the following recommendations are made:

- Maximum (smoothed) urine flow rate should be rounded to the nearest whole number (a recording of 10.25 ml/s would be recorded as 10 ml/s);
- Voided volume and post void residual volume should be rounded to the nearest 10 ml (a recording of a voided volume of 342 ml would be recorded as 340 ml);
- The maximum flow rate should always be documented together with voided volume and post void residual volume using a standard format: VOID: Maximum Flow Rate/ Volume Voided/Post Void Residual Volume.

For example, the automatically detected flows, $Q_{max.raw}$, are 16.6 and 21.3 ml/s with voided volumes 86 and 182 ml, respectively. The smoothed Q_{max} values are 8 and 17 ml/s and should be reported with voided volumes of 90 and 180, respectively, and the estimated residuals as VOID1 = 8/90/0 and VOID2 = 17/180/20 (see Figs. A.1.6.2, A.1.6.5, A.1.6.6).

The adoption of these standards will aid the interpretation of uroflowmetry results. If data are not available, then a hyphen should be used, for example, if only the voided volume is known, VOID:—/340/—or if the voided volume was missing, VOID: 10/—/90.

- If a flow/volume nomogram is used, this should be stated and referenced.

Uroflowmetry data from other than free flow, for example, measured in combination with intravesical pressure should be reported with an additional descriptive index, p, i.e., $Q_{max.p}$, for pressure—flow recording.

Invasive Urodynamics: Filling Cystometry, Pressure-flow Study of Voiding

Introduction

Invasive urodynamic procedures should not be performed without clear indications and the formulation of specific urodynamic question(s). This process will usually be aided by the a priori completion of a frequency volume chart and free uroflowmetry. There are certain key recommendations, which will lead to the performance of a successful urodynamic study.

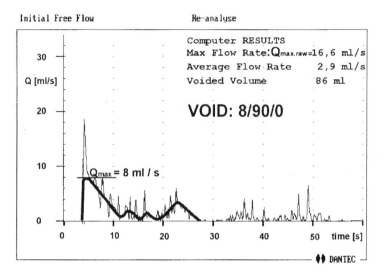

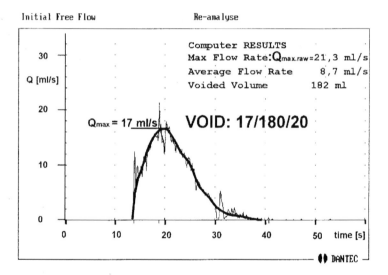

Fig. A.1.6.2 Exclusion of artifactual spikes in the flow curve, $Q_{max.raw}$, and determination of a clinically relevant maximum flow rate, Q_{max}, by manual smoothing. The results from uroflowmetry should be reported in the standard format: $Q_{max}/V_{void}/V_{res}$.

- A good urodynamic investigation should be performed interactively with the patient. It should be established by discussion with the patient that the patient's symptoms have been reproduced during the test;
- There should be continuous and careful observation of the signals as they are collected, and the continuous assessment of the qualitative and quantitative plausibility of all signals;
- Artifacts should be avoided, and any artifacts that occur should be corrected immediately. It is always difficult and is often impossible to correct artifacts during a retrospec-

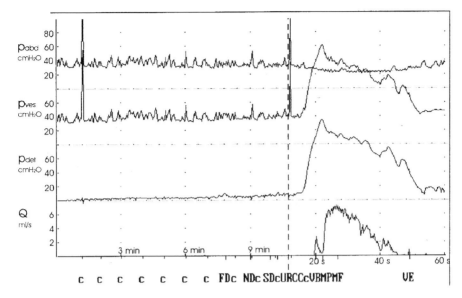

Fig. A.1.6.3 Full recording of filling and voiding. Starting with initial values for p_{ves}, p_{abd} of 32 cmH$_2$O in the typical range for a standing patient with zero p_{det}; testing signal quality with a vigorous cough at beginning, and regularly repeated (here less strong) coughs. Additionally, the pressure recordings show the typical pattern of a talking patient, while the p_{det} trace is unaffected; a weak contraction at first desire FD; another vigorous cough before voiding; beginning of flow shows dyssynergic sphincter activity as proven by decrease in flow with increase in p_{det}.

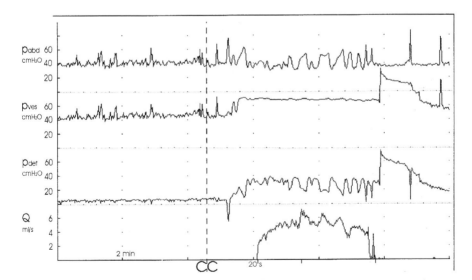

Fig. A.1.6.4 Good recording quality until cystometric capacity CC is reached; at second cough before voding the intravesical signal is lost (no response in p_{ves}, negative spike in p_{det}). Dead p_{ves} – signal during voiding, which is "live" again only at second cough after voiding. Thus, pressure-flow study is lost. Careful observation of signals would have made it possible to interrupt the study immediately when signal failed and correct this problem before voiding starts.

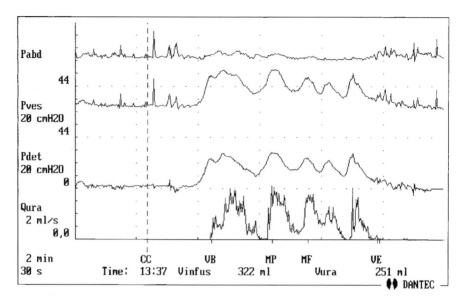

Fig. A.1.6.5 Variable flowrate due to varying detrusor contraction strength. VOID: 7/250/70.

tive analysis. Furthermore, it is more time consuming than if the signals are continuous-ly observed and tested at regular intervals and artifacts recognized during the urody-namic study and corrected.

At present, ambulatory urodynamic monitoring has to rely on retrospective quality control and artifact corrections. However, in principle, the same quality criteria apply for

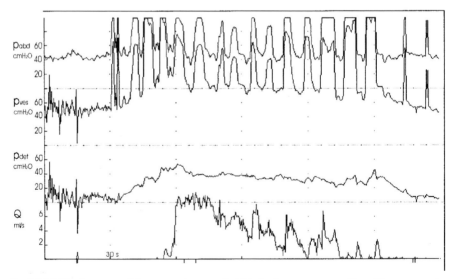

Fig. A.1.6.6 The first part of the traces shows typical bi-phasic movement artifacts. The two coughs before voiding prove good recording quality. The typical picture of a unobstructed voiding: a weak detrusor contraction with p_{det} of 40 cmH$_2$O and a Q_{max} of 9 ml/s is supported by vigorous straining, which causes some variability in flow (VOID: 9/380/100).

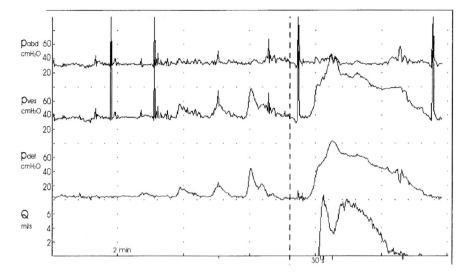

Fig. A.1.6.7 A good recording showing the typical pattern of increasing detrusor overactivity and a dyssynergic event during voiding.

ambulatory urodynamic monitoring as for standard urodynamics [van Waalwijk et al., 2000]. This makes a consensus on quality even more important, because only when such criteria are precisely defined can they be implemented in an "automated intelligent" ambulatory system.

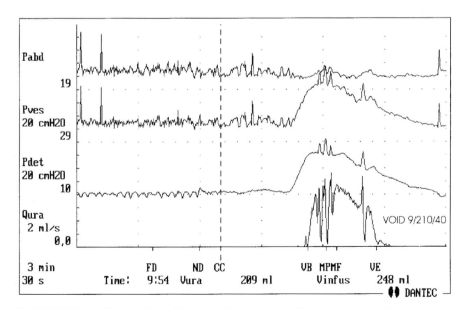

Fig. A.1.6.8 High quality recordings allow detailed interpretation. The typical pattern of rectal activity becomes clearly visible in p_{det}. The flow artifacts can identified as dyssynergic events and manually corrected from $Q_{max.raw} = 11.2$ ml/s to $Q_{max} = 9$ ml/s.

Quality control relies on pattern recognition and a knowledge of normal values as well as prior identification of useful information obtained from noninvasive urodynamics and all other sources relevant for the urodynamic question. Thus, before invasive urodynamics, a frequency volume chart should be completed and multiple free flows should be evaluated. Useful information obtained from noninvasive testing includes typical voided volumes and post-void residual volumes as well as the expected values for Q_{max}. This information should be used for the control of subsequent invasive studies. Only by good preparation can it be assured that (a) the proper answers to the urodynamic questions will be obtained before the study is terminated and (b) necessary modifications, additions, or repetitions of measurements will have been performed in order to derive the necessary information.

The effective practice of urodynamics requires: (a) a theoretical understanding of the underlying physics of the measurement, (b) practical experience with urodynamic equipment and procedures, (c) an understanding of how to assure quality control of urodynamic signals, and (d) the ability to analyze critically the results of the measurements. Because urodynamics deals largely with mechanical measurements such as pressure and volume and their related changes in time, and because many analytical models use mechanical concepts such as resistance to flow or contraction power, it is essential that the nature of these measurements and concepts, in particular for pressure and flowrate, are understood. Therefore, in addition to a comprehensive understanding of anatomy and physiology, some basic knowledge of biomechanics and physics is required.

The quality control of urodynamic measurements must be approached on a holistic basis. Different types and levels of data quality and plausibility control should be used: (a) on a physical and technical level, (b) on a biomechanical level, and (c) on a pathophysiological clinical level. A common problem in urodynamics is that clinicians often proceed immediately to a clinical interpretation, i.e., to level c without a critical analysis of the potential pathophysiological information content, without considering the plausibility of the signals (level a), without considering the biomechanical context of the measurements (level b), and without taking into account the physical properties of the parameters, technical limitations, and accuracy of the signals. Therefore, it is recommended that:

● Invasive urodynamics should not be performed without precise indications and well-defined 'urodynamic questions' that are to be answered by the results of the urodynamic study.

Measurement of Urine Flow Rate During Pressure–Flow Studies

The usefulness of the concept of a FRCZ for data analysis requires that the recorded pressure and flow rate signal be synchronized with respect to the FRCZ [Griffiths et al. 1997]. Normally, no measurable time delay will exist between the intravesical pressure signal and the actual flow at the FRCZ. However, a significant delay is to be expected for the typical urodynamic flow rate recorded extracorporeally. This delay will vary with anatomy, pathology, flow rate, and the set-up for measurement. Our understanding of the actual dynamics of flow rate changes is limited, and the relatively slow response of most flow meters may not be sufficient to match the dynamics of the much-faster pressure signal. The actual time difference may be from 0.5 to 2 s; the time delay between urethral closure and the end of any flow recording may be much longer, particularly in prostatic obstruction and terminal dribbling than between the opening of the urethra and the start of a flow rate signal. Therefore, we recommend the use of more descriptive terminology for synchronizing pressure and flow values, such as $p_{det.Qbeg}$ for the pressure at which flow begins instead of $p_{det.open}$, and $p_{det.Qend}$ when flow ends instead of $p_{det.close}$. The time delay correction needs to be considered when analyzing pressure flow studies [Griffiths et al. 1997].

In average, the maximum flow rate Q_{max} recorded during PF studies, $(Q_{max.p})$, is lower than during free flow (Q_{max}). This, however, is not due simply to a mechanical increase of outflow resistance by the intraurethral catheter, because such a difference is also found in suprapubic PF studies. A difference has also been reported between $Q_{max.p}$ during conventional and ambulatory urodynamics. This indicates more complex causes, possible psychogenic, but also physiologic, for example, that a difference in detrusor contraction strength may be involved, and that the fast filling rate used in clinical studies may lead to reduced contractility. This could also explain the difference in results between conventional and ambulatory studies.

Measurement of Intravesical and Abdominal Pressure

- It is recommended that there is strict adherence to the ICS standardization of zero pressure and reference height. Only then can pressure recordings be compared between patients and centers.

Zero pressure and reference height are concepts which are often confused in urodynamics. For example, by use of the misleading term "zero reference height". As both are independent features of pressure, they must be considered separately, and both must follow recommended ICS methodology.

- Zero pressure is the surrounding atmospheric pressure.

Zero pressure is the value recorded when a transducer is open to the environment when disconnected from any tubes or catheters, or when the open end of a connected, fluid-filled tube is at the same vertical level as the transducer. Only then can a "set zero" or "balance" be performed.

- The reference height is defined as the upper edge of the symphysis pubis.

The reference height is the level at which the transducers must be placed so that all urodynamic pressures have the same hydrostatic component. It is often argued that it does not make a difference for the most relevant parameter, p_{det}, if the same error is introduce to p_{ves} and p_{abd}, as they tend to cancel each other out. This is not an acceptable argument. The hydrostatic pressure is real and important, and inevitably plays a role in any intracorporeal pressure recording. Many important aspects of quality and plausibility control, such as typical resting value ranges at different patient position, are based on the proper recording of pressures, and will not apply if pressures are not recorded according to ICS standards. Also, it is only meaningful to subtract one pressure from the other, for example ($p_{ves} - p_{abd} = p_{det}$), when both are recorded to the same reference level.

Pressure Transducers

Urodynamic techniques were developed using external pressure transducers connected to the patient with fluid-filled lines, allowing easier compliance with the standards of correct zero and reference height. Catheter mounted pressure transducers, so-called microtip transducer catheters have become popular due to their apparent higher accuracy, better dynamic resolution, and their apparent independence from hydrostatic pressure. A catheter mounted pressure transducer is an advantage for dynamic recordings of urethral pressures during coughing (stress profiles) as well as for ambulatory urodynamics in mobile patients. Here only the application of catheter mounted pressure transducers for intravesical and abdominal pressure recordings will be discussed as urethral pressures are dealt with in a separate report [Lose et al., 2002].

All aspects of urodynamic pressure recording outlined in the preceeding section are valid and independent of transducer type. It is impossible to define the precise position of an intravesical and a rectal catheter mounted pressure transducers at to place them at any common level, and impossible to position them at the standard level of the upper boarder of the symphysis pubis. It has become popular to circumvent this problem by setting the catheter mounted pressure transducers to zero pressure when inside the body at the start of pressure recording. This, however, means that both the standard zero pressure as well the reference level are ignored, so that such recorded pressure cannot be compared between patients or centers. The fact is, the initial intravesical and abdominal resting pressures are real, are different between patients, and depend significantly on patient's position. Thus, there are significant potential errors; by ignoring the correct atmospheric zero pressure, an error of up to 50 cmH$_2$O, and as the reference height of the catheter mounted pressure transducers is usually undetermined, another potential error of 10 cmH$_2$O is possible for a full bladder can occur. In addition, when a study starts with zero abdominal pressure then the commonly observed abdominal pressure decrease at pelvic floor relaxation during voiding will evidently result in negative abdominal pressure values, and thus in p_{det} being higher than p_{ves}.

The same problems of apparent independence from the existing hydrostatic pressure also applies to air-filled catheters and/or connection tubings. Due to the absence of a water column between the balloon-covered opening on the catheter and the external transducer, the reference height in an air-filled system will refer to the position of the sensing balloon on the catheter and not to the external transducer.

- It is recommended that for intravesical and abdominal pressure recording external transducers connected to fluid-filled tubings and catheters be used. If microtip or air-filled catheters are used, any deviation from standard zero and reference level should be minimized and taken into account at the time of data analysis.

Urodynamic Catheters

Comparison between patients and urodynamic studies performed in different centers would be facilitated by the use of standard catheters. It is recommended that:

- For the measurement of intravesical pressure and for bladder filling, the standard catheter for routine urodynamics is a transurethral double-lumen catheter.

Only in small children and patients with severe constrictive obstruction (stricture) does suprapubic pressure recording have clear advantages. Intraurethral catheters should be as thin as possible, limited only by the practicality of insertion and by internal lumen sizes, which should be sufficiently large to avoid excessive damping of pressure transmission and to achieve the desired filling rate with standard pumps. A 6-Fr double lumen catheter is the smallest practical size at present.

The major advantage of a double lumen catheter is that the fill/void sequence can be repeated without the need for re-catheterization. Note that the use of a 6-Fr double lumen catheter can limit the infusion rate during cystometry to 20–30 ml/min, as a typical roller pump may not manage to transport a higher perfusion rate through such a small lumen. This can result in a incorrect filling volume being indicated by the machine, when the filling volume is calculated from the pump setting. For example, with a filling rate set at 60 ml/min and an actually achieved filling rate of 30 ml/min, the machine will show double the filling volume. Thus after voiding, a high calculated residual will occur. With some equipment, higher filling rates are possible; it is essential that any system should be critically tested to (a) measure the maximum filling rate that can be achieved by a particular catheter attached to an individual pump and (b) correct or calibrate the indicated infused volume.

The use of two separate tubes for filling and recording is less convenient. Removing the larger filling tube for voiding may appear to be an advantage because only a single small tube is left in the urethra. However, there are no data to suggest that, for example, in a compressive obstruction such as BPO, a 6-F catheter has detrimental influence on the pressure or flow data. There are, however, data suggesting that results from a single study may be misleading. A double lumen catheter facilitates a second fill/void study to establish reproducibility. Re-introduction of the separate filling tube for a repeated study is more invasive and complicated.

- The use of a rectal balloon catheter is recommended for the measurement of abdominal pressure, p_{abd}.

Although there are various methods for the successful recording of abdominal pressures, a flaccid, air-free balloon in the rectal ampulla gives a suitable signal for p_{abd} to determine a meaningful p_{det} when p_{ves} is measured synchronously ($p_{det} = p_{ves} - p_{abd}$). In females, vaginal recording may be more acceptable and provides comparable results. The recording of p_{abd} allows the measurement of any abdominal (i.e., perivesical) pressure component during changes in intravesical pressure. The role of the balloon is to maintain a small fluid volume at the catheter opening and to avoid fecal blockage, which can prevent or impair pressure transmission to the transducer. Additionally, as the rectal ampulla and the vagina are not homogeneously fluid filled spaces, the balloon prevents pressure artifacts arising from contact between the catheter opening and the wall tissue. The balloon serves this function best when it is filled only to 10–20% of its unstretched capacity. Overfilling and elastic distention of the balloon is the most common mistake in abdominal pressure recording. The resultant high balloon (not abdominal) pressure will produce a misleading pressure reading. Such an artificially-elevated balloon distention pressure can be avoided by making a small hole in the balloon, although this is unnecessary if the balloon is filled properly as described above. It is also possible to record reliable abdominal pressure with a very slowly perfused (<2 ml/min) open ended catheter. However, excessive fluid volume in the rectal ampulla may cause problems.

Equipment: Minimum Requirements for Filling Cystometry and Pressure–Flow Studies of Voiding

The ICS has not yet specified definite technical standards in respect of minimum requirements for filling cystometry and pressure flow studies beyond the ICS Technical Equipment Report [Rowan et al. 1997] and the appendix to the ICS document on pressure flow [Griffiths et al., 1997], where an data exchange software standard is recommended. Some further aspects will be discussed in more detail here.

Equipment Recommendations

The minimum recommended requirements for a urodynamic system are:

- three measurement channels, two for pressure and one for flow;
- a display (on printer and/or monitor) and secure storage of three pressures (p_{abd}, p_{ves}, p_{det},) and flow (Q) as tracings against time;
- infused volume and voided volume may be shown graphically or numerically;
- on-line display of pressures and flow, with adequate scale and resolution; scales must be clearly given on all axes; no information should be lost electronically when tracings go off-scale on display;
- possibilities to record standard information about sensation and additional comments (event recording).

Meaningful plausibility assessment and quality control is possible only when the measured and derived signals are displayed continuously as curves over time, without delay (in real time), as the examination proceeds. Each displayed curve and number should be labeled according to ICS standards with clear scaling of amplitudes and the time axis. The following sequential position of tracings is suggested: p_{abd} at the top, then p_{ves}, p_{det} and Q (see Figs. 3–8). It is least important when p_{abd} goes off-scale and is cut off (Fig. 6). Additional parameters such as EMG, bladder filling, and voided volumes can be displayed either as curves or digitally as numbers.

The following minimum technical specifications are recommended:

- Minimum accuracy should be ± 1 cmH$_2$O for pressure and ± 5% full scale for flow and volume;
- Ranges of 0–250 cmH$_2$O, 0–25(50) ml/s, and 1,000 ml for pressure, flow, and volume, respectively;
- The software must ensure that no information for pressures up to 250 cmH$_2$O and for flow rates up to 50 ml/s is lost internally even when not displayed and that off-scale values are clearly identified;
- An analog/digital (A/D) frequency of 10 Hz per channel as the lower limit for pressure and flow;
- A higher frequency (minimum 20 kHz) is necessary for recording EMG;
- Calibration of all measurements should be possible.

The scalings should be kept unchanged as much as possible, because urodynamic data quality control is based on pattern recognition, and the recognition of patterns depend on scaling. Therefore, it is recommended that:

- During recording and for analysis, minimum scaling for pressure be of 50 cmH$_2$O per cm, for flow 10 ml/s per cm, and for the time axis 1 min/cm or 5 s/mm during filling and 2 s/mm during voiding.

To enable a retrospective judgment of the curves, urodynamic measurements should be documented as curves over time with comments and explanations. It is usually insufficient to document urodynamic measurements by a few numerical values alone. The same amplitude of scaling should be used for all documentation, although the time axis may be compressed. Only if there is no relevant information to be lost by reducing resolution, for example, during filling, the time scale can be compressed.

For a print-out, maximum full scale deflections of 200 cmH$_2$O, 50 ml/s, and 1,000 ml are sufficient for pressure, flow and volume, respectively. In most cases, half the maximum full scale will be sufficient to show all relevant parts of curves. Line resolution should be better than 0.10 mm.

During interventions, for example, interruption of bladder filling or manipulation of catheters, the continuation of both measurement and recording must always be possible.

On-line recording of comments should be possible, to complete the documentation.

Calibration of Equipment

The need to calibrate pressure transducers, flowmeters, and pumps cannot be stated; simply "yes" if there is a need or "no" there is not. The specification of the manufacturer should be studied. Two aspects must be considered: the intended accuracy of the system and the investigator's experience with the system. If a new system is installed or new transducers are being used, it is recommended that regular calibration be carried out. If experience with daily calibration shows that the potential error is small (e.g., <2 cmH$_2$O), then it will be sufficient to calibrate once a month. However, calibration should not be ignored and good urodynamic equipment makes it technically possible to perform a calibration. Calibration should not be confused with simple 'zero balancing', which is only one part of a calibration. In addition to setting the zero, it must possible to check and adjust the amplitudes of all measurement channels, i.e., to calibrate all signals.

Calibration of a flowmeter can be achieved by pouring a precisely measured volume at a constant flow into the flowmeter, typically 400 ml in 20–30 s (at 15–20 ml/s) and checking the recorded volume. Special constant-flowrate bottles are available for flow calibration. Similarly, one can test a pump by measuring the time to deliver a known volume, for example, 100 ml into a measuring cylinder. It is recommended that pump calibration be performed with the filling catheter connected. Such a pump calibration can only be as good as the cylinder used, which needs to have good resolution and be accurate. Some measuring beakers that are usually available in clinics are not accurate.

Pressure Signal Quality Control: Qualitative and Quantitative Plausibility

It is very important to observe and to test signals carefully and to correct any problems before starting the urodynamic study. If the signals are perfect at the beginning of the study, they usually remain so without the need for major intervention. If the signals are not perfect, remedial action must be taken. If a quality problem does not disappear at once, when filling commences, it will usually deteriorate further during the study.

Conscientious observation of the patient and of the signals, in particular p_{det}, during all parts of the study, together with continuous signal testing, are the keys to high quality urodynamics. The first aim is to avoid artifacts and the second to correct the source of all artifacts immediately when they occur.

The following three criteria form the minimum recommendations for ensuring quality control of pressure recordings:

- Resting values for abdominal, intravesical, and detrusor pressure are in a typical range (see below);
- The abdominal and intravesical pressure signals are 'live', with minor variations caused by breathing or talking being similar for both signals; these variations should not appear in p_{det};
- Coughs are used (every I min. or, for example, 50 ml filled volume) to ensure that the abdominal and intravesical pressure signals respond equally. Coughs immediately before voiding and immediately after voiding should be included.

When standards are followed, i.e., with the transducer zeros set to atmospheric pressure, and the transducers placed at the level of the upper edge of the symphysis, a typical range for initial resting pressures values for p_{ves} and p_{abd} is (Schäfer, unpublished communications):

- supine 5–20 cmH$_2$O.
- sitting 15–40 cmH$_2$O.
- standing 30–50 cmH$_2$O.

Usually both recorded pressures are almost identical, so that the initial p_{det} is zero, or close to zero, 0–6 cmH$_2$O in 80% of cases and in rare cases up to 10 cmH$_2$O [Liao et al., 1999].

All initial pressure values should be verified and patients' position should be documented on the urodynamics trace.

All negative pressure values, except when caused by rectal activity, should be corrected immediately. It should always be kept in mind that p_{abd} is recorded not to know the actual rectal pressure, but to eliminate the impact of (abdominal) pressure changes on p_{ves}. The principal aim is to determine the detrusor pressure, p_{det}, which is the pressure in the bladder without the influence of abdominal pressure. Therefore, p_{det} cannot be negative.

By talking to the patient during the study, the proper dynamic response in the pressure signals can be observed and is "automatically" documented (see Figs. A.1.6.3, A.1.6.4, A.1.6.8).

Problem Solving

If either detrusor or rectal contractions occur, the recorded pressures in p_{ves} and in p_{abd} will be different. Such changes can be identified and interpreted with sufficient accuracy and reliability only when the patient is observed and the relation between signal changes and patient sensation/activity are checked for plausibility and documented. Any pressure change caused by smooth muscle contractions will show a "smooth" pattern, (Figs. 5, 7, 8) i.e., there should be no rapid ("*stepwise*") changes (Fig. 4). If pressures increase or decrease step-wise, or with a constant slope over a long period of time, a nonphysiological cause, such as catheter movement, should be considered.

If a sudden drop or increase occurs in either the p_{ves} or p_{abd} signal, the usual cause is the movement, blockage (Fig. 4), or disconnection of a catheter. When the patient changes position, sudden changes in resting values occur and are seen equally in both pressure signals. If p_{ves} (without change in p_{abd}) increases slowly—as typical for a low compliance bladder— it is important to test for any other possible cause for a slow pressure increase. One cause could be a problem with the intravesical catheter measurement, for example, the hole for the pressure conducting lumen is slowly moving into the bladder neck region. This should be assessed by asking the patient to cough, if there is no other apparent artifact. Furthermore, it is recommended that bladder filling is stopped, if the filling rate was above a physiological limit of 10 ml/min. If the value of p_{ves} drops after filling is stopped, it is likely that 'low compliance' was, at least in part, related to fast filling.

There are several common problems that must be solved before the study is started or when observed during a study: *Problem: Initial resting p_{det} is negative, for example, – 5 cmH$_2$O Possible explanations:*

- *because p_{abd} is too high*

  Solution: If p_{ves} is in the typical range, and both pressures are 'live', open the valve in the abdominal line and drain 1 or 2 drops from the rectal balloon filling volume. This will usually cause p_{abd} to fall to a proper value. If not, gently re-position the rectal balloon and/or make a small hole in the balloon.

- *because p_{ves} is too low*

  Solution: This may be due to air bubbles trapped in the catheter, the catheter not being in the bladder, or the catheter being blocked/kinked. Gently flush through the p_{ves} line (max. 10 ml). It is very important to flush slowly while observing the pressure signal because pressures above 300 cmH$_2$O may damage the transducer. If this does not solve the problem, add some more volume to the bladder via the filling lumen. If resistance to filling is high and it does not drain easily when opened, it will be necessary to check catheter position, and to re-position the catheter, if necessary.

Problem: Initial p_{det} too high, for example, 15 cmH$_2$O Possible explanations:

  The key problem here is indicated by the measurement of 15 cmH$_2$O. The situation is different from the clear statement that 'p_{det} cannot be negative', as we do not have a definite upper limit for the normal maximum 'resting' value for p_{det}. Thus, we can only follow the present guidelines that in most tests, in an empty bladder p_{det} is between 0–5 cmH$_2$O, and in some 90% it is between 0–10 cmH$_2$O. For any higher value, stringent plausibility checking must be applied. If the patient has no detrusor overactivity, a p_{det} of 15 cmH$_2$O is unlikely to be valid and there may be a signal problem. First check, if P_{abd} and P_{ves} are in the expected ranges. For example, if in a standing patient, initial P_{ves} is 30 cmH$_2$O and P_{abd} is 15 cmH$_2$O, then by experience the value of P_{abd} is too low (because P_{abd} is too low). If in a supine patient P_{abd} is 10 cmH$_2$O and P_{ves} is 25 cmH$_2$O, then the value of P_{ves} is too high (because P_{ves} is too high). Check the zero balance and proper signal response to coughing for both signals.

- *because P_{abd} is too low*
  Solution to P_{abd} being too low: Very slowly flush the rectal balloon with 1 or 2 ml.

- *because P_{ves} is too high.*
  Solution to P_{ves} being too high: This problem can be related to a misplaced catheter, a kink in the catheter, or contact with the bladder wall in an empty bladder, which occludes the eyehole(s) of the catheter. Proceed according to the solution for P_{ves} being too high, in the first example above.

  If no signal problem can be identified, the clinical study may be started, but the P_{det} signal deserves particular attention. If compliance is normal and the bladder normal at filling, *then it is very important to record and check, for some period after the micturition, the post-voiding resting value of P_{det}. Only if an elevated P_{det} is perfectly reproducible for repeated filling and voiding studies can it be accepted. However, it is most likely that a high resting P_{det} will not be reproducible and will be corrected by the measures described above.*

In summary, if any resting value or cough response does not fit the usual values or patterns, it should be corrected before bladder filling is started. If this is not possible, the signals must be observed even more carefully and every effort made to reveal the potential source of error or artifact during the study.

Retrospective Artifact Correction

In principle, a good P_{det} signal requires only that P_{ves} and P_{abd} show the same fine structure and quality of signals before filling, during filling, and after a voiding. (Figs. A.1.6.3, A.1.6.4, A.1.6.7, A.1.6.8) Both P_{ves} and P_{abd} must have the same zero and reference level. The most common mistake is to set *(balance)* the initial pressure values of P_{ves} and P_{abd} to zero with the catheters connected to the patient instead of setting zero to atmospheric pressure. This results in incorrect P_{ves} and P_{abd}. If this is done, urodynamic studies cannot be compared between centers and between patients. Although it may seem convenient and easy to start with a value of P_{det} as zero, this practice will lead to problems later in the test. As soon as pelvic floor relaxation occurs, which is particularly common during voiding, the value of P_{abd}, if starting at zero, becomes negative. With a negative P_{abd}, P_{det} will be higher than P_{ves}, a conceptually meaningless result. Furthermore, it will then be impossible to correct a negative P_{abd}. Cough tests at regular intervals, particularly before voiding and after voiding, document the dynamic response of the pressure channels and are fundamentally important.

A typical physiological artifact that can be easily recognized is a rectal contraction. Rectal contractions are usually of low amplitude and may or may not be felt by the patient (Fig. 8). The value of P_{abd} shows a phasic rise with no change in the P_{det} signal—a potentially confusing fall in P_{det} results from the electronic subtraction, but this is, of course, an artefact. Usually rectal contractions are relevant only because they may be misinterpreted as detrusor overactivity (Fig. A.1.6.8): they have no relevance to voiding.

Biphasic spikes as a response to cough tests are another example of artifacts that are easy to correct. However, any other artifacts such as a signal which is nonresponding (dead), has stepwise changes in pressure, or has negative pressures, often cannot be corrected or can be corrected only with a lot of speculation about the underlying causes of the problem. Studies with such artefacts, should be repeated see the next section).

Retrospective corrections require the same strategies for plausibility control as during recording, but then they are much more difficult and less successful to perform.

A few common artifacts (e.g., rectal activity, biphasic spikes at cough tests, or insufficient P_{abd} response during straining) can be accepted during the study as they can be corrected retrospectively. Usually, this is easier to do manually than through a computerized system.

Urodynamic Computer Software

Computer applications should allow the easy use of even the most complicated analytical algorithms. However, most of the software offered by the urodynamic equipment industry is neither original nor validated. The software may, in fact, not do what the original developer(s) of the algorithm intended. Therefore, it is recommended that:

● When analytical urodynamic software is used to perform data analysis according to any published concept, the source of the software should be specified. It should also be clearly stated if the software has been validated, i.e., proven to provide results consistent with the algorithms to which the analyses are attributed.

Strategy for Repetition of Urodynamic Tests

● It is recommended that a urodynamic test should be repeated if the initial test suggests an abnormality, leaves the cause of troublesome lower urinary tract symptoms unresolved, or if there are technical problems preventing proper analysis.

It may not be necessary, however, to repeat a study, which beyond any doubt, confirms the expected pathology, for example, detrusor overactivity which correlates with the patient's symptoms. However, if the study is inconclusive, then the consequences of not finding a clear answer to the urodynamic question(s) should be considered. If an invasive therapy is planned, the urodynamics should be repeated. Therefore, it is necessary to analyze the signals during the study and document the study immediately upon its conclusion. Only then is it possible to be sure that the urodynamic study is of a quality that answers the urodynamic question and provides an understanding about the patient's clinical problem. Therefore, it is recommended that:

● The urodynamic findings and the interpretation of the results should be documented immediately after the study is finished, i.e., before the patient has left the urodynamic laboratory. Doing so allows for a second test if required.

The analysis of a good study is easy and straight-forward. Indeed, an easy analysis actually is the key criterion for good urodynamics. A good study is one that is easy to read and one from which a any experienced urodynamicist will abstract the same results and come to the same conclusions. For computerized analyses, high data quality is even more important than for manual graphical data analysis. Efforts to achieve urodynamic data of high quality during the study will produce great benefits at the time of data analysis. The future development of urodynamic equipment and software should force investigators to conduct proper on-line data quality control. Analysis of ambulatory studies will remain problematic, as it is less easy to conduct on-line assessment of quality, and analysis is time consuming. Hence, it will be necessary to ask the patient to return, on another occasion, should the investigation require repeating, for whatever reason.

Conclusions

This is the first report of the ICS Standardization committee of Good Urodynamic Practice. The authors are well aware that this is just a first step and many more will have to follow. Only the essential aspects are considered, but if these basic standards are followed, the quality of urodynamic studies will be significantly improved.

Acknowledgements

The Standardisation Committee is grateful for the extensive editing performed by Vicky Rees, ICS Administrator. The committee is also grateful for the detailed comments received from Linda Cardozo, Paul Dudgeon, Guus Kramer, Joseph Macaluso, Gerry Timm, and Alan Wein.

References

Griffiths DJ, Höfner K, van Mastrigt R, Rollema HJ, Spangberg A, Gleason DM. 1997. Standardization of terminology of lower urinary tract function: pressure-flow studies of voiding, urethral resistance, and urethral obstruction. Neurourol Urodyn 16:1–18.

Liao L, Kirshner-Hermanns R, Schäfer W. 1999. Urodynamic quality control: quantitative plausibility control with typical value ranges. Neurourol Urodyn 18(abstract 99a):365–366.

Lose G, Griffiths DJ, Hosker G, Kulseng-Hansen S, Perucchini D, Schäfer W, Thind P, Versi E. 2002. Standardisation of urethral pressure measurement: Report of the sub-committee of the International Continence Society. Neurourol Urodyn 21:258–60.

Rowan D, James DE, Kramer AEJL, Sterling AM, Suhel PF. 1987. Urodynamic equipment: technical aspects. J Med Eng Tech 11:57–64.

van Waalwijk E, Anders K, Khullar V, Kulseng-Hanssen S, Pesce F, Robertson A, Rosario D, Schäfer W. 2000. Standardisation of ambulatory urodynamic monitoring: Report of the standardisation sub-committee of the International Continence Society. Neurourol Urodyn 19:113–125.

Appendix 1, Part 7

The Standardisation of Terminology in Nocturia: Report from the Standardisation Sub-committee of the International Continence Society

Philip van Kerrebroeck,[1] Paul Abrams,[2] David Chaikin,[3] Jenny Donovan,[4] David Fonda,[5] Simon Jackson,[6] Poul Jennum,[7] Theodore Johnson,[8] Gunnar Lose,[9] Anders Mattiasson,[10] Gary Robertson,[11] Jeff Weiss[12]

[1]*Chairman of the International Continence Soceity Standardisation Committee, Department of Urology, University Hospital Maastricht, The Netherlands*
[2]*Bristol Urological Institute, Southmead Hospital, Bristol, United Kingdom*
[3]*Morristown Memorial Hospital, Morristown, New Jersey, and Department of Urology, Weill Medical College of Cornell University, New York, New York*
[4]*Department of Social Medicine, University of Bristol, Bristol, United Kingdom*
[5]*Aged Care Services, Caulfield General Medical Centre, Victoria, Australia*
[6]*Department of Gynaecology, John Radcliffe Hospital, Oxford, United Kingdom*
[7]*Department of Clinical Neurophysiology, University of Copenhagen and Sleep Laboratory, Glostrup, Denmark*
[8]*Rehabilitation Research and Development Center, Atlanta VA Medical Centre, Atanta, Georgia*
[9]*Department of Obstetrics and Gynaecology, Glostrup County Hospital, University of Copenhagen, Denmark*
[10]*Department of Urology, Lund University Hospital, Lund, Sweden*
[11]*Northwestern University Medical School, Chicago, Illinois*
[12]*Department of Urology, Weill Medical College of Cornell University and The New York Presbyterian Hospital, New York, New York*
Key words: ICS standards, nocturia; polyuria

1. Introduction

Nocturia is the complaint that the individual has to wake at night one or more times to void. (International Continence Society Definition from ICS Standardisation of Terminology Report 2002.)

Nocturia is a condition that has only recently begun to be recognised as a clinical entity in its own right rather than a symptom of some other disorder, or classed as one of many lower urinary tract symptoms. Studies that have investigated nocturia have varied in their definitions of the condition and its surrounding terminology, and these discrepancies have been highlighted in the literature [Robertson, 2000; Weiss & Blaivas, 2000; van Kerrebroeck & Weiss, 1999]. However it is defined, prevalence studies show that nocturia is reported to be a very common condition, affecting particularly older age groups [Chute, 1993; Malmsten, 1997; Swithinbank, 1998].

Four per cent of children aged 7–15 years were reported to experience habitual nocturia [Mattson, 1994], whereas the prevalence has been reported to be 58% and 66% in women and men of 50–59 years, and 72% and 91% in women and men over 80 years [Middlekoop, 1996]. It is evident that nocturia may not only present to the urologist, but that the gynaecologist, geriatrician, neurologist, sleep expert, endocrinologist and general practitioner will all be consulted by patients with this problem. Each specialty is likely to approach their patients from a different perspective, and it is important that some of the basic terms surrounding nocturia have specific definitions so that each individual physician is referring to the same condition and managing it appropriately.

In order to further the discussion on nocturia and in particular, how it should be defined and investigated, a series of meetings were held to facilitate discussion and to reach consensus on definitions [Mattiasson, 1999]. These discussions were finalised in March 2000, and are presented here as an aid to primary and secondary care clinicians involved in assessing and treating patients who suffer from nocturia, and to aim towards standardisation in future clinical study design.

These are the first recommendations for the diagnosis of nocturia. Most of the terms used are listed in Table A.1.7.I, along with their existing or newly agreed definitions. When considering 'normal' measurements, an average 70 kg individual who sleeps 8 hours a night is the basis for these values, and ranges are generally considered to be within 2 standard deviations of this. It must be noted that, while these guidelines aim to provide help with diagnosis, each physician must be prepared to use their clinical judgement in individual cases, as the boundaries of the categories presented are not fixed, and a person's nocturia may have mixed aetiology.

2. Clinical Assessment

The assessment of nocturia can be described by a simple algorithm, which is outlined in Fig. 1. This considers the possibility that the patient may present to the physician specifically because of nocturia, or may present with another condition, whilst also suffering from nocturia. It is possible that a physician will be able to determine nocturia as one cause of distress if the correct questions are asked, which enables further investigation as to the course of nocturia. Of course, there will be a proportion of the population with nocturia, who are not bothered by their condition and who do not present to a clinician at all. However, by definition, these individuals should still be classified as having nocturia. Initial

Table A.1.7.I. Definitions of Terms Associated with Nocturia and Derived from the Frequency Volume Chart

Terms	Definition
Nocturia	Is the number of voids recorded during a nights sleep: each void is preceded and followed by sleep
Nocturnal urine volume	Total volume of urine passed during the night including the first morning void (see definition)[a]
Rate of nocturnal urine production	Nocturnal urine volume/time asleep (i.e. night). Measured in ml/min[a]
Nocturnal polyuria	Nocturnal urine volume >20–30% of total 24h urine volume (age dependent)[a]
24 hour voided volume	Total volume of urine voided during a 24 hour period (1st void to be discarded; 24 hours begins at the time of the next void)
Polyuria	24 hour voided volume in excess of 2800 ml (in 70 kg person, i.e. >40ml/kg)
Night[b]	The period of time between going to bed with the intention of sleeping and waking with the intention of arising
Night-time frequency[b]	Is the number of voids recorded from the time the individual goes to bed with the intention of going to sleep, to the time the individual wakes with the intention of rising[a]
First morning void	The first void after waking with the intention of rising
Maximum voided volume	The largest single voided volums measured in a 24 hour period[a]

[a] In the new ICS terminology report these are signs as their derivation is from the frequency volume chart. Symptoms are defined as complaints.
[b] These terms from the definition of nocutira but may be useful in research studies, for example in urine production rate, related to posture.

screening can lead to life-style advice or to further investigations, which will enable the aetiology to be determined and an appropriate management strategy developed.

2.1. Nocturia

Nocturia is waking at night to void. This applies to any number of voids at any time during the night, as long as the person is awake before voiding. When voiding occurs during sleep, this is nocturnal enuresis. Both conditions can be referred to as night-time voiding, although the distinction between the two is clearly determined by the state of wakefulness.

The first morning void is not included as a night-time void since this is a natural expulsion of the urine produced during the night. In addition, although many people may consider one nighttime void to be normal, they are still considered to have nocturia. For some individuals, the trigger for waking may not be a desire to void, yet voiding is perceived to be necessary once awake; however, these individuals are still considered to have nocturia (Fig. A.1.7.1). Those (e.g., the infirm or frail elderly) who wake with the need to void, but are unable to reach the bathroom before voiding, have a mixture of nocturia and incontinence, not nocturnal enuresis. Patients experiencing nocturia may or may not be bothered by this condition and it is the level of bothersomeness that will determine their help-seeking behaviour.

2.2. Night

Night-time is the period of time between going to bed with the intention of sleeping and waking with the intention of arising. It must be noted that this varies with age, and elderly people often spend longer periods of time in bed than younger people. It is important that the sleeping time is considered, not the actual time in bed.

Shift workers may have a variation in their night-time, and the same definition exists for them. The same is true for people who split their sleeping time into two or more periods during the day. Jet-lag and varied shift patterns may disrupt the natural circadian rhythm and this can lead to poor sleeping patterns, disrupted sleep and nocturia.

2.3. Screen

An initial screen should include a detailed history, including questions relevant to voiding behaviour, medical and neurological abnormalities and sleep disturbance, as well as information on relevant surgery or previous urinary infections. A simple urine test, such as

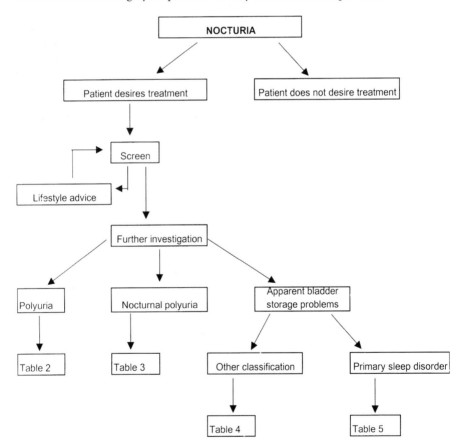

Fig. A.1.7.1 Patients without any bother may present with a different condition, when nocturia is indentified.

dipstick or urinalysis, should be performed to exclude any relevant pathology. A physical examination should also be performed.

2.4. Advice

General lifestyle advice, such as reducing caffeine and alcohol intake, and limiting excessive liquid/food volume intake prior to bedtime can, in some cases, be sufficient to elicit a satisfactory response. However, care should be taken not to impose a general fluid restriction as this could have serious consequences in patients with undiagnosed diabetes insipidus. Patients should be encouraged to return to their doctor for further evaluation if they are not content with the results following their initial advice.

2.5. Further Evaluation

This should begin by asking the patient to keep a frequency/volume chart. The chart should also include a record of the volume and type of fluid ingested as well as the volume and time of each voided urine for 24 to 72 hours. It also should include the time of retiring to bed, time of rising and subjective evaluation of whether each night measured was good, bad or normal in terms of their usual sleeping pattern. In research studies, the impact on quality of life should also be measured using questionnaires such as ICS male [Donovan et al., 1996] or the DAN-PSS in men: [Hald et al., 1991] and the BFLUTS in women [Jackson et al., 1996], which allow the assessment of the occurrence of nocturia and the degree of problem or bother that it causes. No specific measure has yet been devised to evaluate the full impact of nocturia on aspects of everyday life, although one is currently under development.

If a sleep disorder is suspected, a nocturnal polysomnograph should be considered. Examples of sleep disorders with a potential relation to nocturia are presented in Table 5. The pathophysiological causes of these disorders are not fully clarified and may be due to polyuria (e.g., obstructive sleep apnoea syndrome) or arousals with voiding (e.g., insomnia) [Thorpy, 1990].

2.6. Polyuria

A patient with urine output exceeding 40 ml/kg body-weight during a 24 hour period should be considered to be suffering from polyuria. This should be investigated further to determine if the polyuria is due to a solute diuresis (e.g. diabetes mellitus) or diabetes insipidus and, if it is the latter, which type of diabetes insipidus is present (Table A.1.7.II). These distinctions can be made by measuring the glucose, specific gravity and osmolality of a 24 hour urine collection, followed by a variety of more specialized tests best undertaken by the appropriate subspecialist [Robertson, 1995].

2.7. Nocturnal Polyuria

Nocturnal polyuria [Asplund, 1995; Carter, 1992] is defined as the production of an abnormally large volume of urine during sleep. The measurement should include all the urine

Table A.1.7.II. Causes of Polyuria

- Diabetes mellitus
  Insulin dependent (Type I)
  Insulin independent (Type II)
- Diabetes insipidus
  Pituitary
  Renal
  Gestational
  Primary polydipsia (Psychogenic, dipsogenic or iatrogenic)

produced after going to bed and the first void after arising. It can be expressed in several different ways [Robertson, 1999]. If the 24 hour urine volume is normal, the output during sleep can be expressed as a percentage of the total. This value varies considerably from person to person and normally increases with age. Healthy young adults from 21 to 35 years of age excrete around 14 ± 4% or their total urine between the hours of 11 p.m. and 7 a.m. (95% CI = 10–19%) [Robertson et al., 1999], whereas older people excrete an average of 34 ± 15% (95% CI = 30–36%) [Rembratt et al, 2000; Kirkland et al, 1983]. Thus, nocturnal polyuria may be defined as an output greater than of 20% of the daily total in the young and 33% [Carter, 1992] in the elderly with the value for middle age probably falling somewhere between these two extremes. Exceptions to this rule are patients with diabetes insipidus, and those whose sleeping patte-ns vary greatly from the normal eight-hour night-time pattern. There are many causes of nocturnal polyuria that should be considered when carrying out further investigations (Table A.1.7.III).

2.8. Bladder Storage Problems

Patients with nocturia, who do not have either polyuria or nocturnal polyuria according to the above criteria, will most likely have a reduced voided volumes or a sleep disorder. The former can be determined from the frequency volume chart by comparing the night-time voided volume with the maximal bladder capacity that occurs at any time, however a definite range of normal or abnormal volumes is currently lacking, and it is for the physician to evaluate their patients based on the frequency volume charts and their clinical judgement. Some mathematical indices have been suggested in the literature to describe this situation; measurements of the nocturia index (mean measured nocturnal urine volume/functional

Table A.1.7.III. Causes of Nocturnal Polyuria

- Water diuresis

  Circadian defect in secretion or action of antidiuretic hormone
    Primary (Idiopathic)
    Secondary (Excessive evening intake of fluid, caffeine, alcohol)

- Solute/water diuresis

  - Congestive heart failure
  - Autonomic dysfunction
  - Sleep apnoca syndrome
  - Renal insufficiency
  - Oestrogen deficiency

Table A.1.7.IV. Causes of Problems Related to Bladder Storage

- Reduced functional bladder capacity (e.g., significant post void residual)
- Reduced nocturnal bladder capacity
- Detrusor overactivity
  - neurogenic (e.g., multiple sclerosis)
  - non-neurogenic
- Bladder hypersensitivity
- Bladder outlet obstruction with post void residual urine
- Urogenital ageing

Table A.1.7.V. Sleep Disorders Potentially Related to Nocturia

- Insomnia
- Obstructive and central apnoea syndrome
- Periodic legs syndrome
- Restless legs syndrome
- Parasomnias
- Sleep disorders related to medical diseases, e.g., chronic obstructive lung disease, cardiac diseases etc.
- Sleep disorders related to neurological diseases, e.g., Alzheimer's, Alzheimer's, Parkinson's and nocturnal epileptic seizures

bladder capacity*) and nocturnal polyuria index (mean measured nocturnal urine volume/24h voided volume) may be very useful in a clinical trial situation, although an explanation of these is beyond the scope of this document and can be found in other publications [Weiss et al, 1998; Weiss & Blaivas, 2000; van Kerrebroeck & Weiss, 1999]. For patients exhibiting signs of bladder storage problems, further urological investigation should be carried out to determine the classification of the problem (Table A.1.7.IV).

Some patients will have been categorised as having bladder storage problems, which is borne out by their frequency volume chart, yet their real problem is one of sleep disturbance. Patients who are constantly waking at night due to other reasons may feel the need to void at each waking stage, and void a small volume. This might appear to the physician to be a problem with bladder storage, especially if the patient is unaware of the sleep problem. Further investigation in a sleep laboratory may be necessary to determine the cause of nocturia in these patients (Table A.1.7.V).

References

Asplund R. 1995. The Nocturnal Polyuria Syndrome (NPS). Gen Pharmac 26(6):1203.

Carter PG. 1992. The role of nocturnal polyuria in nocturnal urinary symptoms in healthy elderly males. MD thesis, Bristol.

Chute CG, Panser LA, Girman CJ, et al. 1993. The prevalence of prostatism: a population based survey of urinary symptoms. J Urol 150:85–9.

Donovan JL, Abrams P, Peters TJ et al. 1996. The ICS-'BPH' Study: the psychometric validity and reliability or the ICSmale questionnaire. Br J Urol 77:554–62.

Hald T, Nordling J, Andersen JT, Bilde T, Meyhoff HH, Walter S. 1991. A patient weighted symptom score system in the evaluation of uncomplicated benign prostatic hyperplasia. Scand J Urol Nephrol Suppl 138:59–62.

Jackson S, Donovan J, Brookes S, Eckford S, Swithinbank L, Abrams P. 1996. The Bristol Female Lower Urinary Tract Symptoms questionnaire: development and psychometric testing. Br J Urol 77:805–12.

Kirkland JL, Lye M, Levy DW, Banerjee AK. 1983. Patterns of urine flow and electrolyte excretion in healthy elderly people. BMJ 287(6406):1665–7.

Mattiasson A. 1999. Nocturia: towards a consensus. BJU Suppl 1; Vol 84.

Mattsson S. 1994. Urinary incontinence and nocturia in healthy schoolchildren. Acta Paediatr 83:950–54.

Malmsten UG, Milsom I, Molander U, Norlen LJ. 1997. Urinary incontinence and lower urinary tract symptoms: an epidemiological study of men aged 45 to 99 years. J Urol 158:1733–7.

Middlekoop HA, Smilde van den Doel DA, Neven AK, Kamphuisen HA, Springer CP. 1996. Subjective sleep characteristics of 1485 males and females aged 50–93: effects of sex and age, and factors related to self evaluated quality of sleep. J Gerontol A Biol Sci Med Sci 51:108–15.

Rembratt Å, Robertson GL, Nørgaard JP, Andersson KE. 2000. Pathogenic aspects of nocturia in the elderly: Differences between nocturics and non-nocturics. ICS meeting.

Robertson G, Rembratt A, Eriksson KE. 2000. Desmopressin in the Treatment of Disorders of Urine Output in Humans. Arch Int Med (In Press).

Robertson GL. 1995. Diabetes Insipidus, in Endocrinology and Metabolism Clinics of NorthAmerica, 24(3):549–72.

Robertson GL. 1999. Brit J Urol 84(Suppl 1):17–9.

Robertson GL, Rittig S, Kovacs L, Gaskill MB, Zee P, Naninga J. 1999. Scand J Urol Nephrol Suppl 202:36–9.

Swithinbank LV, Donovan J, James MC, Yang Q, Abrams P. 1998. Female urinary symptoms: age prevalence in a community dwelling population using a validated questionnaire. Neurourol Urodyn 16:432–4.

Thorpy MJ. 1990. International classification of sleep disorders: diagnostic and coding manual. Rochester MN, American Sleep Disorders Association (Chairman).

van Kerrebroeck P, Weiss JP. 1999. Standardisation and terminology of nocturia. In: Mattiasson A (ed): "Nocturia towards a consensus." BJU Suppl 1 Vol 84:1–4.

Weiss JP, Blaivas JG. 2000. Nocturia. J Urol 163:5–12.

Weiss JP, Blaivas JG, Stember DS, Brooks MM. 1998. Nocturia in adults: etiology and classification. Neurourol Urodynam 17:467–72.

Appendix 2, Part 1
Frequency-Volume Chart

Please complete the confidential form overleaf as accurately as possible.

Please note the time you pass your water, and the volume passed. Any measuring jug will do for this purpose. Obviously when you are at work it may be inconvenient to measure the volume; In this case record only the time. However, at other times please try to record both.

If you wet yourself at any time record the time and underneath the letter "W".

Day-time means when you are up: Night-time when you are in bed.

An example is provided below to help you:-

EXAMPLE

DAY	time/volume (mls.)	DAY-TIME	NIGHT-TIME	Number of pads used in 24 hour period		
1	7 am/200	1pm/–	6 pm/400	11pm/300	3am/200	6am/W
2	at work, couldn't measure volume	wet at 6 a.m.				
3						

Name	date of appoinment					
DAY	time/volume (mis.)	DAY-TIME	NIGHT-TIME	Number of pads used in 24 hour period		
1						
2						
3						
4						
5						
6						
7						

instructions on other side

AVERAGE DAILY FLUID INTAKE in. cups) =

Patient Information Sheet

SOUTHMEAD HEALTH

Services

A NATIONAL HEALTH SERVICE TRUST

URODYNAMIC INVESTIGATIONS

Urodynamic Unit
Southmead Hospital
Bristol BS10 5NB
Telephone (0117) 9595181

Urodynamic tests will show how well your bladder is working
Why do you need these tests?
- Your Doctor or consultant needs more information about the cause of your bladder problems
- To be sure that you receive the correct treatment
- During your tests, a Doctor, Nurse or Technician will be with you. They will also answer your questions and tell you the results of your tests

Your appointment letter will say which tests you will be having. These may include:-
Flow Studies
- Takes approximately 2 to 3 hours
- This test will show how much your bladder can hold, and at what speed it empties
- After drinking some water you will be asked to wait until your bladder is full

- Then to pass water into a specially adapted toilet
- Afterwards your bladder will be scanned, using ultrasound, to see whether it has emptied completely
- This process will be repeated 2 or 3 times which is why this test takes a long time
- Following the flow studies you will be sent a further appointment to see the Consultant in the Outpatient Clinic

Transport (with flow studies appointments only)

- If hospital transport has been requested this will be arranged for you

Urodynamics (UDS)

- Takes approximately 1 hour
- This test will show how effectively your bladder is working
- A small soft plastic tube is passed into the bladder and used to fill it with fluid
- Pressure recordings are taken from the tube as your bladder fills and empties

Video urodynamics (VIDEO)

- Takes approximately 1–2 hours
- This test is similar to UDS above
- X-rays are taken during the test to show how the bladder is working

Ambulatory studies (LTM)

- Takes 3–4 hours
- A small, soft plastic tube is passed into your bladder and records what happens as your bladder fills
- Your bladder will be monitored whilst you are walking, exercising and relaxing
- You will be asked to fill and empty your bladder twice
- It is best to wear loose fitting clothes and please bring a book or knitting etc to do whilst 'relaxing'

Pad test

- Takes approximately 1–1/2 > hours
- This will measure any leakage of urine that you have
- After drinking some water, you will be given a weighed pad to wear
- Then you will be asked to do some exercises for one hour
- Afterwards the pad will be weighed again and any leakage calculated

After your tests

- The results will be sent to your Doctor and Consultant who will arrange your next appointment
- It is a good idea to increase the amount you drink for 24 hours after the tests
- You may notice a small amount of blood in your urine, and feel slightly uncomfortable
- This is nothing to worry about and should get better within 24 hours
- If it becomes a problem, please contact your family Doctor for advice

ud.1.March 96

Your rights as a Patient

- To know how, and why, you will be treated and what the alternatives are
- To be given enough information to make decisions about your care
- To have access to your health records
- To know that information about you will not be given to anyone who is not involved in your care
- To choose whether or not to take part in research or Medical Student training

If you have any comments on the service provided by the Unit, either good or bad, please speak to a member of staff or you can send them to;
The Clinical Director of the Urodynamic Unit of the Urology Service Manager
Sponsored by
mediplus
Produced by Potten, Baber & Murray Ltd, Tel: 01179661126

Urodynamics Data Sheet: Full Version

URODYNAMIC UNIT

SOUTHMEAD HOSPITAL, BRISTOL

NOTE:–

(a) Number of entries Strictly dictated by number of boxes

(b) Where no information enter

(c) - = not applicable

1. SURNAME:
    FIRST NAME:

2. ADDRESS:
    Post Code   Tel. No.

3. DATE OF BIRTH:

4. SEX: (1 made; 2 female)

5. HOSPITAL NUMBERS(S):

6. INITIAL REFERRAL: 1 Urol   2 gynae   3 Surg   4 Geriatric
    5 G.P.   6 Nurse   7 Other   8 Paediatrics

6a. 1 = in patient   2 = out-patient   3 = not-known

7. CONSULTANT: (Name)

8. G.P.: (Name)
    Address (not coded)

9a. CIU NUMBER   9b. INVESTIGATION NUMBER:
        Presenting Complaint: HEIGHT   cms
        Previous Treatment: WEIGHT   Kg
            SMOKER   YES/NO   …/Day
        Examination:
        Management:
        Report sent to: Follow up arrangement:–
        If enter 'other' in any question please describe on this sheet.

10. DATE:

11. AGE:

12. TRIAL IDENTIFICATION (see code)
    X if not known
    – is not applicable

13. ENTER HISTORY   1 YES
    2 NO
    If NO go to 54

14. INVESTIGATOR:

15. LENGTH HISTORY:
    (Enter figure if   O = less than 1 yr
    1–9 years)   A = more than 9 years
    B = lifelong
    X = not known

16. FREQUENCY OF MICTURITION: (from F/V chart)
    (Waking hours)   X = not known
    – = not applicable (eg retention,
    appliance, conduit)

17. NOCTURIA: XX = not known
    (from F/V chart)   – = not applicable (eg
    retention, appliance, conduit)

18. FLUID INTAKE:
    (litres per 24 hrs)   O = less than 1 L
    (Enter figure if intake   A = more than 9L
    1–9 litres/24 hrs)   X = not known

19. ANALYSIS, VOIDED VOLUME/FREQUENCY/VOLUME CHART
    X = not known
    – = not applicable (eg retention,
    appliance, conduit)
    Maximum voided volume   ml.
    Average voided volume   ml.
    Maximum duration between daytime voids   hrs.

20. PREMICTURITION SYMPTOMS
    1 = normal
    2 = decreased sensation
    3 = absent sensation
    4 = increased bladder sensation
    5 = bladder pain
    6 = urethral pain
    7 = urgency, fear of leakage
    8 = cannot void
    X = unknown
    If 1, 3, 8 or X in 20 go to 21
    FREQUENCY (of premicturition symptoms)
    1 = more than × 1/day
    2 = × 1/day

    3 = more than × 1/week

    4 = × 1/week

    5 = less than × 1/week

    X = unknown

21. HESITANCY   1 = none

    2 = only on full bladder

    3 = occasional

    4 = usually

    5 = always strains to void urine

    6 = cannot void urine

    X = unknown

  if 1, 5, 6 or X in 21 go to 22

    FREQUENCY (of hesitancy)   1 = more than × 1/day

    2 = × 1/day

    3 = more than × 1/week

    4 = × 1/week

    5 = less than × 1/week

    X = unknown

22. INCONTINENCE   1 = none

    2 = present (or under treatment

    for incontinence, eg catheter)

    X = unknown

  if 1 or X in 22 go to 30

23. STRESS INCONTINENCE   1 = no

    2 = yes

    X = unknown

  if 1 or X in 23 go to 24

    FREQUENCY (of stress incontinence)

    1 = more than × 1/day

    2 = × 1/day

    3 = more than × 1/week

    4 = × 1/week

    5 = less than × 1/week

    X = unknown

24. URGE INCONTINENCE 1 = no

    2 = yes

    X = unknown

  if 1 or X in 24 go to 25

    FREQUENCY (of urge incontinence)

    1 = more than × 1/day

    2 = × 1/day

    3 = more than × 1/week

    4 = × 1/week

    5 = less than × 1/week

    X = unknown

25. PATIENT: PRESENT HISTORY OF ENURESIS
    1 = no
    2 = present problem
    3 = yes + past history (with enuresis free interval of years)
    X = unknown
  if 1 or X in 25 go to 26
    FREQUENCY (of enuresis)   1 = more than × 1/night
    2 = × 1/night
    3 = more than × 1/week
    4 = 1/week
    5 = less than 1/week
    X = unknown

26. OTHER INCONTINENCE   1 = none
    2 = post micturition dribbling
    3 = continuous incontinence
    4 = other
    5 = Incontinence during sexual intercourse
  if 1, 3 or X in 26 go to 27
    FREQUENCY   1 = more than × 1/day
    2 = × 1/day
    3 = more than × 1/week
    4 = × 1/week
    5 = less than × 1/week
    X = unknown

27. DEGREE OF INCONTINENCE   1 = drops, wets underclothes
    2 = 'floods', wets outer clothes
    3 = 'floods', on floor
    X = not known

28. MANAGEMENT OF INCONTINENCE
    1 = no protective measures, no clothes change
    2 = changes underwear/clothes
    3 = pads for safety
    4 = pads for necessity
    5 = appliance
    6 = catheter
    7 = urinary diversion
    8 = other
    X = unknown
    complete ONLY if 3 or 4 in 28
    PADS PER DAY
    PADS PER NIGHT

29. INCAPACITY DUE TO INCONTINENCE
    1 = none
    2 = minimal
    3 = social restriction, e.g. length of time out
    4 = physical restriction, e.g. tennis or dancing
    5 = housebound
    6 = hospitalised
    7 = other
    X = unknown

30. PHYSICAL INCAPACITY   1 = none
     2 = minor, walks unaided
     3 = walks with aids (e.g. sticks)
     4 = partial use wheelchair
     5 = wheelchair bound
     6 = bedbound
     7 = limited manual dexterity, otherwise mobile
     X = unknown

31. HISTORY OF ENURESIS
     (i) Patient (includes
     present enuresis)   1 = no
     2 = yes
     X = not known
     (iii) Family   1 = none
     2 = yes, sibs
     3 = yes, sibs & parents
     4 = yes, parents
     5 = unspecified family history
     X = unknown

32. URINARY STREAM   1 = normal
     2 = decreased
     3 = decreased only on full bladder
     4 = interrupted
     5 = decreased and interrupted
     6 = cannot void
     7 = decreased with terminal dribble
     X = unknown

33. POST MICTURITION SYMPTOMS   1 = normal
     2 = persistent abdominal sensation
     3 = persistent perineal sensation
     4 = feeling of incomplete emptying
     5 = cannot void
     X = unknown
   if 1, 5 or X in 33 go to 34
     FREQUENCY   1 = more than 1 ×/day
     2 = × 1/day
     3 = more than × 1/week
     4 = × 1/week
     5 = less than × 1/week
     X = unknown

34. DYSURIA/U.T.I.   1 = none – no proven UTI
     2 = occasional – no proven UTI
     3 = frequent – no proven UTI
     4 = occasional – proven UTI
     5 = frequent – proven UTI
     6 = none – proven UTI
     X = unknown

34a. HAEMATURIA   1 = yes

        2 = no

        X = not known

35. HISTORY OF RETENTION   1 = none

        2 = spontaneous

        3 = acute retention after operation

        4 = acute retention after childbirth

        5 = chronic retention

        6 = retention secondary to acute neurological disease

        7 = other

        X = unknown

    if 1 or X in 35 go to 37

36. PRESENT MANAGEMENT OF RETENTION

        1 = indwelling catheter

        2 = intermittent self-catheterisation

        3 = urinary diversion

        4 = drugs

        5 = other

        X = unknown

37. BOWEL FUNCTION

    (if stoma code -)

    (a) Control   1 = normal

        2 = urgency

        3 = poor control (soiling)

        X = unknown

    (b) Stool frequency   1 = >1/day

        2 = × 1/day

        3 = between alternate days and

        × 2/week

        4 = < × 2/week

        X = unknown

    (c) Mechanics of defecation   1 = normal (no straining)

        2 = strains

        3 = suppositories

        4 = enemas

        5 = manual evacuation

        X = unknown

    (d) Post-defaecation symptoms   1 = none

        2 = feeling incomplete emptying

        (further evacuation gives relief)

        3 = Feeling incomplete emptying

        (further straining no relief)

        4 = Other

        X = unknown

    (e) Bowel diagnosis   1 = normal

        2 = irritable bowel syndrome

        3 = constipation

        4 = diarrhoea
        5 = constipation/diarrhoea
        6 = other
        X = unknown

38. PRESENT DRUG THERAPY   1 = none
        2 = anti-biotics
        (if on more than one   3 = bladder stimulants
        drug, use left hand   4 = bladder depressants
        box for drug with   5 = urethral relaxants
        most bladder/urethral   6 = urethral stimulants
        effect)   7 = anti-depressants
                8 = diuretics
                9 = oral contraceptives
                A = oestrogens
                B = other
                X = unknown

39a. NEUROLOGICAL FEATURES   1 = none
        2 = diabetes
        (if more than one   3 = cervical disc/sp'osis
        feature, use left   4 = lumbar disc/sp'osis
        hand box for condition   5 = paraplegia/tetraplegia
        with most bladder/ 6 = M.S.
        urethral effect)   7 = C.V.A.
                8 = dementia
                9 = other cerebral disorders
                A = spiná bifida
                B = epilepsy
                C = Parkinsons
                D = other neurological disease
                X = unknown

39b. SEXUAL FUNCTION   1 = normal
        2 = abnormal
        3 = unknown
     If 2 state abnormality on front sheet

40. MALE OPERATIONS/TRAUMA
    (i) For outflow tract problem   1 = none
            2 = TUR
            3 = RPP
            4 = urethral dilatation
            5 = artificial sphincter
            6 = other urethral surgery
            7 = bladder neck incision
            X = unknown
    (ii) Surgery with possible denervation
            1 = none
            2 = Heimsteins
            3 = rectal resection
            4 = denervation procedure
            5 = other
            X = unknown
    (iii) Other procedures/factors
            1 = none
            2 = pelvic radiotherapy
            3 = renal failure/transplantation
            4 = cystoscopy
            5 = trauma
            6 = urinary diversion
            7 = other
            X = unknown

Go to 46

FEMALE PATIENTS ONLY

41. *FEMALE OPERATIONS/TRAUMA*
    (i) For stress incontinence
            1 = none
            2 = vaginal repair
            3 = Marshall Marchetti
            4 = colpo
            5 = sling
            6 = Stamey
            7 = Teflon
            8 = artificial sphincter
            9 = other
            X = unknown
    (ii) For gynaecological symptoms including prolapse
            1 = none
            2 = vaginal repair
            3 = abdominal hysterectomy
            4 = vaginal hysterectomy
            5 = laparotomy
            6 = other
            X = unknown

(iii) Surgery with possible denervation effects

    1 = none

    2 = Wertheims hysterectomy

    3 = A.P. resection

    4 = Helmsteins

    5 = denervation procedures

    6 = other

    X = unknown

(iv) Other factors   1 = none

    2 = pelvic radiotherapy

    3 = renal failure/transplant

    4 = cystoscopy

    5 = urethral dilatation

    6 = other urethral surgery

    7 = relevant trauma (spinal injuries & direct urinary tract trauma)

    8 = diversions

    9 = other

    X = unknown

42. HORMONAL STATUS   1 = premenopausal

    2 = probably premenopausal (hyst)

    3 = menopausal

    4 = probably menopausal (hyst)

    5 = post-menopausal

    6 = probably post-menopausal (hyst)

    7 = pre menarche

    X = unknown

if 5, 6 or X then go to 44

if 7 go to 46

43. SYMPTOMS RELATED TO MENSTRUATION

    1 = no relation to cycle

    2 = worse premenstrually

    3 = worse during menstruation

    4 = worse postmenstrually

    5 = worse mid-cycle

    6 = not relevant

    X = unknown

44. PARITY (Number of deliveries)

    if 0 (zero) in 44 go to 46

45. COMPLICATIONS

    OF DELIVERY   1 = none

    2 = > 4 Kg baby

    Code complications   3 = forceps

    NOT each delivery.   4 = breech

    If all code 1 enter 111   5 = lower segment caesar.

    If 1 abnormal,   6 = episiotomy

    eg 6 and others normal   7 = tears

    code 611 etc.   8 = other

    X = unknown

46. SYMPTOMATIC DIAGNOSIS
   (i) Bladder during filling   1 = normal
       2 = unstable
       3 = hypersensitive
       4 = other
       X = unknown
   (ii) Urethra during filling   1 = competant
       2 = incompetent e.g. stress incontinence
       3 = other
       X = unknown
   (iii) Bladder during voiding   1 = normal
       2 = underactive
       3 = other
       X = unknown
   (iv) Urethra during voiding   1 = normal
       2 = mechanical obstruction
       3 = neuropathic obstruction
       4 = urethral syndrome
       5 = other
       X = unknown

PHYSICAL EXAMINATION: if 1 in 4 (Male) answer 47, if 2 in 4 (Female) go to 48.

MALE

47(a). PROSTATE   1 = normal
       2 = BPH +
       3 = BPH + +
       4 = BPH + + +
       5 = malignant
       6 = prostatitis
       X = unknown

47(b). INCONTINENCE SEEN DURING PHYSICAL EXAMINATION
       1 = none
       2 = incontinence observed
       X = unknown
       go to 50

FEMALE

48. VAGINAL EXAMINATION   1 = normal vagina
       2 = atrophic vaginitis
       3 = infective vaginitis
       X = unknown

49(a). PROLAPSE
   (i) Uterine prolapse   1 = none
       2 = uterine prolapse Gd.1
       3 = uterine prolapse Gd.2
       4 = uterine prolapse Gd.3
       X = unknown
   (ii) Cysto urethrocoele   1 = none
       2 = slight cystocoele
       3 = marked cystocoele
       X = unknown

(iii) Gut prolapse   1 = none
         2 = rectocoele
         3 = enterocoele
         X = unknown

(iv) Other factors   1 = none
         2 = deficient perineum
         3 = other
         X = unknown

49(b). INCONTINENCE SEEN DURING PHYSICAL EXAMINATION
         1 = none
         2 = incontinence observed
         X = unknown

FOR ALL PATIENTS

50. NEUROLOGICAL SIGNS
(i) Legs   1 = normal
         2 = LMN
         3 = UMN
         4 = LMN/UMN
         5 = other
         X = unknown

(ii) Anal reflex   1 = normal
         2 = absent
         X = unknown

(iii) Anal tone   1 = normal
         2 = present but lax after p.r.
         3 = reduced throughout
         4 = absent
         X = unknown

(iv) Perineal sensation   1 = normal
         2 = patchy loss
         3 = absent
         X = unknown

51. OBESITY   1 = slim
         2 = slight obesity
         3 = moderate obesity
         4 = gross obesity
         X = unknown

52. BLADDER   1 = not palpable
         2 = palpable
         X = unknown

53. PELVIC FLOOR SQUEEZE   1 = normal
         2 = decreased
         3 = absent
         X = unknown

53a. UPPER TRACT   1 = normal
       DILATATION   2 = present
       Information from) X = unknown
       I.V.P., ultrasound, etc)
       CODE 54–66 as 1 = done
       2 = not done

54. INVESTIGATION
       a = Full UDS
       b = FLOW RATES only
       c = PAD TESTS only
    if 1 in 54a go to 55
    if 1 in 54b complete 67 to 70 then go to end
    if 1 in 54c complete 82 then go to end
    if 1 in 54b and 1 in 54c complete 67 to 70 and 82 then go to end

55. FLOW RATES (initial or multiple)

56. STATIC UPP

57. STRESS UPP

58. SACRAL REFLEXES

59. URETHRAL SENSITIVITY

60. FILLING CMG

61. FLUID BRIDGE TEST

62. VOIDING CYSTOMETROGRAM

63. EMG

64. EMG (single fibre)

65. QUANTITATIVE URINE LOSS (PAD TESTING)

66. VIDEO
    If 1 in 55 answer 67
       FLOW RATES:- (if single flow, ie initial flow in full UDS, then code 67 only and go to 71)
       FLOW RATE   VOLUME VOIDED   RESIDUAL URINE

67. ml/sec   mls

68. ml/sec   mls

69. ml/sec   mls

70. FLOW RATES/ULTRASOUND RUs – DIAGNOSIS DERIVED FROM MULTIPLE FLOWS (67 to 69)
       1 = normal
       2 = obstructed
       3 = equivocal
       4 = dysfunctional voiding
       5 = other
       X = unknown
    go to the end if 1 in 54(b) and 2 in 54(c) otherwise answer 82
    if 1 in 4 and 1 in 56 (*MALE*) then go to 71, if 2 in 4 and 1 in 56 (*FEMALE*) go to 72

71. UPP STATIC (male)

    X = unknown

        Prostatic length   cms

        Prostatic plateau height cmH_2O

        Prostatic area $cm.cm.H_2O$

        MUP cmH_2O

        MUCP cmH_2O

        Prostatic peak

        1 = yes

        2 = no

  go to 74

72. UPP STATIC (female)

    X = unknown

        Absolute length   cms

        Functional length   cms

        MUP cmH_2O

        MUCP cmH_2O

        Total area $cm.cmH_2O$

        Increment on squeeze cmH_2O

  if 1 in 57 answer 73.

73. UPP STRESS   Transmission ratio at 100 mls   %

    X = unknown

        Transmission ratio at capacity   %

  if 1 in 58 complete 74

74. SACRAL REFLEXES

    X = unknown   Anal stimulus, Anal response   m.secs.

        Urethral/BN stimulus, Anal response   m.secs.

        Penile stimulus, Anal response   m.secs.

        Anal stimulus, Urethral response   m.secs.

        if 1 in 59 complete 75

75. URETHRAL SENSITIVITY

    X = unknown   Mean threshold   m.Amps.

        if 1 in 60 complete 76 and 77

76. FILLING CMG

    (Pdet.)

    X = unknown

    − = feature NOT seen

        Filling speed   ml/min

        Empty resting pressure $cm.H_2O$

        FDM   ml

        UDM   ml

        Vol. 1st unstable contraction   ml

        Leakage at (volume)   ml

        Leakage at (pressure) $cm.H_2O$

        Cystometric capacity   ml

        Full resting pressure (if no detr.contr.) $cm.H_2O$

        Pressure at capacity (if unstable) $cm.H_2O$

Old Instability Index (Pves)   cm.H_2O/ml
New Instability Index (Pdet)   cm.H_2O/ml
Compliance $\Delta V \Delta P$

77. OBSERVED INCONTINENCE   1 = none
    2 = stress
    3 = urge unstable
    4 = unstable urethra
    5 = stress/urge unstable
    6 = stress/unstable urethra
    7 = other
    X = unknown
   if 1 in 61 complete 78

78. FLUID BRIDGE TEST   1 = abnormal lying
    2 = abnormal erect
    3 = normal lying
    4 = normal erect
    X = unknown
   if 1 in 62 complete 79

79. VOIDING CYSTOMETROGRAM
    X = unknown   Max. flow pressure (Pves)   cmH_2O
    Max. flow pressure (Pdet)   cm.H_2O
    Max. flow rate (F)   ml.sec.
    P.det.iso   cm.H_2O
    Urethral Resistance (P.ves/F2)
    Volume passed   ml
    Residual urine   ml
    After contraction
    1 = none
    2 = present
   if 1 in 63 complete 80

80. EMG
    (i) Site   1 = pelvic floor
       2 = urethra
       3 = anal
       4 = other
       X = unknown
    (ii) Type   1 = plug
       2 = needle
       3 = surface
       4 = catheter
       5 = other
       6 = unknown
    (iii) Findings   1 = normal
       2 = dyssynergia
       3 = reduced activity
       4 = other
       X = unknown
       if 1 in 64 complete 81

81. EMG (single fibre)
   X = unknown
        1 = normal
        2 = abnormal
        Fibre density
        If 1 in 65 complete 82

82. QUANTIFICATION URINE LOSS PER EXERCISE CYCLE
   X = unknown   mls
        if coded 1 in 54(c) go to end
        ALL PATIENTS
   if 1 in 56 complete 83

83. DIAGNOSIS UPP
   (i) Static profile   1 = normal
        2 = low static UPP
        3 = high static UPP
        4 = increased prostatic area
        5 = other
        X = unknown
   (ii) Squeeze   1 = normal
        2 = weak
        3 = absent
        X = unknown

84. STRESS UPP DIAGNOSIS   1 = normal
   (code severest abnormality)   2 = abnormal at 100 mls
        3 = abnormal at capacity
        4 = equivocal at 100 mls
        5 = equivocal at capacity
        X = unknown
   If 1 in 60 complete 85 & 86
   DIAGNOSIS FILLING PHASE

85. BLADDER
   (i) Sensation   1 = normal
        2 = reduced
        3 = increased (hypersensitive)
        4 = absent
        X = unknown
   (ii) Detrusor activity   1 = stable
        2 = unstable (spontaneous)
        3 = unstable (provoked)
        4 = other
        X = unknown
   (iii) Compliance   1 = normal
        2 = low
        3 = high
        4 = other
        X = unknown
   if 1 in 66 complete (iv) and (v)

(iv) Bladder shape   1 = normal
    2 = trabeculation
    3 = diverticula
    4 = trabec/divertic
    5 = other
    X = unknown

(v) Bladder base function   1 = normal
    2 = bladder base descent
    3 = other
    X = unknown

86. URETHRA

(i) Urethral sensation on
    catheterisation   1 = normal
    2 = increased
    3 = absent
    X = unknown

if no video (2 in 66) complete (ii), if video (1 in 66) complete (iii)

(ii) Urethral behaviour   1 = normal urethra
    2 = incompetent urethra (Genuine Stress Incontinence)
    3 = unstable urethra with leakage
    4 = unstable urethra without leakage
    5 = other
    X = unknown

(iii) Video: BN/urethral
    function (filling)   1 = normal
    2 = BN beaking at rest
    3 = BN beaking on strain
    4 = BN and urethra open at rest with leak
    5 = BN and urethra open on stress with leak
    6 = BN beaking at rest + stress incontinence
    7 = unstable urethra with leakage
    8 = unstable urethra without leakage
    X = unknown

if 1 in 62 complete 87 & 88

DIAGNOSIS VOIDING PHASE

87. DETRUSOR   1 = normal detrusor contraction (normal flow)
    2 = sustained low detrusor pressure (with low flow)
    3 = fluctuating detrusor pressure (with intermittent flow)
    4 = sustained high detrusor pressure (with low flow)
    5 = acontractile detrusor (voids by straining)
    6 = detrusor contraction – with strain
    7 = acontractile detrusor (no voiding)
    8 = detrusor contraction (no voiding)
    9 = normal void – no detrusor contraction
    A = normal void – no detrusor contraction – Piso present
    B = other
    X = unknown

88. URETHRA
   if no video (2 in 66) complete (i), if video (1 in 66) performed complete (ii)
   (i) Standard UDS   1 = normal
               2 = dyssynergic
               3 = obstructed
               4 = other
               X = unknown
   (ii) Video UDS   1 = normal
               2 = BN obstruction
               3 = detrusor/BN/dyssynergia
               4 = detrusor/urethral/dyssynergia
               5 = static distal sphincter obstruction
               6 = mechanical prostatic obstruction
               7 = mechanical urethral obstruction
               8 = other
               X = unknown
   if 1 in 66 complete 89

89. OTHER VIDEO FEATURES   1 = none
               2 = VU reflux
               3 = prostatic duct reflux
               4 = no milk back
               5 = other
               X = unknown

90. URODYNAMIC
   Technical Aspects   1 = no problems
               2 = unable to catheterise
               3 = catheter voided
               4 = undue anxiety (including fainting)
               5 = other
               X = unknown

91. CLINICAL URODYNAMIC DIAGNOSIS
               1 = interstitial cystitis
               2 = urethral syndrome
               3 = prostatodynia
               4 = other
               5 = diagnosis as above
               X = unknown

Appendix 3, Part 2
Urodynamics Data Sheet: Shortened Version

U R O D Y N A M I C U N I T
SOUTHMEAD HOSPITAL, BRISTOL
M 1337
NOTE:–

(a) Number of entries Strictly dictated by number of boxes

(b) Where no information enter

(c) N = not applicable

1. SURNAME:
        FIRST NAME:

2. ADDRESS:
        Post Code   Tel. No.

3. DATE OF BIRTH:

4. SEX: (1 male; 2 female)

5. HOSPITAL NUMBER(S):

6. INITIAL REFERRAL: 1 Urol   2 Gynae   3 Surg   4 Geriatric
        5. G.P.   6 Nurse   7 Other   8 Paediatrics

6a. 1 = in patient   2 = out-patient   3 = not known

7. CONSULTANT: (Name)

8. G.P.: (Name)
        Address (not coded)

9a. CIU NUMBER: 9b. INVESTIGATION NUMBER:
        Presenting Complaint: HEIGHT   cms
        Previous Treatment: WEIGHT   Kg
            SMOKER   YES/NO   …/Day
        Examination:
        Management:

Report sent to: Follow up arrangements:–
If enter 'other' in any question please describe on this sheet.

10. Date

11. Age

12. Trial I.D.

13. Enter Hist.

14. Inv.

15. Length Hist.

16. Freq. (day)

17. Noct.

18. Fluid Intake

19. F/V chart
    Max. vol.
    Av. vol.
    Duration

20. Pre. mict.
    Freq.

21. Hest.
    Freq.

22. Incontinence

23. Stress 1.
    Freq.

24. Urge I
    Freq.

25. Enuresis
    Freq.

26. Other 1.
    Freq.

27. Degree

28. Management
    Pads/day
    Pads/night

29. Incapacity

30. Physical Incap.

31. Hist. Enuresis
    (i) Patient
    (ii) Family

32. Stream

33. Post. Mict.
    Freq.

34. Dysuria

34a. Haematuria

35. Hist. Retention

36. Management Retn.
37. Bowel Function
      (a) Control
      (b) Stool Freq.
      (c) Defaecation
      (d) Post defaec. symp.
      (e) Diagnosis
38. Drugs
39a. Neuro. feat.
39b. Sexual Function.
MALE ONLY
40. Operations/Trauma
      (i) outflow
      (ii) denervation
      (iii) Other
FEMALE ONLY
41. Operations/Trauma
      (i) for stress Inc.
      (ii) gynae. symp/prolapse
      (iii) denervation
      (iv) Other
42. Hormone
43. Symp. Mense
44. Parity
45. Delivery
ALL PATIENTS
46. Symptomatic diag.
      (i) Bladder fill
      (ii) Urethra fill
      (iii) Bladder void
      (iv) Urethra void
PHYSICAL EXAMINATION
MALE ONLY
47a. Prostate
47b. Incont. seen
FEMALE ONLY
48. Vag. exam.
49a. Prolapse
      (i) Uterine prolapse
      (ii) Cysto. urethra
      (iii) Gut prolapse
      (iv) Other
49b. Incont. seen

ALL PATIENTS

50. Neuro. signs
    (i) Legs
    (ii) Anal reflex
    (iii) Anal Tone
    (iv) Perineal sens.

51. Obesity

52. Bladder

53. P.F. squeeze

53a. Upper tract dilatation

54. Investigations
    (a) Full UDS
    (b) Flowrates
    (c) Pad Test

55. Flow rates

56. Static UPP

57. Stress UPP

58. Sacral reflex

59. Urethral sens.

60. Fill CMG

61. F.B.T.

62. Void CMG

63. EMG

64. EMG (single fibre)

65. Pad Test

66. Video

FLOW RATES

       Flow   Volvoid   R.U.

67.

68.

69.

70. Ultrasound/F.R. diag.

71. Static UPP (MALE)
    Length
    plat.
    area
    MUP
    MUCP
    Peak

72. Static UPP (FEMALE)
    Abs. length
    Function length.
    MUP
    MUCP
    area
    sq.
73. Stress UPP
    Tr. 100 ml
    Tr. cap

Appendix 4, Part 1
ICIQ Modular Questionnaire

Introduction

The scientific committee which met at the end of the 1st ICI in 1998 supported the idea that a universally applicable questionnaire should be developed, that could be widely applied both in clinical practice and research.

The hope was expressed that such a questionnaire would be used in different settings and studies and would allow cross-comparisons, for example, between a drug and an operation used for the same condition, in the same way that the IPSS (International prostate symptoms score) has been used.

An ICIQ Advisory Board was formed to steer the development of the ICIQ, and met for the first time in 1999. The project's early progress was discussed with the Board and a decision made to extend the concept further and to develop the ICIQ Modular Questionnaire. The first module to be developed was the ICIQ Short Form Questionnaire for urinary incontinence: the ICIQ-SF. The ICIQ-SF has now been fully validated and published[1]. Given the intention to produce an internationally applicable questionnaire, requests were made for translations of the ICIQ-SF at an early stage, for which the Advisory Board developed a protocol for the production of translations of its modules. The ICIQ-SF has been translated into 30 languages to date.

In addition to the ICIQ-SF, ten modules have been adopted which are direct (unchanged) derivations from already published questionnaires. (Tables A.4.1.I–A.4.1.III)

WWW.ICIQ.net will be used to provide the validation status of the modules under development for urinary symptoms, bowel symptoms and vaginal symptoms.

Table A.4.1.I. Fully validated ICIQ symptom modules

Question Items	ICIQ-MLUTS (ICSmale SF[4])	ICIQ-FLUTS (BFLUTS SF[5])	ICIQ-UI SF[1]	ICIQ-N (ICS male[2]/ BFLUTS[3])	ICIQ-OAB (ICS male[2]/ BFLUTS[3])	ICIQ-MLUTS LF (ICS male[2])	ICIQ-FLUTS LF (BFLUTS[3])
Genders available for use in							
Male	✓		✓	✓	✓	✓	
Female		✓	✓	✓	✓		✓
Storage							
Frequency	✓	✓		✓	✓	✓	✓
Nocturia	✓	✓		✓	✓	✓	✓
Urgency	✓	✓			✓	✓	✓
Bladder pain		✓				✓	✓
Urinary retention						✓	✓
Voiding							
Hesitancy	✓	✓				✓	✓
Straining	✓	✓				✓	✓
Strength of stream	✓					✓	✓
Intermittency	✓	✓				✓	✓
Incomplete emptying	✓					✓	✓
Burning on urination						✓	✓
Urination position						✓	
Urine flow control							✓
Incontinence							
Urge urinary incontinence	✓	✓			✓	✓	✓
Stress urinary incontinence	✓	✓				✓	✓
Unexplained urinary incontinence	✓	✓				✓	✓
Nocturnal enuresis	✓	✓				✓	✓
Post micturition dribble	✓					✓	
Frequency urinary incontinence		✓	✓				✓
Amount of urinary incontinence			✓				✓
Type urinary incontinence			✓				
Protection type/use						✓	✓
Change of clothing						✓	✓
Quality of life			✓				
Bother of each symptom						✓	✓

Table A.4.1.Ia. Available translations of fully validated ICIQ symptom modules

Question Items	ICIQ-MLUTS (ICSmale SF⁴)	ICIQ-FLUTS (BFLUTS SF⁵)	ICIQ-UI SF¹	ICIQ-N (ICS male²/ BFLUTS³)	ICIQ-OAB (ICS male²/ BFLUTS³)	ICIQ-MLUTS LF (ICS male²)	ICIQ-FLUTS LF (BFLUTS³)
Afrikaans			✓				
Arabic			✓				
Australian-English			✓				
Brazilian-Portuguese			✓				
Bulgarian			✓				
Czech			✓				
Danish	✓	✓	✓	✓	✓	✓	✓
Dutch	✓	✓	✓	✓	✓	✓	✓
Dutch for Belgium		✓		✓	✓		✓
Estonian			✓				
Finnish	✓		✓	✓	✓	✓	
French	✓	✓	✓	✓	✓	✓	✓
French Canadian	✓			✓	✓	✓	
German	✓	✓	✓	✓	✓	✓	✓
German for Austria		✓		✓	✓		✓
Greek			✓				
Hungarian			✓				
Icelandic			✓				
Israeli	✓			✓	✓	✓	
Italian	✓		✓	✓	✓	✓	
Japanese	✓		✓	✓	✓	✓	
Korean		✓		✓	✓		✓
New Zealand-English			✓				
Norwegian	✓	✓	✓	✓	✓	✓	✓
Polish			✓				
Portuguese	✓			✓	✓	✓	
Romanian			✓				
Russian			✓				
Slovakian			✓				
South African-English			✓				
Spanish	✓		✓	✓	✓	✓	
Swedish	✓	✓	✓	✓	✓	✓	✓
Taiwanese	✓			✓	✓	✓	
Tamil	✓			✓	✓	✓	
Turkish	✓		✓	✓	✓	✓	
Ukranian			✓				
UK-English	✓	✓	✓	✓	✓	✓	✓
US-English			✓				

Table A.4.1.II. Fully validated ICIQ quality of life modules

Question Items	ICIQ-LUTSqol (KHQ[6])	ICIQ-UIqol (I-QOL[9])	ICIQ-Nqol (N-QOL[7])	ICIQ-OABqol (OABq[8])
Genders available for use in				
Male	✓	✓	✓	✓
Female	✓	✓	✓	✓
Ageing		✓		
Annoyed				✓
Anxiety/nervousness	✓			✓
Bad feeling	✓			✓
Bladder control		✓		
Clothing	✓	✓		
Concentration			✓	
Depression	✓	✓		
Distress				✓
Disturbance of others			✓	
Embarrassment	✓	✓		✓
Energy			✓	
Enjoyment		✓		
Everyday life	✓		✓	
Family	✓			✓
Fluid restriction	✓	✓	✓	
Forward planning		✓		✓
Friends	✓			✓
Frustration				✓
Helplessness		✓		
Household tasks	✓			
Hygiene				✓
Job	✓			
Limited to home		✓		✓
Overall impact				✓
Partner				✓
Perceived health		✓		
Physical activities	✓	✓	✓	✓
Preoccupation		✓	✓	
Productiveness			✓	
Protection use	✓			
Relationships	✓			✓
Sex life	✓			
Sex worry		✓		
Sleep/rest	✓	✓	✓	✓
Smell	✓	✓		✓
Social life/restriction	✓	✓		✓
Tired	✓			
Toilet location		✓		✓
Travel	✓			✓
Worry		✓		
Worry about ageing		✓		
Worry about treatment		✓		

Table A.4.1.IIa. Available translations of fully validated ICIQ quality of life

Question Items	ICIQ-LUTSqol (KHQ[6])	ICIQ-UIqol (I-QOL[9])	ICIQ-Nqol (N-QOL[7])	ICIQ-OABqol (OABq[8])
Genders available for use in				
Afrikaans	✓	✓		
Australian-English	✓	✓		
Brazilian-Portuguese	✓	✓		
Bulgarian	✓			
Canadian English	✓	✓		✓
Czech	✓			
Danish	✓	✓		✓
Dutch	✓	✓		✓
Dutch for Belgium	✓	✓		
Estonian	✓			
Finnish	✓	✓		
French	✓	✓		
French for Belgium	✓			
French for Canada	✓	✓		✓
French for Switzerland	✓			✓
German	✓	✓		✓
German for Austria	✓			
German for Switzerland	✓			✓
Greek	✓	✓		
Hebrew	✓	✓		
Hungarian	✓			
Italian	✓	✓		✓
Italian for Switzerland	✓			✓
Japanese	✓	✓		✓
Korean	✓	✓		✓
Lithuanian	✓			
Mandarin for Taiwan		✓		
New Zealand-English	✓	✓		
Norwegian	✓	✓		✓
Polish	✓	✓		✓
Portuguese	✓	✓		
Romanian	✓			
Russian	✓			
Slovakian		✓		
South African-English	✓	✓		
Spanish	✓	✓		✓
Spanish for Argentina	✓			
Spanish for Chile	✓			
Spanish for Colombia	✓			
Spanish for Peru	✓			
Spanish for Mexico	✓			
Spanish for USA	✓	✓		
Swedish	✓	✓		✓
Turkish				✓
Ukranian	✓			
UK-English	✓	✓	✓	✓
US-English	✓	✓		✓

Table 3 Fully validated ICIQ sexual matters modules

Question Items	ICIQ-MLUTSex (ICS male[2])	ICIQFLUTSsex (BFLUTS[3])
Genders available for use in		
Male	✓	
Female		✓
Ejaculation	✓	
Erections	✓	
Impact on sex life	✓	✓
Pain on ejaculation	✓	
Sex life status	✓	✓
Reasons for no sex life	✓	
Dry vagina		✓
Intercourse incontinence		✓
Pain on intercourse		✓

Table 3a Available translations of fully validated ICIQ sexual matters modules

Question Items	ICIQ-MLUTSex (ICS male[2])	ICIQFLUTSsex (BFLUTS[3])
Danish	✓	✓
Dutch	✓	✓
Dutch for Belgium		✓
Finnish	✓	
French	✓	✓
French Canadian	✓	
German	✓	✓
German for Austria		✓
Israeli	✓	
Italian	✓	
Japanese	✓	
Korean		✓
Norwegian	✓	✓
Portuguese	✓	
Spanish	✓	
Swedish	✓	✓
Taiwanese	✓	
Tamil	✓	
Turkish	✓	
UK-English	✓	✓

References

1. Avery K, Donovan J, Peters T, Shaw C, Gotoh M, & Abrams P. The ICIQ: a brief and robust measure for evaluating the symptoms and impact of urinary incontinence. *Neurourol.Urodyn.* 2004; 23(4): 322-330.
2. Donovan J, Abrams P, Peters T, *et al.* The ICS-'BPH' study: the psychometric validity and reliability of the ICS*male* questionnaire. *Br.J.Urol.* 1996; 77: 554-562.
3. Jackson S, Donovan J, Brookes S, *et al.* The Bristol Female Lower Urinary Tract Symptoms questionnaire: development and psychometric testing. *Br.J.Urol.* 1996; 77: 805-812.
4. Donovan J, Peters T, Abrams P, *et al.* Scoring the Short Form ICS*male*SF questionnaire. *J.Urol.* 2000; 164: 1948-1955.
5. Brookes ST, Donovan JL, Wright M, Jackson S, Abrams P. A scored form of the Bristol Female Lower Urinary Tract Symptoms questionnaire: data from a randomized controlled trial of surgery for women with stress incontinence. *Am.J.Obstet.Gynecol.* 2004;191(1):73-82.
6. Kelleher C, Cardozo L, Khullar V, *et al.* A new questionnaire to assess the quality of life of urinary incontinent women. *Br.J.Obstet.Gynaecol.* 1997; 104: 1374-1379.
7. Abraham L, Hareendran A, Mills I, *et al.* Development and validation of a quality-of-life measure for men with nocturia. *Urology* 2004; 63(3): 481-486.
8. Coyne K, Revicki D, Hunt R, et al. Psychometric validation of an overactive bladder symptom and health-related quality of life questionnaire: The OAB-q. *Qual.Life.Res.* 2003;11:563-574.
9. Wagner TH, Patrick DL, Bavendam TG, Martin ML, Buesching DP. Quality of life of persons with urinary incontinence: development of a new measure. *Urology* 1996;47(1):67-72.

ICIQ UISF (Urinary Incontinence Short Form)

□□□□□□ ICIQ-UI-SF □□□□□□

| Initial number | **CONFIDENTIAL** | DAY | MONTH | YEAR |

Today's date

Many people leak urine some of the time. We are trying to find out how many people leak urine, and how much this bothers them. We would be grateful if you could answer the following questions, thinking about how you have been, on average, over the PAST FOUR WEEKS.

1   Please write in your date of birth:

□□□□□.□□

DAY   MONTH   YEAR

2   **Are you** *(tick one):*   Female □   Male □

---

3   **How often do you leak urine?** *(Tick one box)*

never	□	0
about once a week or less often	□	1
two or three times a week	□	2
about once a day	□	3
several times a day	□	4
all the time	□	5

---

4   **We would like to know how much urine you think leaks.**
   How much urine do you usually leak (whether you wear protection or not)?
   (Tick one box)

none	□	0
a small amount	□	2
a moderate amount	□	4
a large amount	□	6

---

5   **Overall, how much does leaking urine interfere with your everyday life?**
   Please ring a number between 0 (not at all) and 10 (a great deal)

      0 1 2 3 4 5 6 7 8 9 **10**

not at all   a great deal

ICIQ score: sum scores 3+4+5 □□

6 When does urine leak? *(Please tick all that apply to you)*

never – urine does not leak ☐

leaks before you can get to the toilet ☐

leaks when you cough or sneeze ☐

leaks when you are asleep ☐

leaks when you are physically active/exercising ☐

leaks when you have finished urinating and are dressed ☐

leaks for no obvious reason ☐

leaks all the time ☐

Thank you very much for answering these questions.

Copyright © "ICIQ Group"

Index